herbal medicine
trends and traditions

ALSO BY CHARLES W. KANE

HERBAL MEDICINE OF THE AMERICAN SOUTHWEST
A Guide to the Identification, Collection, Preparation, and Use of Medicinal and Edible Plants of the Southwestern United States

herbal medicine
trends and traditions

A Comprehensive Sourcebook on the Preparation and Use of Medicinal Plants

CHARLES W. KANE

Lincoln Town
P R E S S

For Charles F. Kane.
It all started with Jewelweed.

CONTENTS

COLOR PLATES

PREFACE

The foundation for Trends and Traditions was developed while I was deployed to eastern Afghanistan. Writing served as both a distraction and a fruitful process meant to create something pertinent. It took me away from frustration, anxiety, and boredom; a sort of internal respite. Writing was the only thing I had that wasn't part of the collective Army–war experience. I also knew the material would be used for good, and that was inspiring.

Some things experienced while there I was able to synthesize and make work for this material – the Afghan's use of Myrrh or Cannabis for instance. Others, like being in a TIC with the Taliban has little relevance – even though they used Barberry and Walnut for concealment. Jokes about returning fire *around* the plants were endless, but in good fun.

I didn't have the luxury of a quiet study, but when I was able to devote even a scrap of time to writing I always felt accomplished and purposeful. When not outside the wire, on check–point duty, weapon cleaning, or involved in a million other inane goings–on of FOB life, I did get a substantial amount done.

Soon realizing after my return home there is little call for the infantryman's skill–set, I renewed my work in accomplishing what I had started in Afghanistan. Resumption of teaching, wildcrafting, and private practice, meshed well with concluding Trends and Traditions.

Many times while sifting through dozens of journal articles or while putting the finishing touches on a well–worked section I felt spoiled to have it so easy. Sometimes at dusk while writing I would look out at the desert mountains and sense the chaos I had left was not far away. If given the choice I would do it all the same way again...but, once was enough.

Writing has never come easy to me, or rather *good* writing has never come easy to me. It is one of the most introspective processes imaginable, filled with obsessive focus and reinvention. If any work of writing is good it is due to a neglected piece of outward life.

Charles W. Kane
Oracle, Arizona

ACKNOWLEDGMENTS

Along the way in any endeavour there are people whose assistance help bring about an idea or project to fruition. In many ways writing a book is no different than any other relative undertaking. Surely different skills are needed, but the support gathered from others is the same whether the medium is words or sockets and wrenches.

First I'd like to thank family and friends for their letters, e–mail, and care packages while I was overseas. They kept me afloat and inspired faith that the situation was only temporary. To all of you who were pulling for me, something must of worked.

A hearty thanks to the John and Donna Albertsen for driving my Ford truck around the block once a week. Dr. Michael Stone went above and beyond by heading up the dragon skin project. Christy Lazzaretti will always be remembered as a special lady whose love and care during that time were unequalled.

As a community user I am grateful to have had access to the University of Arizona's health and science library's journal collection. Mac MacBride's photographic expertise was important as was my student's willingness to be photographed while wildcrafting. Charles Brock at the DesignWorks Group did a tremendous job in designing a stylish book cover. I couldn't be more pleased.

Certainly there is a whole line of herbalists, doctors, and healers whose works have influenced my own. Eclectic, Physiomedicalist, and lay root doctor traditions from the Victorian era tend to impress me more than current interpretations. That said, it is also important to stay up to date with the latest theory or study.

Ultimately though it is the real–time experience of people getting better from herbs that added most to this work. To all my patients who took the bitter herb: your willingness and faith, through success and failure, contributed most.

INTRODUCTION

The worlds of war and medicine seem as far apart from each other as the realms of destruction and healing. But more often than not these realms exist side by side – sometimes the best healers are terribly fierce or an individual's constitutional strength often turns to his weakness as age progresses. We all live with life and death, creation and dissolution – it's just part of being here.

Using plants to fight disease and sustain health are examples of how we have developed systems over the ages to stave off, or at least modify the enviable – dissolution and death. This branch of medicine, using plants to affect health and disease, is an old one, maybe even the original one. That plants influence us therapeutically is of little dispute; to what degree and how reliably they affect us, is.

With the following work I have attempted to clarify the therapeutic value of the most popular plants currently used in western herbal medicine. Botanicals like Milk thistle, Echinacea, and St. John's wort are popular for the right reasons – they are truly first class medicines. Like most other widely used herbs they are relatively non–toxic, effective in their realms, and have an extensive history of use. I have also included a number of fad herbs, not just because they are popular, but because they also are decent medicines.

Beyond the obvious format, I have used many of the monographs as a staging points for the discussion of related concepts. Applied physiology, constitutional medicine, the nuances of wildcrafting, and even the limitations of herbal medicine are delved into more in–depth throughout the book.

This work includes each plant's botanical description, distribution, medicinal use, collection method, and associated cautions. Of particular relevance is each plant's choice preparation(s) and dosage. For the individual who desires instruction on making herbal medicines, Trends and Traditions is comprehensive. All of the main water, alcohol, and oil based preparations are covered. Even essential oils and hydrosols are discussed.

I have written Trend and Traditions as a manual for both the practitioner and the enthusiast. For the herbalist, doctor, chiropractor, or related practitioner it is my hope this reference cuts away the aloof–theoretical quality often found in similar works. For the "weekend warrior" some of the terminology may seem heady, and to address this I have included an extensive glossary, but know it is better to stretch yourself mentally than stay in the simplistic confines of "if you have xyz ailment take xyz herb". Sure, there is some of that in this work, how can there not be? But after immersing yourself in Trend and Traditions it will plainly be seen this work goes beyond the limited "pin the tail on the donkey" approach.

The usefulness of the this book hinges on two questions: When should I use herbal medicines and how should I use them? The answers to these questions are not easy or even short. But concisely: use herbs when a trip to the emergency room or family doctor is not necessary, when complaints are minor and not a threat. Use them when regular medicines are not working or when their side–effects outweigh their benefits. For the practitioner or the invested learner herbs can be applied more broadly to include ailments that regular medical normally considers its territory. These chronic or functional problems often need initial medical diagnosis and follow up, but when the afflicted individual is dedicated to getting better with herbs, there is much that can be accomplished. Herbs can be used to supplant a whole range of pharmaceuticals. With proper application an individual can replace many conventional medications used for metabolic, inflammatory, pathogenic, and neurobiological issues.

Do not use herbal medicines as a replacement for ambulatory care. Herbs preform poorly if used for organic problems when an organ or tissue group is broken beyond repair. They are simply outclassed in these situations. Lastly if on a slew of pharmaceuticals adding an herb or two to the mix is just going to make an uncertain situation a little more so. Get off the non–essential drugs first, then work herbs into the fray.

I often hear among the inexperienced, "they are unproven and dangerous" or "herbal medicines are natural and can do no harm". Dangerous? Try "proven" conventional medicine. Through unnecessary surgeries and dosing errors it is a leading cause of death in America.

Natural and gentle? Just because something is natural doesn't mean it's weak. Some herbs rival pharmaceuticals in their strength...and toxicity.

Herbs are simply tools. Each one better at one thing than the other. Some are food–like in their strength, others are stronger and drug–like. Each herb should be approached individually.

The point of this work is to relay how plants help people. For that to occur useful information must be presented in a way that is relevant and approachable. For these reasons the style of Trends and Traditions is a departure from the "quoting of study results", the "1960s–esque ramble", or "it will cure whatever ails you" flavors. I think what you as the reader really wants is an authentic communication that cuts through the crap.

Whatever your skill level or reason for using herbal medicines I believe you will be rewarded by the pertinent and applicable information contained within Trends and Traditions. Above all consider it a genuine rendering from someone within the field, designed to change a vague subject into a useful tool.

FORMAT EXPLANATION

PLANT NAMES

Common and scientific names are given for both the plant and family. Each profile is headed by the main common name, followed by a current scientific name and synonyms. Secondary common names follow. The main common name assigned to each plant is generally accepted as the most common, i.e. Bayberry not Waxberry, Black cohosh not Bugbane, Yarrow not Milfoil, etc. One notable exception to this is Creosote bush, popularly known in the medicinal herb world as Chaparral. Even though Chaparral has name recognition, it adds no coherent descriptiveness to the plant; on the contrary, it is misleading, as it refers to a vegetation zone found throughout the mid–mountain West. Arctostaphylos and Ceanothus are typical inhabitants, not Larrea.

With all of that said, do not get stuck in the name game. Most common names as well as many scientific names for any given plant change from generation to generation. No name is set in stone. Botanical classifiers can be fickle in applying and reapplying nomenclature depending on the classifying systems/politics of the day. When you know the plant, you know the plant, names be damned.

DESCRIPTION AND DISTRIBUTION

Look to these sections for the plant's botanical description and growth tendencies. Going against the conformity of the metric system all measurements are in standard. Emphasis is placed on where the plant grows in this country. Of course many plants are native to other regions of the world; if this is the case then its distribution is discussed equally. Elevation ranges, topographies, and environments are covered for profiled plants.

CHEMISTRY

Each plant's chemical composition is listed. Many species are well–researched; others are not. This is reflected in each plant's listing.

MEDICINAL USES

Each plant's effect on organ systems, tissue groups, and occasionally symptoms are described. Application to disease syndromes has been keep to a minimum but occasionally it is pertinent – how the plant affects stress patterns and its mechanism of action are preferred.

Plants are multi–directional. Rarely do they affect just one area of the body. They influence the body by how an organ or tissue group eliminates or detoxifies the compounds comprising them. It is not the plant that is the remedy for the ailment or discomfort, but it is what the plant does to the body, organ system, or group of tissues that then affects the manifested problem. Only after knowing that an aromatic–bitter herb stimulates secretion and dilates vasculature of the stomach lining will its effect on quieting indigestion make sense.

INDICATIONS

A synopsis of medicinal uses. The indicated medicinal use for each plant. If "(external)" is not by the indication then that application is designed for internal use.

COLLECTION

It is not practical to suggest the collection of every plant listed in this book. Besides the monumental amount of work involved, an individual would need to travel the world around. Pick the ones you can collect. For the others, commercially available crude material or refined preparations are common.

Depending on the plant, virtually any part can be medicinally potent. Mostly though roots, bark, leaves, flowers, seeds, and sap or exudate provide the strongest medicines. Stems, branches, and core wood are less likely to give benefit. The former parts are functional, having an array of chemical processes taking place within them. The latter parts are structural, serving mainly as a skeletal support for the functional parts – much like our bodies.

There are two main polarized attitudes encountered concerning the collection of wild plants for medicine. The ideologies that these attitudes spring from have an effect on our perspectives concerning both nature and society. Whether it is the big–money, corporate–consumption mentality or the tendencies that go along with most environmental groups out to "save" the natural world through law an bureaucracy, neither world–view is helpful to the respectful wildcrafter who takes only what he needs…which may not be what he desires. The first attitude: take all that you can if it is of any value regardless of environmental impact. This tendency and its effects are noticeable on a number of medicinal plants in commerce. This same attitude enables consumption for its own sake at many levels of our society. No need to go into our voracious appetites for all things new and environmentally burdensome.

The second attitude is the exact opposite – it is one of containment and cordoning nature off with red tape, charging to get in, leaving no trace, and then exiting back to the city or suburbs. One sees the natural world existing solely to be exploited, the other sees the same as godlike and more important than people. Ironically both attitudes are opposite sides of the same coin. They alienate and remove us from meaningful interaction with our natural surroundings. Meaningful interaction hinges on having something to do in the natural world. Want to save nature? Then interact with her; know her through involvement – hunt, fish, build a log cabin, collect some plants. These activities foster common–sense respect.

Aside from the philosophies that revolve around our interaction with nature and plant collection, because of the times we live in some activities may need to be curtailed. If you are collecting imperiled root medicines; if you are collecting for profit, or to stock a product line, step back and really look at the impact of your activities. Do you really need to be digging up quantities of Echinacea, Goldenseal, American ginseng, Wild yam, etc. all to supply the consumer, who probably isn't taking the herb properly anyway? I am not suggesting the total halt of this type of plant collection, but a serious reevaluation by

involved individuals. As a wildcrafter there are some plants that I will not collect, period. There are others that I will not collect in certain areas. Let the plant and its overall population and health make the decision. "I need it, so I am collecting it regardless", is the wrong answer.

Inversely, there are a large number of medicinal plant species that are listed on "risk" or "watch" lists by various organizations that really have no business being there. By listing plants like Oregongrape, Yerba santa, or Squaw vine, all regionally abundant, there is an over-reaching environmentalism that is created. This fosters an over-protective air of false concern, ultimately leading to misunderstanding.

Plant collection for yourself, your family, or even for a small patient group occurs on a different scale. Endangered and scare plants aside, this type of wildcrafting usually does not pose any problem.

GUIDELINES

Make an objective and educated choice on whether or not to collect a particular plant. Is the plant threatened or endangered? Can the stand support collection? Are seasonal conditions proper?

1. Have positive identification.
2. Collect away from roadsides, city and town areas, industrial sites, agricultural areas, and heavily traveled foot trails.
3. Become familiar with the overall plant populations in your area. If only a small stand exists in one area, move on and collect where it is more abundant.
4. Do not collect more than 10% of any stand.
5. Clean up before leaving; fill in holes and if preparing medicines in the field then spread around core wood and other unusable plant materials to lessen visual impact of your activities.
6. Have respect. If done right, without greed, you are supported by the plants – the natural world, and they are supported through your understanding of them.

DRYING PLANTS

1. Dry plant materials out of direct sunlight. Herbage can be placed loosely in paper bags or laid well–spaced on cardboard flats. Small bundles of leafing tops, with the topmost portions of the plant hanging down are secured from ceiling rafters until dry.
2. Once dry, garble the leaves and flowers from the stems; discard the stems (unless otherwise mentioned).
3. Chop roots into ¼"–½" pieces or longer longitudinal strips. Both these and bark strips dry adequately if well spaced.
4. For quicker drying or to ensure no mold growth occurs if in a humid environment a dehydrator can be used.

PREPARATIONS

Any herb can be of high quality and collected in a pristine environment, but if the delivery method is inferior, its quality will not amount to much. The best way to internally benefit from a medicinal plant is to eat it, preferably fresh. For most of us, this is cumbersome, if not impractical, hence the reason for preparation development in the first place. Do not be fooled by elaborate preparation technique and designer products. Generally speaking the simpler the preparation, the more potent the end result.

DOSAGE

The listed dosage is a good starting point for an average–weighted adult. Depending on weight and sensitivity, it may be decreased or increased accordingly. For children and infants reduce the dose according to weight. If a dose for a 150lb. adult is 30–60 drops 3 times daily, then for a 50lb. child, 10–20 drops 3 times daily is the correct reduction. All percentages apply to alcohol and glycerin contents.

CAUTIONS

If the following precepts are adhered to when using medicinal plants there will be little to fear from potential adverse reactions.

1. Quantity: a little will help, a lot may harm. Any plant properly dosed can be medicinal. The same plant may be toxic in larger amounts.
2. As a society, we are over medicated. If taking pharmaceuticals for a particular problem, throwing an herb or two into the mix to affect the same organ or tissue group may be OK…or not. Do some homework first, or see a professional versed in such matters.
3. If any herb makes you sick, causes a headache, diarrhea, nausea, dizziness, or other unwanted sensations then lessen the dose or discontinue the herb.
4. If an herb affects the mother to be, then it is affecting the fetus. The herb's activity is usually delivered to the baby through breast milk as well. While pregnant or nursing limit herbs that have strong physiologic activities. In these times think of food as medicine.
5. Aside from the fundamental social and moral wrong of abortion, and the medical procedure's link to breast cancer, a number of herbs discussed in this book have abortifacient potential. As a rule, they are unreliable and if used in sufficient quantity are apt to cause harm to the "mother" as well.

A NOTE ON FORMULAS

This book is lacking formulas for a reason – one size does not fit all. If you think the situation calls for a formula then keep it simple. A formula comprised of over five or six herbs is likely to cause more physiologic chatter than therapeutic direction. A well–formulated mixture should be direct, elegant, and unfettered. Keep in consideration the multi–systemic nature of herbs; they usually affect more than one organ system.

Excessive polypharmacy is rampant in the natural supplement industry. Look at the label of most herbal supplement combinations; if the ingredient list is filled with numerous herbs then that formula has absolutely no direction, and only can help someone through placebo or by creating a little physiological "noise" in the body by its elimination through various pathways.

PREPARATIONS

Imagine a plant that has been optimally potentiated through proper preparation. Its effect will be more distinct and the effective dose will be less. How an herb is prepared is equally important to what herb is prepared. Superior medicines are made that way by quality material and a delivery method that suits that particular plant.

In determining which methods are optimal for delivery, each plant should be taken on a case by case basis. That said, groupings or corollaries are evident when focus is placed on a particular plant's family or related constituent groups. Chances are Marshmallow, Mallow, and Hollyhock, all Mallow family plants, will be best prepared through water–based preparations. Not only are they closely related botanically but they are closely related chemically, therefore preparations will be similar, if not identical. Torchwood family plants (Myrrh, Frankincense, Guggul, and Elephant tree), due to their resins and non–polar compounds, should be tinctured with a higher percentage of alcohol.

It is easily forgotten that up to the mid–20th century, half of what doctors prescribed and pharmacist's filled, were plants or derivatives thereof. Prior to WWII, the national formulary and US dispensary (both standard references for doctors/pharmacists) had more print related to whole plants, their derivatives, and related preparation, than synthetically created drugs.

It is a misconception that the area of herbal preparation (herbal *medicine* for that matter) is uncertain and untried. For over a span of two centuries, preparation (and use) was developed, expanded upon, and peaked (then withered due to neglect). Just as there is no need to reinvent the wheel, there is no need to alter traditional and effective plant preparation technique.

What follows are main preparations standard in past and present–day herbal medicine. They are simple, time–tested methods designed to get the most from each plant.

BATH
1. Draw a hot bath.
2. Add 1 gallon of tea to water.
3. Soak.

CAPSULE

Capsules come in various sizes with 'o' (250 mg.), 'oo' (500 mg.), and 'ooo' (1000 mg.) being the most common. To fill simply immerse the two halves in an herbal powder, then fit the capsule together. Encapsulation machines speed up the process. They are available in various designs.

COUGH SYRUP

METHOD 1: HONEY STEEP
1. Take 5½ oz. of finely chopped, fresh plant material; pack into a pint mason jar and fill to the top with honey.
2. Secure lid and set aside for several weeks. Squeeze or press the honey from the herb and bottle the infused honey.
♦ Ratio: 1 part herb (weight) to 2 parts of honey (volume).

METHOD 2: TINCTURE IN HONEY/GLYCERIN BASE
1. Mix together 8 oz. of appropriate tincture(s) with 4 oz. of honey and 4 oz. of glycerin.
2. Bottle.
♦ Ratio: 2 parts tincture (volume) to 1 part honey (volume) to 1 part glycerin (volume).

METHOD 3: TINCTURE WITH SIMPLE SYRUP
1. Mix together 8 oz. of tincture(s) and 8 oz. of simple syrup.
2. Bottle.
♦ Ratio: 1 part tincture (volume) to 1 part simple syrup (volume).

CONSIDERATIONS
None of these preparations need to be refrigerated. Method 2 and 3 are basically diluted tinctures and are stronger than the honey steep. 1–2

teaspoons will be an average adult dose; 1 table-spoon for the honey steep.

DOUCHE

1. Make a half–strength tea.
2. Cool until warm.
3. Add ½ teaspoon of table salt per pint of tea.
4. Use as directed.
5. Make fresh daily.

EYEWASH

METHOD 1
1. Make 1 pint of tea with distilled or filtered water through the properly designated method (infusion, decoction, etc.)
2. Strain well through a paper towel or cloth.
3. Add ½ teaspoon of table salt.
4. Stir until dissolved.
5. Apply as needed.
6. Make fresh daily.

METHOD 2
1. Add 10 drops of appropriate tincture to 2 oz. of isotonic water (¼ teaspoon of table salt to 1 cup of distilled or filtered water).
2. Apply as needed.
3. Make fresh daily.

FLUIDEXTRACT

First introduced into the U.S.P. of 1850, the fluidextract is an official pharmaceutical preparation. More concentrated than a tincture it is 1:1 in strength, meaning each milliliter of extract contains a representation of 1 gram of dried herb (1 oz. of fluidextract will be derived from and have the potency of 1 oz. of dried herb).

Not all plants lend themselves well to fluidextracts, but the ones that are suited for the preparation are mentioned in each plant profile. To make a fluidextract a basic tincture needs to be made through percolation; it is then concentrated to a 1:1. Essentially fluidextracts enable a lower dose, and are convenient if making formulas.

MATERIALS
♦ Gather all materials designated under Dry Plant Tincture/Percolation.
♦ Extra container to catch the second batch.
♦ Double boiler.

METHOD 1: WATER SOLUBLE PLANTS
1. Use Method 1 with plants that are mostly water soluble; they will call for 50% alcohol or less.
2. Make a normal base menstruum as described under Percolation. If needed use Appendix D worksheets.
3. Set up and drip as described under Percolation.
4. The first catch is composed of ¾ of the FFV (final fluidextract volume). Example: If the FFV is 8 oz., then the first catch will be 6 oz.
5. Remove the "first catch" and set aside.
6. Place the extra container under the cone to collect the second catch.
7. Drip the remaining base menstruum.
8. Place the second catch in the double boiler and heat slowly until the fluid volume reaches the remaining ¼ part of the FFV.
9. Let cool; combine the two catches; bottle.

CONSIDERATIONS
♦ Nearly all of the necessary preparation and set up are the same for both the standard percolation and fluidextract.
♦ The main differences are:
1. "The catch" is being separated into two batches. The first catch is the most concentrated and the more medicinally active part of the percolation. This is purposely not reduced through heat due to its density of compounds – and even a minimal amount of heat degradation is unacceptable for this part of the extract.
2. If desired more menstruum can be made and run through the herb to increase the second catch. Normally 6–7 parts (1–2 parts to moisten, 5 parts to be dripped

through) total will be used, but it can be increased to any amount, because it will be reduced through the double boiler anyway. If desired 100 parts of menstruum can be run through; but know it will all have to reduced in the end. It is a time consuming process.

♦ When reducing the second catch be sure to do so with least amount of heat possible. It should be hot enough to where subtle evaporation, not boiling, occurs.

METHOD 2: ALCOHOL SOLUBLE PLANTS

1. Use method 2 with plants that are mostly alcohol soluble; they will call for 51% alcohol or more.
2. The base menstruum will be made into two separate batches – first batch is called HAM (high alcohol menstruum); second batch, LAM (low alcohol menstruum).
3. To make the HAM, increase the alcohol percentage by 20% and decrease the water percentage by 20%. Example: if the plant normally calls for 60% alcohol/40% water, then ratios for the HAM will be 80% alcohol/20% water. The HAM is composed of the volume taken up by the compressed herb and ¾ of the FFV.
4. LAM ratios are the exact opposite. If 60%/40% alcohol/water ratio is called for then the LAM will be comprised of 40%/60%. The LAM is composed of the remaining base menstruum.
5. Example using 8 oz. of Astragalus root: Its compressed volume is 12 oz. The base menstruum of 52 oz. (8 oz. x 5 = 40 oz. + 12 oz.) calls for 60% alcohol/40% water. The HAM is composed of 18 oz. (12 oz. [volume of compressed herb] + 6 oz. [¾ of FFV]. Of this 18 oz., 80% or 14.4 oz. is alcohol and 20% or 3.6 oz. is water. The LAM is made separately. It is composed of 40% alcohol or 13.6 oz. and 60% water or 20.4 oz. equalling 34 oz. or the remaining base menstruum.
6. With the HAM, moisten and digest (at least 24 hours). If there is insufficient HAM to cover the herb completely for proper digestion then add a small amount of LAM.
7. Start the drip process. When the HAM is in danger of falling below the top layer of saturated powder then add the LAM.
8. To conclude, follow from #4 under method 1.

CONSIDERATIONS

♦ The idea of this method is solve out most of the non–polar compounds with a higher alcohol content so they are caught in the first catch. Follow up with a higher water percentage for the remaining polar constituents, which generally hold up better through the heating/double boiler process.
♦ Same as method 1.

FOMENTATION

1. Soak a cloth or towel in a warm herb tea.
2. Squeeze excess tea from the cloth.
3. Apply the cloth to the affected area.
4. Re–soak and apply as needed.

HYDROSOL

Also called floral water, a hydrosol forms during essential oil distillation. Considered a by–product of the distillation process, it is composed of the condensed steam (water) that was initially in contact with the plant material. Filled with hydroscopic volatile compounds and traces of colloid–formed essential oil, hydrosols share some therapeutic characteristics with essential oils; the main exception being potency. Dilute and mild, hydrosols can even be used as a replacement for standard teas. Often they are used as facial sprays or washes. They make a fine replacement for the water portion when making ointments.

LINIMENT

An externally applied tincture. Isopropyl alcohol can be used instead of ethyl alcohol for this preparation. Do not use isopropyl alcohol internally.

OIL, ESSENTIAL

Typically prepared through steam distillation, essential oils represent the volatile or aromatic fraction of a particular plant. Essential oils differ greatly from herbal oils. Two very different processes are employed to reach two very different finished products. The two are not interchangeable.

Pure essential oils can be used both externally and internally. Because they represent a potentiated fraction of a plant care should be taken when they are used, especially when ingested. Undiluted they represent some of the strongest topical medicines we employ. As antiinflammatories, analgesics, and antimicrobials/antivirals they excel. Applied undiluted to sensitize tissue/mucus membranes they may cause some irritation; diluting 100-200% with a carrier oil (olive, almond, etc.) usually is sufficient to reduce this tendency. They can be added to an herbal oil in a wide range of ratios – just enough to impart a fragrance, or enough to be the main topical agent.

Ingested, essential oils should be approached with some caution as toxicity due to overdose is a pertinent issue. Unlike tinctures, where 30–60 drops (for many plants) is a normal therapeutic dose, 2–3 drops for an essential oil is roughly equal in potency. For this preparation several drops are placed in a gelatin capsule and then swallowed. See Spirit for another internal preparation utilizing these potent oils.

Most plants with a distinctive smell can be used as essential oils: many plants in the Mint, Sunflower, Cypress, and Pine families are well utilized. Although this preparation excludes many other constituents, due to their nonvolatile nature – vitamins/minerals, glycosides, and most alkaloids – if used properly the right plant can be better directed and potentiated.

Essential oils are easily added to tinctures; they are particularly useful, like fluidextracts, when keeping volume low is important.

When purchasing essential oils the label will typically say "not for internal use". This is due to their innate concentrated form. Check that they are not preserved or diluted with synthetics (some "natural" perfumes).

For those of you who want to distill your own essential oils, there are many decent distillers on the market today. Most fall into two camps – the "lab equipment" type and the old–school copper type. Both work; if nothing else the decision to purchase one or the other is often based on size and visual appeal.

See Hydrosol for a useful distillation by–product.

OIL, HERBAL

Herbal oils are usually applied to unbroken skin for their interaction with the epidemic/keratin (surface) layers. They soften the skin, retain the active medicine, and provide a limited protective coating. This enables skin conditions to better respond and more fully heal. Herbal oils are the base for both ointments and salves. Ointments are better at penetrating; salves at protecting.

Vegetable oils can be broken into several classes depending on viscosity or thickness and to what degree they dry or thicken when exposed to air. Olive, almond, and peanut oils are thicker than most, and create less of a film when exposed to air. Mustard seed, canola, sesame, sunflower, pumpkin, soy, and corn oils thicken to a moderate degree, but are less viscous. Hemp, linseed (flax), safflower, sunflower, and walnut oils are the least viscous, and upon air contract, produce a gummy film.

Rancidity is a factor with all fats. If an herbal oil is being stored for over several months use olive as the base oil. It is greatly resistant to oxidation and rancidity. Even compared to grapeseed, known for its high antioxidant activity, olive oil will be found more stable.

Once made store the oil in an air–tight, darkened glass container. Refrigeration is not necessary, but nonetheless should be kept at cool temperatures.

METHOD 1: ALCOHOL INTERMEDIATE

Best for herbs that are high in volatiles, resins,

and other non–polar constituents. It stands out as one of the better herbal oil techniques, demonstrated by the vibrant color imparted to the oil.

1. Mix 1 oz. of dried, coarsely powered herb with ½–1 oz. of 190 proof ethyl alcohol.
2. Cover and let stand for an hour.
3. Pour 7 oz. of olive oil into a blender.
4. Add the alcohol–saturated herb.
5. Blend on high for 15 minutes or until blender container is very warm to hot.
6. Strain the oil/herb through a piece of cloth.
7. Discard the herb, bottle the oil.
♦ Ratio: 1 part herb (weight) to ½–1 part 190 proof ethyl alcohol (volume) to 7 parts olive oil (volume).

METHOD 2: WILTED HERB

This method works best for herbs that become less potent upon fully drying. We are taking advantage of their fresh state but need to reduce their water content to lessen possible fermentation.

1. Wilt the plant to half of its original weight; this often takes 8–12 hours.
2. Chop or dice the herb being careful not to make a puree, as this will release too much water into the oil, encouraging fermentation.
3. In a jar combine 1 oz. of chopped herb in 7 oz. of olive oil.
4. Mix thoroughly.
5. Seal and let stand in a warm (90–100 degrees) place, out of direct sunlight, for 14 days. Covered, exposed to the sun or next to a stove or heat duct, are some good places.
6. Strain, but do not press the oil from the herb.
7. Let stand until any residual water and the oil completely separate. Pour off the oil, or with a basting syringe collect it apart from any water layer. Bottle the oil; discard the water.
♦ Ratio: 1 part herb (weight) to 7 parts olive oil (volume).

METHOD 3: OLD STANDARD

1. Combine 1 oz. of dried, powdered herb with 7 oz. of olive oil.
2. Using a blender thoroughly mix the combination.
3. Pour into a sealable jar.
4. Seal and let stand in a warm (90–100 degrees) place, out of direct sunlight, for 14 days. Covered while exposed to the sun or next to a stove or heat duct are some good places.
5. Agitate several times a day.
6. After 14 days, in a blender, blend until the container is very warm–hot.
7. Strain; bottle the oil.
♦ Ratio: 1 part herb (weight) to 7 parts olive oil (volume).

METHOD 4: HEAT

This method is particularly useful when the alcohol intermediate method is not preferred. Use with plants high in stable oleoresins, such as Cayenne pepper, Ginger, or Myrrh.

1. Combine 1 oz. of dried, powdered herb with 7 oz. of olive oil.
2. Mix thoroughly and tighten lid
3. Submerged in a heated pot of water, heat to 140–160 degrees for 4–5 hours.
4. Remove from heat and let stand for an additional 4 hours.
5. Strain and bottle.
♦ Ratio: 1 part herb (weight) to 7 parts olive oil (volume).

OINTMENT

Ointments are best used when there is a need of a penetrating topical medicine. They affect a deeper array of tissues (compared to salves) but need to be applied more often.

1. Combine 7 parts base oil (almond/olive/pre–made herbal oil) with 1 part beeswax.
2. Slowly heat until beeswax is dissolved in oil.
3. Cool until wax starts to faintly harden on the sides of the container. At this point you should be able to put your finger into the oil without it being too hot.

4. In a blender pour 12 parts of distilled water/herb tea/hydrosol.
5. Blend on low.
6. Slowly pour the oil/beeswax mixture into the blender.
7. Do not blend for too long – 10–15 seconds.
8. The mixture should have a creamy consistency.
9. Blot any extra liquid from the top of the ointment.
10. Mix in any additional essential oils at this point (1 ml. per 5–7 oz. or so).
11. Scoop into containers and refrigerate.
♦ Ratio: 7 parts herbal oil (volume) to 1 part beeswax (weight) to 12 parts water/tea/hydrosol (volume).

CONSIDERATIONS

Depending on what tea/hydrosol or essential oil is added, the refrigerated ointment will last without spoilage, for several months, some longer.

POULTICE

METHOD 1: BASIC

1. Moisten the needed amount of dried and powdered herb with warm water until a porridge–like consistence is reached.
2. Apply directly to the affected area, or cover the area first with muslin cloth, then apply.
3. Secure poultice with a covering and/or bandage.
4. Change 2–3 times daily, or when cool.

METHOD 2: FIELD POULTICE

1. Bruise and/or puree the fresh plant.
2. Apply to affected area and secure.
3. Change 2–3 times daily.
4. A "spit poultice" can be quickly made by chewing the intended herb (make sure it is internally non–toxic) and applying it to the affected area.

POWDER

Depending on the part of the plant some materials are harder than others to powder. Roots, bark, and stems are more difficult than leaves, flowers, and lightweight parts. For lighter materials an average blender with a metal or glass container is adequate; for tougher materials a vita–mix works well, or an industrial grinder/mill. Once the plant is powdered it can then be used as a dust, or as a starting point for DPTs, poultices, etc.

SALVE

Salves will be best applied when there is need of a protective coating covering the skin.

1. While slowly heating 7 oz. of an herbal oil add 1 oz. of beeswax.
2. Let wax slowly dissolve.
3. While still hot, pour into containers.
4. As the salve cools, it will solidify.
♦ Ratio: 7 parts herbal oil (volume) to 1 part beeswax (weight).

SITZ BATH

Using ½ strength or full strength tea apply/soak until tea is cool.

SPIRIT

A spirt is simply an essential oil diluted with a specific amount of alcohol. This preparation is mainly designed to make essential oils more palatable for internal use. It also makes essential oils more suitable as formula ingredients.

1. Take 1 part essential oil and dilute with 9 parts 190 proof ethyl alcohol.
2. Mix; bottle; store.
♦ Ratio: 9 parts alcohol (volume) to 1 part essential oil (volume).

SUPPOSITORY

Suppositories are preparations made for either vaginal or rectal insertion (less commonly for the urethra). Two types of suppositories are covered here. The first has a glycerin/gelatin base and works well with tinctures and fluidextracts as the added medicinal agent. The second type is Cocoa butter based and is better suited for added herbal oils and essential oils.

METHOD 1: GLYCERIN/GELATIN

1. Mix together 6.5 parts glycerin with 2.1 parts of tincture or fluidextract.
2. Heat for several minutes using low temperatures.
3. Add 1.4 parts of powdered gelatin.
4. Mix thoroughly and remove from heat.
5. Pour into suppository molds and let cool.

- Ratio: 6.5 parts glycerin to 2.1 parts tincture/fluidextract to 1.4 parts gelatin (all totaling 10 parts).

METHOD 2: COCOA BUTTER

1. Using low heat melt 1 part Cocoa butter.
2. Add ½ part herbal oil and mix together.
3. Add any essential oil at this point. 1ml. per 5–7 oz. of oil.
4. Pour into suppository molds and let cool.

- Ratio: 1 part Cocoa butter to ½ part herbal oil.

CONSIDERATIONS

- The ratios presented here are meant as guides and can be altered if the suppository's consistency needs to be changed.
- Placing the suppositories in a refrigerator or freezer for a short period of time can help in their solidification.
- Suppositories are best used before bed when the body is in a horizontal position.
- If at any time the suppository causes any irritation discontinue or change recipe.
- Pharmaceutical grade gelatin, suppository molds (both the disposable plastic type and the aluminum/metal block type) are available through pharmacy suppliers. Check on-line or with compounding pharmacies.

SYRUP, SIMPLE

Simple syrup is called for in some respiratory formulations and in any other formula where a preparation's sweetness and soothing qualities are part of its effect.

1. In a pot combine 32 ounces of refined white sugar and 16 oz. of water.
2. Slowly heat and stir until the sugar is fully dissolved. Occasionally 1 or 2 additional ounces of water will be needed to full dissolve the sugar.
3. Let cool and bottle. The syrup does not need to be refrigerated.

- Ratio: 2 parts sugar (weight) to 1 part (volume) water.

CONSIDERATIONS

- Any tea can be converted into a syrup by simply adding sugar in the proper ratio. Senna, Marshmallow, Wild cherry, Rhubarb, and Ginger are a number of classics. Tinctures/fluidextracts can also be added to simple syrups, usually in a 1 part to 1 part ratio.
- Other sweeteners will ferment and spoil if used without added alcohol.

TEA

Tea preparations are best applied to plants that have a large array of water–soluble compounds. Plants that are being used for tannins, starches, minerals, and other polar compounds are best taken as teas. All plants are dried first then infused or decocted.

Making tea with a fresh plant is a waste. Intact, living plant cells are adept at holding on to their vital cellular compounds, not giving them up to water. Through drying this force is disrupted – cell walls are broken making the plant's various constituents permeable to water. Make tea or any water–based preparation fresh daily.

INFUSION

1. Bring 1 quart of water to a boil.
2. Turn off heat.
3. Stir in 1 oz. of dry, fragile plant materials – leaves, flowers, thin stems, etc.
4. Cover and steep for at least 15 minutes.
5. Uncover and strain.
♦ Ratio: 1 part herb (weight) to 32 parts water (volume).

DECOCTION

1. Bring 1 quart of water to a slow simmer.
2. Stir in 1 oz. of thicker, dried plant materials – bark, roots, stems, pods, etc.
3. Cover and simmer for at least 15 minutes.
4. Turn heat off.
5. Steep for 15 minutes.
6. Uncover and strain.
♦ Ratio: 1 part herb (weight) to 32 parts water (volume).

COLD INFUSION

1. Suspend in a mesh tea bag or colander 1 oz. of dried plant materials in 1 quart of water.
2. Steep over night at room temperature. Strain.
3. Make fresh daily.
♦ Ratio: 1 part herb (weight) to 32 parts water (volume).

TINCTURE

♦ Plants that are high in volatile oils, complex starches, and other non–polar constituents are best prepared through tincturing.
♦ A 1:2 FPT (fresh plant tincture) means that in each fluid oz. of tincture produced there is contained the therapeutic constituents of ½ oz. of fresh herb. The herb/menstruum ratio generally corresponds to this as well: 1 part of fresh herb to 2 parts of menstruum. A 1:5 DPT (dry plant tincture) means 1 part of dried herb to 5 parts of menstruum or in each fluid oz. of tincture produced there is contained the therapeutic constituents of ⅕ oz. of dried herb.

♦ A 1:2 FPT is equal in strength to a 1:5 DPT. Since the dried plant lacks water it is being added back into the menstruum to properly extract the plant's constituents.
♦ The alcohol percentage of the FPT is high. What is being relied upon in this tincture preparation is the hydroscopic (hygroscopic) activity of alcohol. The alcohol literally dehydrates the fresh plant. It pulls all of the plant's constituents/cytoplasm out into the surrounding alcohol. The result is a highly potent, intact representation of the fresh plant. FPTs with lower alcohol contents are inferior; water limits the pulling activity of alcohol.
♦ 1:2 for a FPT and 1:5 for a DPT are standard ratios originated by chemists in western medicine's past when plants were the main medicines.
♦ Depending on the plant, lower tincture and extract ratios (1:1 or 2:1, etc.) are not necessarily better or stronger. One characteristic of a good quality tincture is its lack of particulate matter, or sediment. Often many plants respond poorly to a 1:1 or more concentrated preparations because their constituents are not able to remain in suspension and "salt out" through being too concentrated. This limits the body's ability to properly absorb the preparation.
♦ All tinctures are made with 190 proof ethyl alcohol, commonly called Everclear. Look to liquor stores or the liquor section of grocery stores. Availability varies from state to state.

FRESH PLANT TINCTURE

METHOD I: OLD STANDARD

1. Place 2 oz. of fresh, chopped plant material in a glass jar.
2. Add 4 oz. of alcohol.
3. Secure the lid. There is no need to shake the mixture. After 14 days, press or squeeze the tincture from the herb.
4. Discard the marc (spent herb).
5. Bottle the tincture.

♦ Ratio: 1 part fresh herb (weight) to 2 parts 190 proof ethyl alcohol (volume).

A SIMPLIFIED METHOD

1. Place 5½ oz. of fresh, chopped plant material in a pint mason jar.
2. Fill to the top with alcohol.
3. Secure the lid and follow the instructions mentioned previously.

♦ Ratio: 1 part fresh herb (weight) to 2 parts 190 proof ethyl alcohol (volume).

CONSIDERATIONS

♦ Filling the jar to the top with alcohol will not amount to exactly 11 oz. (or 2 parts), but it will be close enough.

♦ After the jar is sealed and several days have passed often the alcohol fully settles to where the level is below the jar's lip. Remove the jar's lid and top–off with alcohol. Secure lid. Press after the initial 14 days.

DRY PLANT TINCTURE

METHOD I: MACERATION

1. Place 2 oz. of dried and powered plant material in a glass jar.
2. Add 10 oz. of alcohol/water mixture – see each plant's preparation/dosage for the correct alcohol/water percentage. (If a plant calls for 60% alcohol then add 6 oz. of grain alcohol and 4 oz. (40%) of water).
3. Combine together with the powdered herb in a glass jar. Secure lid and then shake well for several minutes.
4. Let stand for 2 weeks – shaking everyday for 5 minutes.
5. Press the tincture from the marc. Or squeeze by hand using a large piece of flannel or cheese cloth.
6. Discard the marc.
7. Bottle the tincture.

♦ Ratio: 1 part dried herb (weight) to 5 parts menstruum (volume).

CONSIDERATIONS

♦ When using this tincture method with high tannin–content plants the menstruum should consist of 10% glycerin. This inhibits the tannins from binding together and with other constituents.

METHOD 2: PERCOLATION

Percolation is a tincturing technique regarded as superior to maceration. Fresh menstruum with full extractive potential is always in contact with the powdered herb; by the time it drains from the cone to be caught below it is "full" with compounds.

The concept is the same when percolating coffee. Powdered and moistened herb is packed into a glass cone or funnel. This is suspended over, via a stand, or inserted into, a suitable receiving container. Menstruum is added topside into the large opening of the cone. As it descends, the menstruum's flow rate is controlled by a cap or valve. The menstruum that is caught in the receiving vessel is now the percolate (or tincture).

MATERIALS

♦ Powdered herb.
♦ Premixed menstruum. See specific plant profile or Appendix B for alcohol/water percentages.
♦ Glass percolation cone/glass funnel/improvised glass bottle. Original percolation cones, used up until around the early part of the 20th century are scarce. Glass funnels are still abundant and can be found at reasonable prices at antique shops or on–line. A large 40+ oz. malt liquor bottle can be converted to a percolation cone by removing the base with a glass cutter. Make sure to sand the sharp edges. With the converted bottle the screw cap serves as the drip control. To fabricate a drip control for the glass funnel, an irrigation drip valve, a couple of inches of suitable poly tubing, and plumping tape are all that are needed.
♦ Receiving vessel: quart, ½–gallon, or gallon mason jar.
♦ Filter: basket or cone–type coffee filter (2).

PREPARATION

1. Use the percolation worksheet (Appendix D).
2. Determine the preparation's ratio of strength (almost always 1:5, although there are several exceptions).
3. Weigh the powdered plant.
4. Put the powdered plant in a measuring cup or mason jar with side measuring increments. Lightly compress the plant, and record its volume.
5. Determine the FTV (final tincture volume). Example: If the ratio of strength is 1:5, and 5 oz. of powdered herb is being percolated then FTV is 25 oz. (The ratio of strength can also be viewed as a simple weight to volume formula. 1:5 (1 part of plant (5 oz.) to 5 parts of menstruum–or FTV (25 oz.).
6. When calculating the base menstruum make sure to include the volume of the compressed plant. This is necessary because a certain amount of menstruum will always remain behind in the marc after the percolation is complete. It is *not* pressed from the marc.
7. Example: If the ratio is 1:5, the powdered plant weights 5 oz., its volume is 8 oz., the FTV is 25 oz., and the tincture calls for 50% alcohol and 50% water, then, the base menstruum is (25 oz. + 8 oz.) 32 oz. and composed of 16 oz. alcohol and 16 oz. water.

MOISTEN AND DIGEST

1. Place the dried, coarsely powdered plant material in a bowl.
2. Moisten: add about ⅔ of the plant's volume in menstruum to the powered plant and mix thoroughly. If needed more can be used to adequately moisten the powder (should be formable without excess dripping).
3. Place a menstruum–moistened filter (cone or basket–shaped) inside the glass funnel or percolation cone. With your hands flatten out as many wrinkles as possible.
4. Gently add the moistened herb, placing it on top of the filter, inside the cone.
5. Tamp and evenly compress the moistened

herb. Fingers work well for this. If the material hardly packs, use more force; if you are straining, use less. Ideally you want the material to be uniformly compressed, where after adding the menstruum it will slowly travel to the lower opening. Air pockets and channels (some can form next to the lower filter) are not wanted. An overly packed cone, where the menstruum struggles to decent is not wanted either.

6. Place another filter on top of the compressed material. This is mainly used so the compressed herb does not stir when adding menstruum.
7. Pour enough menstruum onto the compressed herb (actually pouring the menstruum onto the top filter) to fully saturate the herb. As you pour watch the compressed herb; you should be able to see the liquid–layer of menstruum filtering downward. When the herb is fully saturated, and a drip occurs at the small lower opening, close the opening (cap or valve).
8. Add enough menstruum so that a ¼–½ inch layer is covering the compressed herb.
9. Digest: set aside for 24 to 48 hours.

PERCOLATE

1. Open the cap/valve until a steady drip occurs.
2. In very small increments through tightening the cap or valve reduce the drip to 1–2 drops per second.
3. Place or suspend the dripping cone over a suitable receptacle. Various sized mason jars work well, as they are clear and have mouths that serve as stands.
4. Pour the remaining menstruum onto the compressed herb/filter. Depending on how large the cone is this may need to be done in several installments
5. Keep careful watch on the menstruum level. Do not allow it to contact/fall below the compressed herb. If so, air pockets will be created reducing the proper decent of the menstruum.

6. Drip enough menstruum to "catch" the FTV. (This is not a precise science: it is not uncommon to be off by 10% or so; more than that indicates a calculation error).

7. Some menstruum will always be left in the marc. Do *not* press the marc. It contains only menstruum–moistened spent material.

8. Bottle, cap, and label the percolate, which is now a properly made tincture.

CONSIDERATIONS

♦ Do not agitate or disturb the herb once compressed with menstruum filtering downward.

♦ When the percolate starts to rise to the level of the dripping cap/valve, switch containers as to not submerge the cap/valve in the percolate.

♦ If the tincturing process goes array for any reason – excessive air pockets, over or under packed herb – pour the remaining menstruum and the moistened herb in a jar together and proceed with a standard maceration. This will probably occur a number of times when starting out. It's just part of the learning process.

METHOD 3: VINEGAR (ACETUM TINCTURE)

Using either the maceration or percolation technique vinegar (apple cider vinegar is fine) is used as a solvent. Only useful for several herbs such as Artemisia and Lobelia, its main drawback is a short storage time.

WASH

Topically apply an herb tea to the affected area.

WASH, NASAL

The principal use of this preparation is as wash for the sinuses. It is a somewhat bizarre experience that goes against instinct (sucking water in through the nose, instead of blowing it out). But the result is worth the strangeness, particularly if there is a sinus infection.

1. Make an isotonic solution adding ½ teaspoon of table salt to 1 pint of warm water or an appropriate tea.

2. Pour the solution into a bowl. It should be shallow enough so liquid is close to the bowl's lip.

3. While plugging one nostril, submerge the open nostril into the solution.

4. *Slowly* inhale through the submerged nostril.

5. The solution will be drawn in through the nostril and collect in the mouth.

6. Spit solution out.

7. Change nostrils and repeat.

CONSIDERATIONS

♦ In acute conditions this wash can be repeated every hour or so.

♦ A special container called a "neti pot" is made for this application. It is basically a miniature watering can. It holds no significant advantage over simply using a bowl.

MATERIA MEDICA

AGRIMONY
Rosaceae/Rose Family

Agrimonia gryposepala
Common agrimony

Agrimonia striata
Roadside agrimony, Woodland agrimony

DESCRIPTION

A member of the Rose family, Agrimony is an herbaceous sub–shrub. Blending into the surrounding understory, the plant's leaves are its most unique feature. Consisting of varying sized toothed leaflets they are arranged along the leaf stem in an odd–pinnate pattern. Here, sets of significantly undersized leaflets separate larger leaflets. The pattern is distinctive and helpful in identifying the plant. The small, 5–petaled, yellow flowers form in elongated racemes. They are followed by small, seed capsules covered by hooked prickles.

DISTRIBUTION

Agrimony is common throughout much of North America – look to stream margins, pastures, and woodlines where some sunlight is able to pass through the taller trees and shrubs.

CHEMISTRY

Coumarins; flavonoids; tannins; terpenoids.

MEDICINAL USES

As an astringent, Agrimony affects the urinary tract. The plant's array of tannins constrict surface tissues. In addition, the tannins have an underlying antiinflammatory effect on local vascular tissue. One of the plant's specific indications is mucus in the urine. Relatedly if the urine is cloudy and/or strong smelling (typical symptoms of a urinary tract infection), the plant's soothing and astringent qualities will likely give relief. As a lithotropic agent, it is an old remedy. Combined with Lobelia and Gravel root, obstructions of the urinary tract are more easily passed. Corresponding tissue trauma is quieted. Occasionally,

Agrimony is of use to the aged who are troubled by incontinence. In these situations, if urinary tissues are lax and without tone, the tea again will prove useful.

Women will benefit from Agrimony, as most other Rose family astringents, if used to curb menorrhagia. Again it is the plant's tannin group that is responsible for its menses–diminishing effect. Minor postpartum bleeding also will abate due to the plant's mild uterine lining astringency. There is probably little Agrimony will do if the situation is caused by diminished levels of estrogen/progesterone upon entering menopause.

Mild vaginitis responds well to the tea when it is applied using a douche or sitz bath. Although not particularly antimicrobial it will be found soothing to inflamed tissues.

INDICATIONS

♦ Cystitis/Urethritis/Nephritis, all chronic with cloudy–odiferous urine
♦ Lithiasis
♦ Incontinence, in the aged
♦ Menorrhagia, idiosyncratic
♦ Postpartum bleeding/As a postpartum tonic
♦ Vaginitis (external)

COLLECTION

Gather Agrimony with or without flower development in the spring or summer when new leaf growth is apparent.

PREPARATIONS/DOSAGE

♦ Herbal infusion: 4–8 oz. 2–3 times daily
♦ FPT/DPT (50% alcohol): 1 teaspoon 2–3 times daily
♦ Douche/sitz bath: as needed

CAUTIONS

Agrimony is a mild plant. There are no significant cautions for its use. If drunk to excess mild stomach upset is possible.

Alfalfa

Fabaceae/Pea Family

Medicago sativa
Lucerne

DESCRIPTION

Alfalfa is a 2′–3′ tall, herbaceous, short–lived perennial. Erect to decumbent, the plant's stems are variable in pattern. Its trifoliate leaf arrangement is typical of many plants of the Pea family. Each leaflet is between ½″ to 1½″ in length and is lanceolate to obovate. At branch ends flower clusters are arranged in racemes. Individual flowers are bilaterally symmetrical and are a shade of purple. The corolla is ¼″–½″ in length.

DISTRIBUTION

Due to the plant's significant world–wide distribution its exact native range in Eurasia remains uncertain.

CHEMISTRY

Crude protein; lignins; isoflavones; miscellaneous nutrients.

MEDICINAL USES

As a mild remedy for nutritional deficiencies, Alfalfa is an excellent source of absorbable minerals. It combines well with Red raspberry leaf or Horsetail as a tea used when there is tissue wasting due to gastrointestinal–centered illness. Regional ulcerative conditions, functional or organic issues, and even the psychosomatic involvement of anorexia, all of which may lead to weight reduction, will be buffered by the plant. That is, Alfalfa will keep the body better nourished so tissues are more apt to heal. Whenever malnourishment is a factor, Alfalfa will do some good.

Some find that the encapsulated seed reduces arthritic inflammation, the herb tea stimulates lactation, and on occasion diminishes the hot flashes of menopause. The last two effects probably can be attributed to some sort of hormonal influence produced by many plants of the Pea family. However, there are other plants better suited for these issues – see Therapeutic Index.

INDICATIONS

- Anorexia
- Deficiency, nutritional
- Malnourishment, due to organic or functional issues

COLLECTION

Gather the herbage; dry normally. Personally wildcrafted Alfalfa will almost always be superior to commercial grades. The plant does not have a long shelf life. Its vibrant green color will begin to diminish in several months.

PREPARATIONS/DOSAGE

- Herb infusion: 4–8 oz. 2–3 times daily

CAUTIONS

Just as Alfalfa is a superb tea for nutritional deficiencies, its primary advantage – recovering trace minerals from soil – can also be a problem if collected in contaminated areas. Alfalfa picks up a fair share of copper, lead, cadmium, and nickel. Therefore it is best to know where the material comes from before using.

OTHER USES

The plant is important as a silage crop and in soil conditioning.

Aloe

Liliaceae/Lily Family

Aloe barbadensis (Aloe vera, A. vulgaris, A. perfoliata var. vera)
True aloe

Aloe ferox
Cape aloe, Bitter aloe

DESCRIPTION

Aloe barbadensis or Aloe vera, as it is more commonly known, is a succulent plant that stands between 2'–4' tall. At the plant's base form large rosettes of lance–shaped leaves. A well–hydrated leaf is stout and weighty; at maturity, leaves can reach lengths of 30" and weigh 2–3 lbs. Leaf skin is smooth, rubbery, and grayish–green with re-curved teeth lining its margins. Tall flower racemes originate from the center of the plant. Individual flowers are tubular, yellow, and droop downwards. The lower flowers mature and open first.

In many respects, Aloe ferox and A. barbadensis are very similar. However, A. ferox is a much larger plant, reaching 6'–10' at maturity. The central stem crown bares a rosette of thick, succulent green leaves. Mature plants can develop impressive trunks which become covered by older leaves if they are left unpruned. Reddish–brown teeth are arranged along leaf margins and occasionally on both the upper and lower surfaces. Flower stalks can be branched. The central stalk stands several feet tall and supports a cluster of reddish–orange tubular flowers. Like A. barbadensis, the lower flowers are the first to mature and open.

DISTRIBUTION

Aloe barbadensis appears to be originally from the eastern Mediterranean area, but like Corn and Cannabis, it has been cultivated and trans-ported for thousands of years making the exact location of its native region difficult to ascer-tain. Now though, the plant is widely distrib-uted throughout the Middle East, northern Af-rica, and peninsular India. Here in the West it is found throughout Central America, Mexico, Florida, Texas, and throughout the low–eleva-tion Southwest where it is grown with some ex-tra care. A. ferox is a South African native, but like A. barbadensis, it is extensively grown as an ornamental. In the past, it was widely cultivated for its dried exudate.

CHEMISTRY

Anthraquinones: barbaioin (aloin), which breaks down into aloe–emodin–9–anthrone; isobarba-loin; lignins; saponins; sterols.

MEDICINAL USES

There are essentially two different medicines derived from Aloe. Both have diverging physi-ologic activities, modes of action, and collection techniques.

Aloe leaf exudate, which is yellowish–brown when fresh, is mainly contained between the rind and inner leaf within a layer of specialized cells. Collected and dried, it is the historical Bit-ter aloe of the old drug trade. Even up to 2002, some over–the–counter and pharmaceutical preparations were comprised mainly of Aloe leaf exudate.

The fresh or dried exudate is useful primar-ily as a stimulant laxative. If constipated, use it internally for short periods. Aloe exudate stimu-lates peristalsis and fluid secretion by the large bowel. Curiously, these activities are largely achieved only after colonic bacteria transform the anthraquinone aloin into an active metabo-lite, aloe–emodin–9–anthrone. Like Senna, the addition of carminative herbs such as Ginger or Peppermint will offset potential griping caused by Aloe alone.

Arthritis that is dependent upon poor bow-el health and related constipation will also im-prove under the use of Aloe exudate. Like other stimulant laxatives, Aloe can be habit forming if taken for lengthy periods. Address liver health, stress patterns, and diet before relying on Aloe or any stimulant laxative for regular bowel move-ments.

Topically it is significantly inhibiting to a number of fungal and bacterial strains. There-fore, as a paint or dust, it is well applied to infec-tions that are non–resolving and tenacious.

Aloe's leaf pulp is also used topically for wound healing but its mode of action differs from the leaf exudate. The leaf pulp diminishes inflammation through its inhibitory effects on thromboxane and bradykinin. Both compounds are mediators of inflammation. Aloe's polysac-charide content enhances the synthesis of con-nective tissue and skin repair. A fresh leaf poul-tice applied to burns is one of Aloe's foremost applications. Its speed in diminishing pain and redness verges on remarkable.

Secondarily the leaf pulp facilitates wound healing by its absorbent quality. Like all succulent plants, Aloe's internal structure is hydrophilic; it absorbs polar fluids and holds on to them. Placing an open leaf poultice on a damaged area facilitates the absorption of disorganized surface tissue fluids, which speeds healing. To maximize the advantages of Aloe's absorbent qualities, change leaf poultice often.

The leaf pulp taken internally reduces blood glucose levels. Aloe's array of hydrophilic constituents slows simple carbohydrate breakdown and absorption[1]. To benefit from Aloe's blood sugar lowering effect, take several tablespoons before meals. Lastly the leaf pulp soothes stomach inflammation and is healing to peptic ulcers.

INDICATIONS

- Constipation, chronic, dry feces (leaf exudate)
- Infections, bacterial and fungal (external–leaf exudate)
- Burns, heat and sun (external–leaf pulp)
- Wounds, injuries (external–leaf pulp)
- Hyperglycemia (leaf pulp)
- Ulcer, peptic (leaf pulp)

COLLECTION

To begin, clip a number of large, hydrated leaves from the lower main stem. Place the clipped leaves, with the cut ends facing down, in a large strainer or colander; pack enough leaves into the strainer as to keep them upright. Place the strainer in a large bowl or pot. Let the exudate drain from the leaves until the flow has ceased. Larger yields will occur if the leaves are well hydrated from recent rains or watering. The collected leaf exudate then can be preserved with 20% alcohol. Alternatively, the exudate can be heated slowly until it thickens considerably, then dried and stored. It is then reconstituted or ground to

a fine powder as needed. The overall anthraquinone concentration is greatest throughout the summer months.

After an incision has been made in the leaf, the mucilaginous pulp is scraped out. It can then be stored unpreserved in a refrigerator for 1–2 weeks at a time.

Gels and juices that are commercially available are refined. Typically, they contain preservatives. Both are derived from the internal leaf. Most of the anthraquinones, cellulose, and leaf material are removed during processing.

PREPARATIONS/DOSAGE

- Leaf exudate: 10–20 drops 1–2 times daily or externally as needed
- DPT (50 alcohol) or leaf exudate: 30–60 drops 2–3 times daily
- Leaf pulp: 1–2 tablespoons 2–3 times daily or externally as needed

CAUTIONS

Pregnant women should not take the leaf exudate internally – the plant has the potential to stimulate uterine contractions. Nursing babies may experience a laxative effect due to anthraquinone's transmission through breast milk.

When used as recommended, leaf pulp taken internally will not cause gastrointestinal problems. However, excessive pulp intake can cause intestinal cramping and diarrhea, which is typical of anthraquinone containing plants.

OTHER USES

Aloe (or more specifically its polysaccharide fraction) has a cult–like following among multi–level marketers and the impressionable. Touted as being capable of healing almost any affliction through its immune system "modulation", these formulations are expensive and exaggerated.

---

1   It is reasonable to assume that the cactus Prickly pear has a similar mode of action due to its pectin content.

AMERICAN GINSENG

Araliaceae/Ginseng Family

Panax quinquefolius (Panax quinquefolium, P. quin-quefolia, Aralia quinquefolia)
Ginseng, Seng

DESCRIPTION

American ginseng is an herbaceous, aromatic perennial. The plant develops from a light–colored, thickened tap root, which often branches with age. To some, the tap root even may appear to have arms and legs, thus, according to the anthropomorphic Doctrine of Signatures, denote Ginseng as a medicine/tonic for Man (in my experience, plants with roots that appear to have a human–like form are common but few are adequate tonics). Ginseng is a superb tonic not because of its outward configuration but because of its internal attributes.

The plant consists of a single stem that arises from the root's crown. On the stem are borne 3–4 whorled leaves. Each leaf is composed of 3–5 leaflets. Each leaflet is 2½"–6" long, 3" wide, oblong to obovate, with pointed tips and serrated margins. The inconspicuous greenish–white flowers form in a single small umbel. Like other members of the Ginseng family, each flower is unisexual and is composed of 5 petals and 5 sepals. The subsequent bunched fruit cluster is bright red; each small drupe contains 2 seeds.

DISTRIBUTION

American ginseng has a significant disbursement given its commercial value and over–harvesting history. Locally look for American ginseng in rich, broadleaf–hardwood forests. A plant of the mountains and woodlands, it is reclusive. It ranges from South Dakota and Oklahoma east to Maine and Georgia, encompassing the entire east coast (except Florida) and inland eastern states.

CHEMISTRY

Saponins: ginsenosides; polysaccharides: arabinose, rhamnose, mannose; amino acids; poly-acetylenic alcohols; fatty acids.

MEDICINAL USES

As an adaptogen and tonic American ginseng shares a majority of effects parallel to the most widely used and well known Ginseng, that of Panax ginseng. Proportionally American ginseng holds lower amounts of ginsenosides. However, its particular combination of ginsenosides give the plant slightly different physiological effects. Qualified by the Chinese as a "cooler" Ginseng, American ginseng tends to be slightly more pronounced in its effect on mood and mental imbalances.

Most likely due to the plant's influence the on central and autonomic nervous systems, both waking and sleep patterns tend to stabilize under its use. Sufferers of fatigue–related insomnia, if long–term stress is the main disrupting influence, will find the plant corrective. And this is where American ginseng, like other ginsengs, really shines. Long–term stress syndromes, when organ and tissue groups are beginning to suffer from continually elevated stress hormones, particularly the catecholamine group, will show improvement. The plant is uncanny in its ability at producing a subtle but perceptible sense of betterment shortly after normal dosing.

As a promoter of endurance and stamina the aged and weak will see profound effects from the plant. Known as an adaptogen or a tonic it is excellent at filling voids in individuals who lack vitality. It particularly is indicated when long–term chronic stress or deficiency is related to a wasting state of the body.

As an aphrodisiac, American ginseng is often found just as useful as its more popular eastern relative, Panax ginseng. Men, whose libido is compromised by the effects of stress, will find it enhancing. Noticeable improvement will be seen in arousal response, vascular stimulation of erectile tissue, and stamina. Women too will benefit in this area, particularly those who suffer from stress–related diminished libido. For both men and women American ginseng affects a majority of physical/cerebral parameters.

Like uncured Panax ginseng, American ginseng has stabilizing effects on metabolic excesses. In conjunction with chronically elevated insulin levels, post–prandial hyperglycemia is easily remedied. In addition, cholesterol levels and blood pressure also may be lowered. Relatedly American ginseng has been found to retard LDL oxidation, ultimately lessening the atherosclerotic potential of this cholesterol. Known as "syndrome x", the plant will be of use to sufferers of this all–too–common genetic or diet–lifestyle metabolic picture.

American ginseng is a valuable restorative of energy and well–being in the face of conventional cancer treatments, i.e. chemotherapy and radiation. The regeneration that is felt shortly after taking the plant has complex origins: the plant's adaptogenic, red blood–cell stabilizing, antioxidant, and immune modulating properties combine to reduce the unwanted side–effects of these conventional treatments.

As a cancer preventative, American ginseng shares a majority of attributes with Panax ginseng. Like its Asian relative, the plant inhibits various malignant cell lines. Through several immunological enhancements, mainly elicited by cytokine stimulation, the internal environment better reacts to counter malignancies. Use American ginseng as a buffer against a cancerous potential that unfortunately accompanies some people due to genetics or lifestyle. American ginseng's prophylactic and modifying activity comes to us mainly through three constituent groups: ginsenosides (adaptogenic/immunologic), phenolics (antioxidant), and polysaccharides (immunostimulatory).

As a neuroprotectant, American Ginseng is a useful cerebral–spinal stabilizer. The plant's antioxidant compounds help protect neuronal cell membranes. In addition, premature apoptosis is retarded keeping cellular communities more intact. It is specific in stabilizing cellular functionality. Thus, the plant can reduce the dementia, memory–loss, and disorientation that commonly follow a cerebral stroke or ischemia. At the heart of the plant's protective effect is its inhibition of sodium channel activity, particularly when stroke–related trauma occurs. It is also well used in this arena as a preventative. In fact, most age–related cognition/cerebrovascular issues will improve. Students with increased cognitive needs will notice improvements in focus and retention. American ginseng, like Panax ginseng, will lift the mental fog that can be induced by intense study. It will often give thought processes a renewed strength and vitality.

Virtually any autoimmune disturbance that affects nerve fiber has the potential of being influenced beneficially by the application of American ginseng. Specific results have been seen with beginning–stage multiple sclerosis; the plant tends to slow lymphocyte–mediated demyelination. Consider it stabilizing to the nicotinic acetylcholine receptor and autoantibody disarray that is associated with myasthenia gravis. Combined with Ginkgo, its cerebral/neuronal influence will serve an individual well as a preventative/inhibitor of these two debilitating diseases.

The plant's cellular protectant properties also extend to the liver and to the blood. The membranes of both hepatocytes and erythrocytes show stabilization from the plant's influence. This specifically has value to individuals who are under area–specific oxidative stresses that are caused by viral infection, exposure to solvents or heavy metals, harsh pharmaceutical therapies, or immunological disturbances affecting these regions.

In conclusion, American ginseng serves as a excellent tonic and protectant, differing only subtly from Asian ginsengs. In the areas of metabolic excess, oxidative stress, and sleep/fatigue/vitality issues, the plant will be seen as a therapeutic gift.

INDICATIONS

♦ Insomnia/Fatigue from long–term stress
♦ Weakness/Diminished vitality from age or illness
♦ Lowered libido, male or female, with associated stress factors
♦ Hyperglycemia with elevated insulin levels

- ◆ Elevated cholesterol levels
- ◆ Fatigue from chemotherapy or radiation
- ◆ Cancer, general preventative
- ◆ As a neuroprotectant
- ◆ Stroke/Ischemia
- ◆ Multiple sclerosis
- ◆ Myasthenia gravis
- ◆ Liver and red blood cell oxidative stress

COLLECTION

Within most states American ginseng exists precariously. Excessively collected for centuries, mainly to supply a voracious Chinese herbal market with a billion–plus subscribers, it is amazing the plant still remains. Beginning in the early 1700s American ginseng collection was a major economic activity, and in some cases surpassed a man's ability to profit through the fur trade. Even famous frontiersman Daniel Boone collected for the Chinese market.

Since 1973 the plant has been placed on the CITES (Convention on International Trade in Endangered Species of Wild Fauna and Flora) list; still most native populations continue to decline due to poor harvesting practices.

State and federal laws are easily circumvented and will continue to be due to market demand, which in itself is not a morale or abiding entity, but a consuming process. What will change Ginseng's status though is proper understanding leading to stewardship. On a local level, people who live around the plant, particularly the harvesters, must generate a sense of responsibility in collection practices. Individuals who interact with the plant must understand the slow growing nature of American ginseng, as well as its growth patterns and what interconnected/isolated groups need to thrive. Know the stand that is being collected from, and know if others are collecting from that stand as well.

Planting practices are a substantial equalizer. If done properly stands will maintain and even increase in size and overall health. Only seed bearing plants should be collected, and only when the fruit is mature as to ensure successful propagation after sowing seeds an inch or so in the soil. Disperse the seeds locally to increase that stand's population. Also some can be taken and planted a distance away; a truly rewarding experience is creating a new stand of plants, and here you become part of the solution, not the problem.

The 10% rule – collecting no more then 10% of a particular stand, is conservative, but applies well to American ginseng. Of course if more then one collector is harvesting from a particular group, 10% becomes relative, as the stand will diminish quickly if everyone takes 10%. The answer to this is know your territory, take care of it, and protect it. I saw an extreme example of this while in Afghanistan; the residents of the Zadran region took their pine nuts so seriously turf–war gun battles were not uncommon during the collection season. We never were sure if the gunfire was Taliban related or pine nut related. Extreme, yes, but the principle, being that concerned about a little piece of land and what flourishes on it, is a breath of fresh air compared to the industrial attitude of take all you can while not minding the consequences.

If performed correctly, wildcrafting the plant for personal use is reasonable enough. Unfortunately, most collectors of American ginseng gather the plant to supplement their income. Too often they are indifferent to the overall environmental impact of their activities.

The cultivation of American Ginseng, like Panax ginseng, is tedious but frequently successful. This practice has substantially reduced the pressure on wild populations. The difference in therapeutic value between wild and cultivated American ginseng (real or imagined) is inconsequential. Let us take a lesson from the Chinese, whose wild ginseng is nearly extinct, entirely as a result of over harvesting. In the majority of situations, wild American ginseng needs a rest from human hands.

PREPARATIONS

Like most other members of the family, American ginseng has limited solubility in water. Alcoholic and powdered preparations will give the best results. It is easy to get used to the taste of the plant: slightly sweet, slightly bitter, and aromatic. A small piece (½" or so) of the whole dried root can be chewed and swallowed. Although this is a crude approach, it often is the most effective preparation when administered 2–3 times a day.

Although less potent, the leaf tea makes a fine substitute for the root. Often it is used after therapeutic stabilization has occurred – after several months of using the root, switch to a continued maintenance dose of the leaf tea.

DOSAGE

- Capsule (00): 1–2, 1–3 times daily
- DPT (70% alcohol): 15–30 drops 1–3 times daily
- Dried whole root: 2–3 small pieces daily
- Cold infusion of leaf: 4–6 oz. 2–3 times daily

CAUTIONS

Although less common than with red or cured Panax ginseng, "ginseng abuse syndrome" with large amounts is possible. This can be avoided knowing that smaller tonic doses are more effective than larger "mega doses". Also the plant is not recommended during pregnancy due to its mild saponin–derived hormonal influence.

ARNICA

Asteraceae/Sunflower Family

Arnica montana
Leopard's bane, Fall herb

Arnica cordifolia
Heartleafed arnica

DESCRIPTION

Arnica montana is a small perennial herb. The plant's basal leaves are ovate to obtuse; stem leaves form in opposite pairs and are more lance–shaped. Both have upper surfaces that are somewhat pubescent. Stems are between 2'–3' high and terminate with the plant's distinctive

yellow–orange ray/disk flowers. Roots are horizontal, from 2"–5" long, and somewhat aromatic.

Arnica cordifolia is an herbaceous perennial, growing to 2' high at maturity. Basal leaves are petioled, cordate, and have toothed margins. The leaves along the plant's stems are arranged in pairs and are near–clasping; they are 1½"–4½" long and ¾"–3½" wide.

The plant's flower heads are typical of the Sunflower family: each inflorescence is divided between disk and ray florets. Rays are ½"–1¼" long, making the flower head's circumference between 1" and 2".

DISTRIBUTION

Arnica montana is native to the mountainous regions of western and central Europe. A. cordifolia is found throughout much of the western U.S. and Canada. Seen in temperate zones, both are meadow–woodland plants.

CHEMISTRY

For Arnica montana: sesquiterpene lactones: guaianolides: helenalin; pyrrolizidine alkaloids: tussilagine, isotussilagine; flavonoids; caffeoylquinic acids; polysaccharides: fucogalactoxyloglucans, arabinogalactans; terpenoid: loliolide.

MEDICINAL USES

Although not found in commerce, Arnica cordifolia is offered here as a native substitute. It is virtually interchangeable with official Arnica montana.

Topically Arnica is a well–known remedy for a number of painful conditions. Those that are treated most effectively with the plant are characterized by subacute/chronic inflammation and pain. Arnica stimulates tissues and excites immunological mediators, such as white blood cells. Consequently, it is less suited for the treatment of new injuries, which are characterized by an array of heightened immunological responses.

With that said, Arnica can reduce acute pain,

although its influence is less reliable. If it does not bring relief in these acute situations, then try Lobelia or Tobacco liniment. Arnica salve, ointment, or liniment is best applied in cases of tissue trauma where the skin is unbroken, such as poorly healing sprains, muscle pulls/strains from overexertion, contusions, and bruises. One exception is the diluted ointment – use it on bed sores, poorly healing wounds, post–operative incisions, and on other breaks that would benefit from the plant's tissue–stimulation and healing properties. Although the application is frequently overlooked, the plant remedies arthritis pain, especially if it is aggravated by the cold. Another indiction for its application is a lack of proper vascular circulation, particularly among surface tissues.

For chronic sore throats, or pharyngitis, 5–10 drops of Arnica tincture in an ounce of water is gargled. Hoarseness from stressed vocal cords, a common problem of singers and orators, is addressed by the mixture; the addition of Ligusticum or Jack–in–the–pulpit will be of benefit as well.

Lastly, Arnica's almost forgotten use is as a cardiovascular stimulant. Use small doses of the tincture to treat acute heart weakness linked to age, cardiovascular disease, or other episodes when there is diminish heart function – being bed ridden or sedentary for long periods, etc. Arnica, in this respect can be used for 1–2 weeks at a time.

The plant's affinity for vascular tissue dictates its internal use. In actuality, when using Arnica internally, we are utilizing its irritant properties in a therapeutic way. As a jump–start, so to speak, Arnica prepares the system for kinder medicines. For deeper–seated weaknesses use Hawthorn; not only is the plant a heart tonic, it is also nutritive.

INDICATIONS
♦ Pain/Inflammation, subacute (external)
♦ Muscle pulls/Strains/Contusions/Bruises (external)
♦ Poorly healing wounds/Bed sores (external)
♦ Pharyngitis, chronic (gargle)
♦ Cardiovascular weakness, acute

COLLECTION
The flowers are the official medicinal portion but with most local varieties, the whole plant can be collected – small root and all. Arnica montana is widely cultivated. A. cordifolia is locally abundant, but like any plant if found on the edge of its range it is less abundant and less tolerant of disturbance. In Michigan, the plant is listed as endangered.

PREPARATIONS
The fresh plant, especially the fresh flower, is the strongest and most potent form but is more apt to cause irritation when applied topically as a poultice or liniment. The dried flowers and fresh/dried roots, used topically in various forms, are less apt to cause discomfort.

Depending on source, age, and the method of drying, the commercially purchased flower is usually of only adequate potency. As stated before, collect your own if possible, but if that is not an option, use the following dosage recommendations when preparing the commercially sourced tea. Also be warned that the off–the–shelf tincture will undoubtedly say "not for internal use". If you do intend to take the product internally make sure it contains ethyl alcohol and not isopropyl alcohol. Beyond that, the label will state this caution because Arnica tincture, taken improperly, will cause digestive upset and short–term cardiovascular irritation.

DOSAGE
♦ FPT/DPT: (65% alcohol): 3–8 drops 1–3 times daily
♦ Liniment/Ointment/Oil/Salve: as needed

CAUTIONS
Be aware of tissue irritation when using topical preparations. For internal use dilute the tea or the tincture in a moderate amount of water; this will ward against gastrointestinal upset. Discontinue internal use if restlessness or excitability

develops. Arnica should not be taken internally by children or by women who are nursing or pregnant.

OTHER USES

Homeopathic Arnica, which is a tame cousin of "herbal" Arnica, is a different substance. The homeopathic form can be used more liberally and in a slightly different fashion because "stronger preparations" may contain no discernible Arnica constituents. Homeopathic Arnica can be used without caution internally, as well as externally. In most cases, the use of the two different types overlap. However, homeopathic Arnica is commonly used when trauma is acute but rarely is it employed for any cardiovascular effect.

Explaining how homeopathic medicines actually work, without inspiring confused looks in the listener, is beyond the author.

ARTICHOKE

Asteraceae/Sunflower Family

Cynara scolymus
Artichoke, Globe artichoke

Cynara cardunculus
Cardoon, Artichoke thistle

DESCRIPTION

Both species presented here are perennials, as are all varieties of Cynara. At maturity C. scolymus is a bushy, coarse plant. Its large lanceolate leaves are deeply lobed, typically without (occasionally with) minute spines. Leaf surfaces, especially the lower sides, are whitish–woolly. Involucre heads are 3"–6" in diameter and narrowed above; each phyllary is occasionally notched. If not collected before flowering the corollas are 1½"–2" in diameter and generally blue–purple. C. scolymus is the official variety of Artichoke.

Of similar statue or slightly smaller, Cynara cardunculus has very spiny leaves and is thistle–like in appearance. The lower sides are densely whitish–gray. The 1"–2½" involucres have spine-

tipped phyllaries. Flowers are bluish–purple.

DISTRIBUTION

Both plants are native to the Mediterranean region, and are cultivated (especially Cynara scolymus) for their edible involucres, roots, or in the case of C. cardunculus, fleshly leaf ribs. Artichoke is mostly relegated to the garden, although in warmer western regions, certainly parts of California, both varieties are escapees, with C. cardunculus considered a troublesome weed.

CHEMISTRY

Caffeoylquinic acids; glycosides of luteolin and apigenin; β–sitosterol, taraxasterol, scopolin, scopoletin, cynarin, chlorogenic acid, cynarasaponins a, b, and k.

MEDICINAL USES

Artichoke shares many therapeutic (and morphologic) characteristics with Dandelion and Milk thistle. Think of them as reflections of one another, each having a specialized area of influence. Artichoke's more prosaic quality is as a bitter stimulant. The tea or tincture held in the mouth, having its bitterness tasted, then swallowed, increases the digestive prowess of both the mouth and gut. Artichoke's bitterness stimulates saliva secretion from the area's secretory glands, which release amylase, a chief enzyme responsible for carbohydrate breakdown. By stimulating its release from gastric glands within the stomach's wall, Artichoke increases gastric juice[2] quantities.

Artichoke, like other bitters, is useful for an array of digestive problems. Straight–forward indigestion, if a simple lack of stomach secretion results in fullness and bloating, is Artichoke's most reliable application. Even the uncomfortable heartburn associated with gastritis can be a symptom of insufficient digestive juice. Here the mucus component, which serves as a stomach wall protectant, is lacking. If this is the case,

2   HCL (hydrochloric acid), pepsinogen (cleaved by HCL into pepsin), and mucus are the main components of the stomach's, gastric or digestive juice.

due to Artichoke's augmentation of gut secretion, the tea's correcting effect will be notable. On the other hand if there is a true excess of digestive secretion, particularly hydrochloric acid, active inflammation/ulceration, or severe cardiac sphincter atonicity, Artichoke will do little good. Here look to soothers like Marshmallow and Slippery elm, which will be topically beneficial to the distressed tissue.

There are other factors, mainly constitutional or stress issues, that have a direct bearing on the body's ability and quality of digestion. Using Artichoke, or any bitter tonic alone, will only be partially effective if the dyspepsia is caused, for example, from a cardiac insufficiency or continued adrenalin stress. Addressing the underlying issue, as opposed to the surface symptom, ideally, will bring sustained relief.

Not only does Artichoke stimulate gastric secretion, but also succus entericus (intestinal juice) by the small intestine, as well as pancreatic juice by the pancreas. Although the plant's effect on these two areas are lesser than its effect on gastric stimulation, it is notable.

Artichoke's influence of the liver is multi–faceted. The plant is well utilized as a long–term preventative/therapy for gall stones[3]. Because artichoke can behave as a choleretic and as a chologogue, the plant should be taken by those who are troubled by gall stone formation or by associated feelings of nausea, fullness, and pain. One reason that the plant provides relief is through its thinning of bile. Super–saturated bile contributes to stone formation; Artichoke's thinning effect enables deposits to slowly dissolve in a less saturated bile medium. This approach is inadvisable for an active gall stone blockage but is appropriate when a long–term maintenance is wanted. For this application, Artichoke combines well with Chelidonium. The plant is doubly indicated if blood cholesterol levels are elevated: the plant inhibits the liver's production of this sometimes over–produced building block and most common gall stone ingredient.

Lesser known are Artichoke's hepatoprotective effects. Similar to Milk thistle, yet not as potent, Artichoke can safely be taken in most cases when there is liver inflammation.

3 Be wary of "liver/gallbladder flushes" containing olive oil and lemon juice. They stimulate bile production and release intensely. I have seen them help as well as harm. In response to the great amount of oil entering the small intestine, both the liver and gallbladder increase bile synthesis/release. Often smaller stones will be expelled in the hepatic/biliary upheaved that occurs; larger stones either will not pass or may become lodged. A main sales point of the olive oil/lemon juice combination: afterwards, when looking at the stool, what appear as expelled gall stones are in reality globules of partly–saponified olive oil. This occurs because there is no way the quantity of ingested oil can be properly digested.

INDICATIONS

- Dyspepsia
- Gastritis, from insufficiency
- Gall stones, non–acute
- Cholesterol levels, elevated
- Liver disease, inflammation

COLLECTION

Artichoke's bitter principals, and therefore activity, are highest before and after flowering. Although leaf effects are better known, the roots are active as well. If grown to capacity in the garden, only several plants will be needed for personal use.

PREPARATIONS/DOSAGE

- Leaf infusion/Root decoction: 4–6 oz. 2–3 times daily
- DPT (60% alcohol): 30–90 drops 2–3 times daily
- Fluidextract: 15–25 drops 2–3 times daily

CAUTIONS

There are few cautions with Artichoke use. With excessive amounts, mild gastrointestinal–hepatic irritation is possible. Do not use if there is an active biliary–gall stone blockage.

OTHER USES

The fleshy phyllaries and the involucre bases of Cynara scolymus are eaten as a vegetable. C. cardunculus is cultivated especially for its leaf ribs, which are favored throughout the Mediterranean region. The fleshy portions are an excellent source of inulin, which is a plant–derived carbohydrate commonly known as a "prebiotic". In the colon, it has a beneficial effect on resident flora populations, therefore improving gastrointestinal and immunological functions.

ASTRAGALUS
Fabaceae/Pea Family

Astragalus membranaceus (Astragalus membranaceus var. mongholicus, A. propinquus)
Milk vetch, Huang qi

DESCRIPTION
An herbaceous perennial reaching sizes of 2'–3', Astragalus forms sizable leaves comprised of 12–24 leaflets. Yellow flowers develop from leaf axils. Seed–containing pods follow after fertilization.

DISTRIBUTION
Astragalus is found throughout much of temperate Asia: Korea, China, Mongolia, and many ex–Soviet satellites, comprising the Far East and Siberia.

CHEMISTRY
Saponins: mongholicoside a and b, astragalosides, acetylastragaloside; isoflavonoids: calycosin, ononin, formononetin; miscellaneous glucosides; arabinogalactans.

MEDICINAL USES
Although an addition from TCM (Traditional Chinese Medicine), Astragalus joins Echinacea and Wild indigo as one of western herbal medicine's most commonly used immune stimulants. Each has its own unique secondary influence, but of the three, Astragalus works best as an immune system tonic: over the vast area of host defense its effects are strengthening, yet gentle.

Astragalus' influence on innate immunity is principally directed towards monocytes/macrophages and their defensive products. Particularly in response to immune suppression, activity and number of both cell types are increased with the plant's supplementation.

One explanation for Astragalus' diverse activity is its leucocyte stimulation. Macrophage[4] phagocytic activity is increased as is these cell's acquired immunity signaling. Considering this, there is little reason why Astragalus' historical (and modern) influence is deemed wide.

The plant influences NK (natural killer) cell activity significantly. Being a special type of lymphocyte able to destroy foreign bodies without prior sensitization (unlike T–lymphocytes), their enhanced activity, stimulated by Astragalus, is a great boone to individuals whose immune systems are suppressed due to prolonged sickness, excessive steroid use, or even chemotherapeutic agents. Interleukin–2, a cytokine produced by NK cells and other lymphocytes, which is involved in enhancing functionality and proliferation of these cells, is also increased.

IgA, IgE, IgG, and IgM (most likely IgD as well), the five main classes of immunoglobulins[5]

---

4   After maturation in various organs and tissues these cells preform area specific immunological functions. Residing in the liver they are called kupffer cells, in the lungs – dust cells, brain – microglia, etc.

5   IgA resides in epithelial tissue of the gastrointestinal tract. Intrinsic to the region's immunity this immunoglobulin contributes the key antibody mediated response to various pathogens affecting the area, which are numerous considering the amount of bacteria that enters the body orally through food and drink.

IgE is the key immunoglobulin group involved in allergic reaction. From mild skin reactions to life threatening anaphylaxis, they are largely responsible. IgE triggers basophils and mast cells to release histamine and other substances which influence local tissue, prompting smooth muscle contraction, capillary fluid leakage, itching, redness, and other indicators of an allergic reaction. These effects we are all familiar with to one degree or another, and to most they are a source of annoyance. But know our bodies would not of developed this group of antibodies and reactions if there were no essential reason.

IgE influences eosinophils, a type of phagocytic white blood cell, responsible for the defense against a large range of parasites. Without our tendencies towards allergic reaction, our ability to neutralize parasites would be hindered. Maybe a trade off, but a life preserving one.

The ability to have a normal allergic reaction, besides its discomforts, indicates immune system vitality. Often essential to humoral immunity are amplified or at least modified by Astragalus. Each class has a select physiological purpose intrinsic to the body's defense through antibody–antigen recognition.

Even though Astragalus is broadly defined as an immune stimulant (in this work it is mostly considered as such) it should be noted that there is virtually no record of the plant triggering pathological basophil or mast cell release, whether related to sensitivity, allergy, or severe autoimmunity. It is not far–fetched to consider the possibility that Astragalus, although directly stimulating to some immunologic parameters, modifies others in more subtle ways.

As an immune system tonic Astragalus' effect will not be noticed immediately upon ingestion. Because of the plant's influence of macrophages (second line of innate immune defense) and a number of slow–responding lymphocytes and their immunoglobulins, Astragalus should be taken longer to appreciate its full benefit.

In conjunction with chemotherapy and/or radiation, both conventional cancer treatments known to cause immune suppression, Astragalus will have a noticeable stabilizing effect on both red and white blood cell parameters. Astragalus will help individuals better tolerate these programs so they are more effective at fighting the cancer. The main drawback of conventional cancer therapies is their harshness to the system – "if you survive the treatment, you'll beat the cancer". Astragalus helps the individual survive the treatment, so hopefully the cancer has a better chance of being beaten.

The plant is useful against any bacterial or viral infection, but it is especially well employed against those that tend to linger. Often Astragalus is combined with other area specific botanicals when suffering from upper or lower respiratory tract infections. Bronchial, urinary, and gastrointestinal tract infections are only some regional crisis' that will respond to the plant. Septic conditions of the blood, leading to fever, abscess, and tissue ulceration, are also indications for Astragalus use. The plant will be best applied as a counter to the tendency. Of course in acute situations conventional antibiotics probably will be necessary.

Of interest to individuals who suffer from virally induced hepatitis, especially hepatitis C, is the plant's hepatoprotective influence. Serum GPT (glutamic–pyruvic transaminase) level is one of several parameters that typically show improvement after treatment with Astragalus. Relatedly hepatic fibrosis, which often leads to cirrhosis, is usually diminished. The plant is generally thought to have a regional antioxidant or antiinflammatory effect.

Another interesting influence of the plant is its synergism with interferon therapy. Combined with standard protocols, results show the two work better than either the plant, or interferon used solely. Suffers of hepatitis C will especially find the duo useful.

Astragalus' activity becomes more confounding in its modulation of a number of autoimmune conditions. It is possible that the plant's effect is through some sort of free radical scavenging property and not direct suppression. Specifically Astragalus is of benefit to suffers of myasthenia gravis, a syndrome effecting nicotinic acetylcholine receptor sites. The plant has been found to reduce the amount of antibodies, which if allowed to progress unchecked leads to the destruction of these cholinergic sites, thus disrupting some normal muscle function.

Sufferers of lupus erythematosus may find Astragalus' protective effect on red blood cells of benefit. Research has shown it to prevent unhealthy alterations in these cells, subsequently relieving symptoms of inflammation and autoimmune aberration. Though there is promise, application is still in its infancy.

Second to Astragalus' immune system activity is its gentle cardiovascular effect. Although

---

in severe immune system depression, possibly a result of chemotherapy/radiation treatment, debilitating illness, or old age, immune mediated inflammation is virtually non-existent. In these cases, the individual's health is typically poor; weakness and deficiency are apparent. Immune system hypersensitivity is altogether different; although paradoxical this type of reactivity also stems from weakness.

not a powerful medicine in this department, its influence here usually is noticed by the elderly and the infirm. The heart's blood moving ability becomes more efficient, as the plant has a positive inotropic effect on the organ. A small decrease in blood pressure is common with its usage. Left ventricle function is strengthened and the plant has modest vasodilatory effects.

As a general tonic for the aged and weak, the plant is worthwhile. Numerous parameters are affected, creating a broad influence over the body. Not only are cardiovascular and immune functions influenced, but even microscopic cellular functions are altered, resulting in a number of betterments: memory, quality of sleep, sense of vitality, and even improvement of vision are some common factors that point to Astragalus' anti–aging/strengthening qualities. It is well combined with one of several Ginseng varieties.

INDICATIONS
- Immune system suppression
- Bacterial/Viral infection
- Bronchial/Urinary/Gastrointestinal tract infection
- Septic conditions of the blood
- Hepatitis, viral
- Cardiovascular weakness
- Myasthenia gravis/Lupus erythematosus
- Weakness/Debility from age or sickness

COLLECTION
Astragalus is extensively cultivated in China and typically harvested when 4–5 years old. Roots in commerce are dried and sliced, appearing tongue depressor–like.

PREPARATIONS
Like many other herbs, Astragalus too is plagued by standardization[6]. With only several excep-

---

6   This two–decade old phenomenon of standardization takes part of its philosophy, that of the magic–bullet pharmaceutical, from the allopathic symptom–suppression approach. Just when many of us thought herbs were safe, maybe not from false discredit or legal status, but from the gripping hands of allopathic–reductionist application... not so!

tions, Ginkgo being one, this herb to drug–like process takes a fine plant and turns it into a botanical Frankenstein's monster.

Crude preparations are fine and effective. Tea, being the traditional preparation is preferred but fluidextract and tincture preparations are fine as well. In traditional Chinese cuisine several slices of Astragalus are added to soups as they are stewing – a simple and effective way of receiving the benefit from this potent tonic.

DOSAGE
- Cold infusion or standard decoction: 4–6 oz. 2–3 times daily
- Fluidextract: 10–30 drops 2–3 times daily
- DPT (60% alcohol): ½–1 teaspoon 2–3 times daily

CAUTIONS
Theoretically Astragalus is contraindicated in any autoimmune condition, but in reality the plant will probably due little harm, and in some cases will led to the condition's betterment. Do not use the plant if dealing with organ transplant issues or severe autoimmune sequela. Beyond these theoretical concerns Astragalus is very well tolerated and can be used safely in ample doses.

Fortunately Astragalus membranaceus contains little selenium (toxic forms or amounts) and swainsonine, a poisonous alkaloid (and potential anti–mutagenic agent). Both elements have been linked to "the staggers", a set of physical and neurological symptoms associated with Locoweed poisoning, mainly affecting stock feeding on related Astragalus and Oxytropis species.

BARBERRY
Berberidaceae/Barberry Family

Berberis vulgaris
European barberry, Common barberry

DESCRIPTION
A large, bushy shrub, growing to heights of 12',

Barberry tends to be untended and deciduous. The plant's leaves are ovate, ¾"–2" long and ½"–¾" wide with serrated margins. They develop in clusters of 2–5 and originate from alternating nodes, where there is a confluence of items: Barberry's 3–parted spines originate from the area, as do the flowers, which are arranged in 1¼"–2¾" long, drooping panicles. Individually they are 6–petaled, yellow, and ¼" wide and across. The berries ripen from late summer to autumn, are oblong, red, and ¼"–½" in length.

DISTRIBUTION

Barberry's native distribution is from Europe and western Asia to northwest Africa. The plant's range has expanded greatly due to ornamental planting and subsequent escapees throughout much of western and northern Europe and temperate North America.

CHEMISTRY

Berberis/Mahonia general: isoquinoline alkaloids: oxyacanthine, berberine, columbamine, corydine, isocorydine, glaucine, jatrorrhizine, magnoflorine, obaberine, obamegine, palmatine, thaliporphine, thalrugosine; lignan: syringaresinol.

MEDICINAL USES

As a berberine containing plant, Barberry is nearly identical in use to Oregongrape and Coptis – herbal siblings of sorts. Although not an exact match to Goldenseal, Barberry is similar enough to serve as a decent replacement for this overused, yet potent plant. With Bayberry or Yerba mansa added, Barberry's influence will be found nearly identical to Goldenseal's.

There are not many other botanicals that rival Barberry's broad antimicrobial activity. Dozens of bacterial and fungal strains are inhibited by the plant. Some of the more common strains that are known to present clinical symptoms that call for Barberry's use are: several Bacillus varieties known to cause food poisoning; Escherichia coli – urinary tract and intestinal infections; both Staphylococcus and Streptococcus strains – re-sponsible for a myriad of systemic and local infections; at least four Salmonella varieties – also a causative factor in food poisoning and intestinal infections. Candida albicans, Trichophyton mentagrophytes, and Microsporum gypseum are several fungal strains that Barberry inhibits.

For systemic infections Barberry combines well with Echinacea or Myrrh; for local or topical involvements, the same applies, although the plant can be used solely with good results. Of course serious infections (systemic infections usually are) will be most efficiently treated with conventional antibiotics, barring allergy or bacterial resistance.

Although bitter, it makes an effective gargle for bacterial–derived pharyngitis. The nasal wash or repeated gargle is a sound treatment for sinusitis as well. Combined with internal use (along with Echinacea or Myrrh) its upper–respiratory cold–fighting power should not be underestimated.

Applied to vaginal Candida infections, as a wash or douche, it will be found effective. Likewise thrush in babies and children will be remedied with topical application. Fungal infections that affect the skin and nails respond particularly well to long soaks in the root decoction.

Food poisoning from a variety of pathogens will be remedied. Not only is Barberry, like Oregongrape, directly inhibiting to these microbes, it also reduces the harmful effects of related endotoxins. Combine Barberry with Peppermint or Ginger if there is nausea or intestinal cramping; with Slippery elm or Marshmallow if irritative diarrhea is evident.

Although Simaruba family plants such as Castela emoryi or Ailanthus altissima, due to their array of quassinoids and tannins, will prove better medicines for traveler's diarrhea (amebiasis) and even giardiasis, Barberry is a worthy second choice. The plant is inhibiting to both Entamoeba histolytica and Giardia lamblia.

The tea or tincture is a simple bitter tonic, stimulating gastric secretions, ultimately being of use in simple indigestion. Take it to stimulate gastric response several minutes before meals.

Like many other bitter herbs, Barberry is overtly a hepatic stimulant. As a chologogue/choleretic the plant triggers bile manufacture, ultimately providing more of this digestive substance for lipid breakdown and assimilation. If plagued by general feelings of sluggishness, frontal headache, and nausea, all upon eating a high–fat meal, the tea will particularly be of use. Occasionally the plant will benefit suffers of anorexia by enlivening the gastrointestinal tract, therefore promoting hunger sensations. Of course psychological issues should be addressed in tandem.

Underlying the plant's bile augmentation is its hepatic sedation. At cellular levels it will be found reducing to inflammation, being decidedly useful to hepatitis sufferers; elevated hepatic enzyme levels tend to lower with the plant's use. Although Barberry's hepatoprotective influence is not as strong as Milk thistle's, still the plant can be used with therapeutic results in many situations if there is liver distress.

Through Barberry's effect over the liver, it has a marked influence over inflammatory skin conditions. Poorly healing skin, reactive dermatitis, including eczema, and acne are the plant's main indications. Most likely Barberry's healing effects are due to its influence over hepatic detoxification pathways, ultimately neutralizing hepatic/systemic/local metabolites and toxins. Topical use of the ointment/oil/salve will compound the plant's benefit to these conditions. Even psoriasis with its related scaly patches of skin responds well to Barberry application due to its reduction of dermis over–proliferation.

Another interesting effect the Berberis–Mahonia group of plants is its influence over liver suppression in mild cases of hypothyroidism. In overt and particularly sub–clinical hypothyroidism liver functions are often slowed due to insufficient or ineffective T3 (triiodothyronine) and/or T4 (thyroxine) levels. Proper activity upon the liver by these thyroid hormones are important for normal hepatic function. Numerous liver–centered metabolic insufficiencies become evident with thyroid deficiency. Poorly healing skin and nails, slowed intestinal movement, and in-

creased allergic reaction, are several of the more common presentations. Use Barberry as a stimulant when thyroid suppression has influence over the area. It can be used with conventional thyroxin therapies. As an eyewash the isotonic tea is useful for bacterially–derived conjunctivitis.

INDICATIONS

♦   Food poisoning
♦   Infections, systemic/local
♦   Pharyngitis
♦   Sinusitis/Common cold
♦   Candida infections (external and internal)
♦   Thrush (external and internal)
♦   Fungal infections affecting skin and nails (external and internal)
♦   Amebiasis/Giardiasis
♦   Indigestion/Poor protein and fat digestion, assimilation
♦   Hepatic sluggishness or inflammation
♦   Poorly healing skin/Dermatitis/Eczema/Psoriasis (external and internal)
♦   Hypothyroidal induced hepatic deficiency
♦   Conjunctivitis, bacterial (eyewash)

COLLECTION

Barberry, being a substantial woody bush, will have similar semi–woody roots. Its subterranean mass is composed of one or several larger tap roots and many secondary spreading lateral or semi–lateral roots. On larger bushes lateral roots can be gathered, ensuring the plant's continuations and future harvests.

Drier locales will produce roots with less water content. For these, dry and use for tea and/or dry plant tinctures. Hydrated roots, collected in wetter seasons/soils, can be dried and used in the aforementioned way, or prepared through tincturing fresh.

PREPARATIONS

Both tea and tincture are fine methods for internal delivery. Although not the official portion, recently collected leaves are fine for making external preparations (oil, salve, ointment, etc.).

DOSAGE

♦ Root decoction/Cold infusion: 2–4 oz. 2–3 times daily
♦ FPT/DPT (40% alcohol): 30–60 drops 2–3 times daily
♦ Capsule (oo): 1–2, 2–3 times daily
♦ Fluidextract: 10–30 drops 2–3 times daily
♦ External preparations: as needed

CAUTIONS

There are few cautions considering Barberry's significant therapeutic activity. Normal doses will not create any problem. One exception is Berberine's possibility of causing hemolysis in babies with G6PD (glucose–6–phosphate–de-hydrogenase) deficiency. Also extremely high doses may erratically affect blood pressure, and common sense tells us – do not use if there is a biliary blockage.

OTHER USES

Barberry is commonly planted as a hedge–divider shrub. The fruit is mildly sour–sweet, and very refreshing. It is a useful edible and jam/jelly base.

BAYBERRY

Myricaceae/Wax Myrtle Family

Myrica cerifera (Myrica carolinensis, M. pusilla, M. mexicana, Morella cerifera, Cerothamnus cerifera, C. pumilus)
Waxberry, Candleberry, Waxmyrtle

DESCRIPTION

As an evergreen small tree or large bush Bayberry's leaves are lanceolate, serrated, and covered with red–golden glands. Due to volatiles held within these glands, when crushed they are pleasantly scented. Being dioecious, male and female flowers form on separate plants; they are diminutive, form in catkin–like spikes, and are also gland dotted. The small fruit are round and green, but appear bluish due to a conspicuous covering of wax.

Bayberry is adept at both sexual and asexual reproduction. The fruit must first pass through the digestive tract, of usually birds, in order to sprout; this removes the inhibiting waxy coating from the seed. As a successful cloner, root crowns and runners are capable of multi–stem growth. Lastly the plant's root nodules are home to a nitrogen–fixing, symbiotic fungus.

DISTRIBUTION

From southern New Jersey, Delaware, and Maryland, south to the Florida Keys, and west to Texas, Bayberry thrives in a number of diverging habitats. In the United States its main range includes the inland coastal plain of the temperate south. It does equally well in subtropical regions including Mexico, south to South America, Bermuda, Cuba, the Bahamas, Puerto Rico, and the British West Indies.

CHEMISTRY

Tannins: catechin, epicatechin, epigallocatechin, gallocatechin, myricitrin; triterpenes: myricadiol, taraxerol, taraxerone; myriceron caffeoyl ester.

MEDICINAL USES

Bayberry is a number of only several plants in the herbal world that have both astringent and stimulating properties. This unique combination of attributes makes Bayberry applicable to a whole range of subacute and chronic conditions which need both tissue stimulation and tightening to initiate healing.

For several common oral problems there is often no other herb that helps like Bayberry. The gargled tea, or tincture in warm water, is superb at tightening spongy and bleeding gums. The powdered plant can even be gently brushed with, and if combined with Myrrh, the tooth powder will have a significant antibacterial quality. Use daily if periodontal disease is a problem.

Chronic pharyngitis that tends to linger responds well to the oral gargle. Combined with Sage steam inhalation, chronic strep throat will often resolve in a more timely manner. If there is attending tonsil involvement with ulceration of the surrounding mucosa use Bayberry alone, or in combination with internal Echinacea or Wild Indigo. Other oral afflictions such as mouth sores/ulcers or aphthous stomatitis, particularly when in tandem with surrounding pale mucosa, will be treated well by the mouth wash. Also sinusitis with copious mucus discharge will be benefited by the gargle or specifically the nasal wash.

Internally the tea or tincture is indicated in chronic or subacute conditions of the gastrointestinal tract. Any gastrointestinal condition that involves hypersecretion and debility will be positively influenced by Bayberry. It is of definite value in curbing chronic diarrhea and intestinal spasm if atonic underpinnings exist. Intestinal irritability, with semi–formed, mucus–tainted stools will also be quieted.

Chronic indigestion in which blood movement to the stomach is lacking, be it from age, constitutional factors, or even alcohol abuse, is often remedied by the plant. Sufferers of gastritis, if the general environment is debilitated, will be pleasantly surprised to find the plant able to give relief. Not as well known is Bayberry's reputation for healing peptic ulcers. If ulceration is long–standing the plant is doubly indicated. Nausea is often quickly settled by the tincture, particularly if there is copious stomach mucus.

At least one constituent (myriceron caffeoyl ester) found in Bayberry is ascribed with vasoconstrictive qualities. This could at least partially account for the plant's tonifying effect on lax and congested tissue.

INDICATIONS
♦ Gums, bleeding, spongy (external)
♦ Pharyngitis, chronic (gargle)
♦ Ulcers, oral (gargle)
♦ Diarrhea, chronic
♦ Intestinal spam, chronic, with irritability
♦ Indigestion/Gastritis
♦ Ulcers, peptic
♦ Nausea, with copious mucus

COLLECTION
Gather Bayberry's root bark, as this portion will be the most potent. In commerce it is not uncommon for aerial stem bark or core material to be present as well, enfeebling the plant's effect.

PREPARATIONS/DOSAGE
♦ FPT/DPT (60% alcohol): 30–60 drops 2–3 times daily
♦ Cold infusion: 2–4 oz. 2–3 times daily
♦ Gargle: as needed
♦ Nasal wash: as needed

CAUTIONS
Do not use Bayberry if pregnant due to its possibility of stimulating menses.

OTHER USES
The waxy outer fruit coating was once utilized in making candles and soap.

BILBERRY
Ericaceae/Heath Family

Vaccinium myrtillus (Vaccinium myrtillus ssp. oreophilum, V. myrtillus var. oreophilum, V. oreophilum) Blueberry, Huckleberry, Whortleberry

DESCRIPTION
As a small understory bush, Bilberry stands from 1' to 2' high. It often appears sparse and weedy due to its shade–adaptive structure. Leaves are distinctly angled, ¾"–1" long, and ovate with serrated margins. Urn–shaped flowers are solitary and develop from leaf axil areas. The juicy dark blue fruit are about ¼" to nearly a ½" in diameter.

DISTRIBUTION
Bilberry can be found in montane and subalpine Spruce–Fir/Lodgepole pine forests. In North America the plant ranges from British Columbia to Arizona and New Mexico. It is additionally abundant throughout Europe and parts of Asia.

CHEMISTRY

Anthocyanidins: cyanidin, delphinidin, peonidin, petunidin, malvidin; flavonols: kaempferol, quercetin, myricetin, isorhamnetin; hydroxycinnamic acids: *p*–coumaric acid, caffeic acid, ferulic acid.

MEDICINAL USES

Bilberry's traditional use, which tends to be overshadowed by the fruit's recently discovered effect on blood vessels and capillary beds, is as an astringent tonic for the gastrointestinal and urinary tracts. For loose stools and diarrhea the leaf or berry tea is sufficiently astringent to act as a binding agent. In simple cases in which poor quality food or other dietary indiscretions are at fault Bilberry will prove reliable. The fruit tea sets well with children and infants due to the mildly sour–sweet taste of the preparation. Both the tannins and anthrocyanins (found within the fruit) also are mildly inhibiting to bacteria, furthering the plant's scope towards microbial derived diarrhea. The leaf tea is somewhat stronger than the fruit is these cases, but both are useful.

Bilberry leaf is a specific renal astringent. It lacks the harshness and antimicrobial strength of other Heath family plants, such as Uva–ursi, but when there is low–grade renal inflammation of a constitutional nature, causing low specific–gravity urine, the tea has a corrective influence. Use the plant if abnormally high levels of vital elements are found within the urine, such as protein and glucose, which if persistent has a weakening effect on the body.

The fruit is indicated in a number of vascular disorders. Due to its anthocyanin fraction it has a marked influence over smaller blood vessels, especially capillary beds. Fruit preparations can be used in nearly any microvascular disability. They stabilize vascular membrane surfaces in the face of injury or oxidative stress.

Moreover Bilberry fruit will be applied with good results to peripheral vascular disorders. Vascular ulceration, extremity pain, heaviness, edema, and even hemorrhoids will shown improvement. The lack of circulation and resulting symptoms of Raynaud's syndrome is also a good application for Bilberry.

Bilberry fruit is best known today as an eye–centered preventive medicine. Its antioxidant activity can applied to any ocular disturbance which involves free radical/oxidative damage (most autoimmune/age–related problems). Macular degeneration and cataract formation may not be corrected by Bilberry, but their progressions are certainly slowed. On a more prosaic note, Bilberry supplementation has been shown to improve night vision, and may in some individuals enhance visual acuity of colors and reduce sensitivity to normally bright light. The herbal legend of RAF pilots during WWII bombing runs having better night vision than their counterparts due to eating Bilberry jam seems to be well established as a sales point. Whether true or not, it makes sense.

Like other flavonoid and anthocyanin containing fruit, Bilberry speeds the healing of damaged tissue. Taken internally, the fruit modifies inflammation and reduces collagen breakdown – two important factors in wound/injury healing.

For the diabetic its application towards lowering blood sugar levels is probably overstated, but on occasion even type–1 diabetics may be able to reduce exogenous insulin injection – care should be taken here. But more concretely Bilberry will retard the progression of diabetic neuropathy through its antioxidant properties.

INDICATIONS

♦ Diarrhea
♦ Urine, low–specific gravity
♦ Vascular disorders, especially peripheral
♦ Raynaud's syndrome
♦ Ocular disorders, as an antioxidant
♦ Night vision, to improve
♦ Wounds
♦ Neuropathy

COLLECTION

The leaves should be gathered in the spring or early summer before fruit development. Simply prune the upper foliage from the plant. Once dry, garble the leaves from the stems. Discard the stems. The berries are hand picked once ripe. A dehydrator will assist in drying, otherwise mold growth is likely.

PREPARATIONS

The infusion method will be best for both leaf and fruit. Other preparations are considered secondary, but serviceable, as listed under Dosage. Standardized extracts are commercially available, but whole–plant preparations will prove just as effective, more so if applied towards gastrointestinal and urinary complaints. If the fresh fruit is available, in place of other supplementation, 1–2 oz. can be eaten daily. The fresh fruit (and the encapsulated powdered fruit) may have a laxative effect, so is inappropriate if used for diarrhea.

DOSAGE

- Leaf/Fruit infusion: 4–8 oz. 2–3 times daily
- FPT/DPT (50% alcohol) of leaf: ½–1 teaspoon 2–3 times daily
- Fluidextract of fruit: 30–60 drops 2–3 times daily
- Capsule (00) of powdered fruit: 2–4, 2–3 times daily

CAUTIONS

Loose stools may be a problem with excessive intake of the fresh fruit.

OTHER USES

Jams, jellies, and juices are common.

BLACK COHOSH
Ranunculaceae/Buttercup Family

Actaea racemosa (Cimicifuga racemosa)
Macrotys, Black bugbane

DESCRIPTION

Black cohosh is an herbaceous perennial. Its above ground portion is comprised of ternately arranged leaves along a single stem. Large, incised, and toothed the leaflets are loosely ovate to oblong. Small white flowers form in terminal racemes. They are followed by small, ovoid, semi–fleshy, capsules. Roots are comparatively small, tapering horizontally with a mass of corresponding smaller anchoring rootlets.

DISTRIBUTION

Wildly distributed throughout the eastern part of the country, the plant prefers rich forest soils with hardwood tress providing dappled shade. The core of Black cohosh territory is generally considered to be the east–central mountain ranges of Virginia, Pennsylvania, and Tennessee; Canada to Georgia, to Missouri.

CHEMISTRY

Triterpene glycosides: actein, cimigenol, cimiracemoside a, cimicifugoside h–1; phenolic constituents: cimicifugic acids a and b, fukinolic acid, cimifugin, cimiracemates a and b, piscidic acid, caffeic acid, ferulic acid, isoferulic acid.

MEDICINAL USES

Black cohosh, brought to us through Eclectic introduction via American Indian usage deserves its significant reputation. The plant is both chemically interesting and medicinally potent.

Use Black cohosh for the relief of mild to moderate pain dependant on weak circulation particularly if there is an underlying sense of bodily chilliness. Arthritis–like discomfort throughout the body, often from the onset of a cold or flu, is alleviated as is diffuse muscular pain sometimes described as fibromyalgia. Black cohosh is a mild cardiac/vascular stimulant, so its effect on pain syndromes is especially applicable when vascular deficiency underlies any painful episode.

Women are benefited by taking the plant through its ability to lessen menopausal discomforts. Hot flashes, heart palpitations, sleeplessness, and moodiness have all been shown to lessen under the plants use. It is also well used as an uterine stimulant when menses is sluggish, and warmth to the area feels beneficial.

Early on in Black cohosh's phytochemical revival, there was some speculation that the plant was estrogenic. According to the lasted round of studies this apparently is untrue. Supposedly the inverse applies – Black cohosh is mildly anti–estrogenic. The plant seems to be somewhat of a paradox. It is unclear exactly how Black cohosh exerts it's anti–proliferative effect. Some studies suggest the plant does indeed block various estrogen receptors (at least associated with uterine and mammary tissue stimulation), others rule against it suggesting an effect disassociated from any hormonal influence, all the while being successful in relieving complaints dependant upon diminished estrogen. Ultimately though Black cohosh's influence of the reproductive environment is not totally clear. To err on the side of caution I recommend against taking it in concordance with any related breast or uterine hyperplasia or cancer.

Considering its main audience, Black cohosh is thought of as a women's herb; but no longer. Men too may benefit from the plant's influence. It has been recently discovered that prostrate cancer cells are inhibited by the plant, apparently through several mechanisms. One of these being 5–α–reductase inhibition, which also speaks to Black cohosh's application to BPH (Benign prostrate hypertrophy).

How the prostrate enlarges is well understood. As men age 5–α–reductase production increases, converting testosterone to 5–α–DHT (5–α–dihydrotestosterone). This converted testosterone then triggers excessive cellular proliferation within the prostrate and seminal vesicles, which leads to BPH, and in some men, prostrate cancer.

For migraines, like relatives Clematis, Anemone, and Pulsatilla, Black cohosh is beneficial. Although not typically as strong as the latter plants, it too is vasodilatory. Dosed properly, as a preemptive, Black cohosh will relieve vascular constriction and therefore the following heightened vasodilation that normally coincides with the intense pain episode of a migraine. As an adjunctive treatment for glaucoma it is of value;

Black cohosh, like its relatives, has an uncanny effect on cerebral spinal fluid pressure, ultimately reducing intraocular pressure. Like Cannabis, used alone Black cohosh will not be as reliable as standard pharmaceuticals but may be useful in conjunction when standard approaches are not working.

Consider the lesser–known Western cohosh or Red baneberry (Actaea arguta) an equivalent to Black Cohosh. Morphologically and therapeutically the two plants appear nearly identical. Although there is no particular study to confirm the two plant's correspondence, empirical observation, confirms this. American herbalists familiar with under–utilized native plants have been using Western cohosh as an equivalent to Black cohosh for a number of years. It rivals the latter's potency and therapeutic sphere.

More broadly speaking, Buttercup family plants that are used therapeutically, typically have some useful overlap. Western cohosh is to Black cohosh, what Desert anemone is to Pulsatilla. Not only are all four plants found within the Buttercup family, but they all share sedative and vasodilatory properties.

INDICATIONS
♦ Pain, arthritis–like
♦ Pain, muscular, with vascular enfeeblement
♦ Menopausal complaints
♦ Amenorrhea/Dysmenorrhea
♦ Depression, dependant upon hormonal fluctuations and vascular deficiency
♦ Headache, migraine type, to preempt
♦ Glaucoma/Cerebral spinal fluid pressure, elevated

COLLECTION
Although the herbage is about half the strength of the root, it too can be collected – or just the herbage if the stand is not large. If collected in season, make sure to replant the fruit by covering with a small amount of forest litter.

Before collection confirm the stand is large enough to support wildcrafting. If the plant grows around you make several scouting trips to ascertain the quality and quantity of that population. If good harvesting practices are followed local stands usually support individual use. Due to over–harvesting and urbanization of forest-lands, the plant is listed as endangered in Illinois and Massachusetts.

Black cohosh populations are dwindling due to a huge transatlantic demand for the plant. Indigenous, home–grown use, most plants can support. Supply and endangerment problems develop when "the whole world" catches on to a therapeutic activity of a relativity isolated perennial...Europe should use its own Actaea as a menopause remedy.

For the commercial sector, wildcrafted stock far surpasses what is grown; much of what is labeled organic, like Ligusticum, is collected from the wild on "certified organic" land – a convenient loophole.

PREPARATIONS

Black cohosh is remarkable in that its potency is well preserved even after drying. Besides minimal constituent degradation, all major triterpene glycosides within the root remain intact, even after decades. The roots, being more resilient, take well to both fresh and dry methods of tincturing. Tincture the herbage fresh, or for tea use the recently dried material. The root tincture and tea both have subtle Licorice–like tastes, which may point to some similarities in chemistry with Licorice.

Standardized products abound; side effects are more often noted with these forms than with whole pant preparations.

DOSAGE

- ♦ FPT/DPT of root (80% alcohol): 20–30 drops 2–3 times daily
- ♦ FPT/DPT of leaf (70% alcohol): 30–50 drops 2–3 times daily
- ♦ Fluidextract of root: 10–20 drops 2–3 times daily
- ♦ Capsule (00) of root: 1–2, 2–3 times daily
- ♦ Leaf infusion: 2–4 oz. 2–3 times daily

CAUTIONS

In clinical practice I have observed, with over use, the development of a particular deep–seated vascular irritation. The discomfort is primarily localized to the arms and legs, and is akin to an internal burning sensation within these areas. Most likely this effect is due to the plant's vasodilatory excitation over a number of vascular groups or some sort of nerve irritation. It is not permanent and dissipates shorty when dosage is stopped or less is taken of the plant. It is not advised to take Black cohosh during pregnancy, due to its effect on the uterine environment and luteinizing hormone.

Do not use if there is existing liver inflammation or with pharmaceuticals that irritate the liver (the majority of them).

OTHER USES

Cultivars abound for ornamental garden use, which most likely are decent medicines as well.

BLACK WALNUT
Juglandaceae/Walnut Family

Juglans nigra
Walnut

DESCRIPTION

Black walnut is a large, handsome tree. With age its brownish bark becomes rough and fissured. Like most others in the genus, its odd–pinnate leaf arrangement is notable. Each leaf is usually composed of 11–23 large leaflets, with one terminating the bunch. Male and female flowers form separately on the same tree, with male catkins reaching 4¾" in length. Female flowers are smaller, usually no more than ½"–¾" long. The tree's oval fruit are distinct. The transitory outward fleshy layer is greenish–yellow when developing. Eventually this gives way to a hardened brown shell, containing an inner edible kernel.

DISTRIBUTION

Black walnut is an abundant hardwood forest

tree. Its range is extensive, flourishing through-out much of the East and Great Plains regions of the United States.

CHEMISTRY

Juglone, α–hydrojuglone, β–hydrojuglone, ellag-ic acid, gallic acid, caffeic acid, neochlorogenic acids, germacrene d.

MEDICINAL USES

One hundred years ago Juglans cinerea, or But-ternut, was the most popularly used Juglans. Today it is Black walnut. Fortunately nearly all varieties can be used in similar ways.

In small, sub–laxative doses, Black walnut is tonifying and soothing to the gastrointestinal tract. Its main tonic use is in quieting gastritis, irritative diarrhea, and intestinal inflammation with associated ileocecal irritation. Use the tea or tincture when chronic intestinal inflammation is causing nutrient malabsorption, particularly of fats. Black walnut is moderately antispasmod-ic. Its use is called for when there is intestinal spasm with flatulence. Internal use of the plant also clears the skin of acne–like eruptions par-ticularly when there is fat malabsorption depen-dent on poor diet.

In larger doses, Black walnut is laxative and is indicated in constipation when there is liver sluggishness. Equally, the plant is called for if constipation easily ensues when attention is not diligently maintained in keeping elimina-tion regular. Interestingly it is of note that con-strictive respiratory disturbances and systemic inflammatory issues sometimes are benefited by Black walnut through its tonifying effect on intestinal walls. Through this influence metabo-lites and toxins are less apt to enter the systemic circulation where they are likely to cause harm.

Although not systemically useful in limiting Candida infections, Black walnut can be helpful if the issue is limited to the gastrointestinal tract. Even though the plant is somewhat antifungal, berberine–containing plants such as Barberry or Oregongrape are more so, making Black walnut over–rated in this area.

Sometimes recommended in diminishing fungal infections, the fresh plant applied topi-cally as a poultice, whether from the green hulls, bark, or leaves, is rather caustic and can cause redness and blistering in even short exposures. Black walnut's juglone content is largely the causative factor. When the fresh plant is crushed larger juglone–like complexes are oxidized and broken down to juglone, which is responsible for the resulting brown pigmentation and charac-teristic smell.

The plant, alone or in combination, is of-ten touted as a vermifuge. Like so many other semi–laxative herbs with unique aromatics, in large amounts Black walnut occasionally gives positive results (pinworm or tapeworm). But all to often its influence is widely exaggerated, par-ticularly by writers[7] with "Cure" in the book's title.

INDICATIONS

♦   GI tract inflammation with attending diar-rhea or constipation
♦   Nutrient/Lipid malabsorption
♦   Cramps, intestinal
♦   Candida albicans infection, GI tract involve-ment

COLLECTION

Collect the green leaves when available; the hulls of the fruit should be harvested when they are just starting to turn brown. Collect the bark in long strips from secondary branches with little thickened–outward bark. Be aware that juglone

---

7   Much of today's herbal writing falls into several camps. One: the "hippy–dippy ramble". Some of these guides con-tain decent information...digestible if the reader is able to get past the author's long–in–the–tooth 1960s viewpoint. Two: "just the facts". Reads like a pharmacology textbook; nearly every sentence is referenced like the author had no original thought. In trying to get the Lancet or New Eng-land Journal of Medicine to pay attention the point is lost. Three: "buy the book; it will cure whatever ails you". Often authored by individuals with no background in the field, these are easy to spot. Glib, over–the–top, and sensational, by far this group does the largest disservice to the field. They are a cheap hustle intending to feed off of people's desire to believe.

makes a nice, brown stain, and when on the skin does not remove well with soap and water.

PREPARATIONS/DOSAGE
♦ FPT/DPT (50% alcohol): 30–60 drops 2–3 times daily
♦ Infusion: 4–6 oz. 2–3 times daily

CAUTIONS
Do not use during pregnancy or topically on abraded or sensitive tissues.

OTHER USES
The kernels of the ripe fruit, like English walnut, are edible. As a stain or dye, the tincture or tea may be only rivaled by Desert rhubarb in its impermeability.

BLUE COHOSH
Berberidaceae/Barberry Family

Caulophyllum thalictroides
Squaw root, Papoose root

DESCRIPTION
Blue cohosh is a long–lived herbaceous perennial, arising from a tangle of hair–like rootlets, anchored to a laterally situated rhizome. Placed only inches below the ground its subterranean root structure is nearly identical to Black cohosh's. Another close relative, Western cohosh, also shares morphological qualities with these two plants..

The arising stem is solitary, 2'–3' in height, terminating with a large (1⅔' wide) triternately compound leaf. Leaflets are obovate and display a 2–3 lobed termination, often appearing like a rounded duck's foot. Flowers form in panicles; each is star–like and is composed of 6 sepals and 6 petals. The whole arrangement is propped on a long stem originating below the leaf. When ripe the fruit are blue and spherical.

Blue cohosh is typically a colony plant – where there is one, there will be others closely gathered. A stand is pleasing to see; the leaves of each plant seem to merge into each other, forming a horizontal leafy plain.

DISTRIBUTION
Like Black cohosh and Goldenseal, Blue cohosh needs a stable, deciduous, damp, and dark forest to flourish. The plant is found from Canada to South Carolina, west to the Dakotas and central plains states.

CHEMISTRY
Quinolizidine alkaloids: n–methylcytisine, baptifoline, anagyrine; aporphine alkaloid: magnoflorine; other alkaloids: caulophyllumine a, caulophyllumine b; triterpenoid saponins: cauloside a, cauloside d, cauloside h.

MEDICINAL USES
In use and also floristically Blue cohosh is related to the better known Black cohosh. They both belong to the same order and both affect the female reproductive system. Although Blue cohosh has not been analyzed in a clinical setting, it is an unpredictable yet potent plant.

If Blue cohosh does have a hormonal effect on the reproductive environment it is yet undiscovered, but such an activity would shed light on the plant's influence. Unquestionably Blue cohosh is vasodialating to the pelvic region, specifically, the female reproductive area. It is therapeutic for a whole range of disturbances that initiate from poor uterine circulation.

Use Blue cohosh if menses is sluggish and there are accompanying menstrual cramps. Being emmenagogue and antispasmodic the plant will be beneficial specifically if menstrual pain is strangely rheumatoid–like and is relieved by warmth. In chronic inflammatory conditions such as PID (pelvic inflammatory disease) and endometriosis Blue cohosh often imparts a needed quality of tissue stimulation. Even long–standing vaginitis and cervicitis is helped by Blue cohosh – especially in combination with a regional antibacterial or antiviral agent.

Women in the throws of menopause often find Blue cohosh quieting to uterine discomfort especially if it is of a congested, arthritis–like quality. In these cases Blue and Black cohosh combine well together.

The plant has a strong following in present–day midwifery. Its current use, to stimulate labor, is surely connected to the past when labor facilitating agents were largely herbal. And for a time Blue cohosh and other herbs were safer than once popular ergot. Today though, unless conditions exclude conventional birthing care, Blue cohosh should be viewed as unnecessary and unpredictable. Used alone in normal amounts the plant can act ideally, but at labor initiating doses trigger erratic contractile waves, leading to a disorganised birth. There is at least one well–documented case of excessive amounts of Blue cohosh used as a labor facilitator by the mother–to–be. After vaginal delivery the newborn received emergency care due to threatening cardiovascular symptoms. He eventually recovered with hospital care, but as a toddler heart impairment was still notable. Other similar undocumented cases are not uncommon.

We in the modern world have low birth mortality rates because of conventional pregnancy and neonatal care. Herbal medicines are needed today because they work in many situations. In some realms though they should be noted, and then left behind (again) for tools that are more reliable.

By far the safest, home–based, "user–friendly" way to stimulate labor is through endogenous oxytocin release. This is achieved through sexual arousal and climax...nipple stimulation and orgasm.

In conclusion, the overall picture for Blue cohosh use is reproductive–centered vascular debility resulting in congestion and sluggishness. Chronic inflammation or at least irritation are typical symptoms. Used solely the plant can be overly energetic. It is best combined with other plants in formula.

INDICATIONS

♦ Amenorrhea
♦ Dysmenorrhea
♦ Vaginitis/Cervicitis, chronic
♦ PID/Endometriosis

COLLECTION

Given that they are fairly close to the surface, the roots of Blue cohosh are not hard to gather. Look for a cluster of stems arising in close proximity to each other. Start digging about 1' out from where the stems join the ground and work inward. In this manner a fairly decent root cluster can be gathered.

PREPARATIONS

Well spaced roots dry adequately even if kept whole. Drying the root is important. Used fresh Blue cohosh tends to be an overt irritant.

DOSAGE

♦ DPT (60% alcohol): 10–25 drops 1–3 times daily
♦ Fluidextract: 4–8 drops 1–3 times daily

CAUTIONS

Blue cohosh should not be used during pregnancy or while nursing. Children also should not use the plant. Excessive use may lead to break–through bleeding and uterine irritation.

BURDOCK

Asteraceae/Sunflower Family

Arctium lappa
Lappa, Greater burdock

DESCRIPTION

Burdock is a comely biennial. Like most plants in its class, its first year's growth is decidedly basal. At maturity the leaves can reach 1⅓' in length. They are ovate and cordate at their bases, green above, and gray and hairy below. Beginning the plant's second year's growth a flower stalk develops, upon which smaller dispersed leaves form. The grouped flowers develop in rounded flat–topped clusters and are dispersed along the upper stalk. Corolla color varies from pink to purple. After drying, the seed heads quickly fall apart. Each hooked seed easily finds purchase on animals or cloths, or is often borne a short distance by the wind.

DISTRIBUTION

Indigenous to Eurasia, Burdock is now distributed throughout temperate regions world–wide. In the United States look to disturbed soils, drainage ditches, and fallow fields. It is rarely found in warmer locales, where lack of cold winters inhibit the plant's continuation.

CHEMISTRY

Polysaccharides: inulin (among others); phytoalexins; chlorogenic acid, caffeic acid; lignans: arctiin, arctigenin, diarctigenin (seeds).

MEDICINAL USES

Burdock is an internal medicine for the skin. Its influence is noted when applied to surface disorders that have their roots in a disturbed internal metabolism. It is an excellent remedy for individuals whose liver and kidneys are not eliminating wastes as they should. Burdock influences both organs, but especially the kidneys to optimally remove waste material and metabolites from the blood. For both psoriasis and eczema, chronic acne and boils, and other non–resolving skin conditions the plant will have merit if the internal situation fits for its use.

Burdock is somewhat diuretic in nature, but specifically it is useful in removing elevated uric acid levels within the blood and related tissues. Alone, or combined with Dandelion it is an excellent gout treatment. Uric acid forming foods, such as legumes and organ meats should be removed from the diet in order to expedite the deposit's elimination. Likewise if there is a tendency for acid–based kidney stones, Burdock will be helpful in their dissolution. For this application it combines well with Corn silk.

Underlying nearly all of Burdock's therapeutic uses is the plant's antioxidant/free radical scavenging attributes. Like so many other plants, Burdock is a potent quencher of ROS (reactive oxygen species). Not only are the hydroxyl radical, superoxide, nitric oxide, and peroxyl groups affected, but non–radicals, such as hydrogen peroxide, ozone, and singlet oxygen are affected as well. Glutathione, a potent cellular antioxidant is better preserved with Burdock supplementation. These antioxidant effects have wide reaching influences over numerous degenerative/inflammatory states. At the heart of Burdock's influence is its preservation of cellular components like proteins, phospholipids, and cholesterols. Essentially it protects against cellular injury.

Burdock retards LDL (low density lipoprotein) oxidation and its subsequent harmful interaction with arterial tissue, ultimately serving as a cardiovascular protectant. Use it if there is a history of atherosclerosis–cardiovascular illness. The plant generally will not correct a heart or vascular condition, but it will serve as a preventative for such things.

Like its relatives, Dandelion, Jerusalem artichoke, and Chicory, Burdock has a substantial inulin content within its roots. Due to the body's inability to digest this complex carbohydrate inulin enters the colon intact promoting beneficial microflora growth, particularly of bifidobacteria. This in turn stabilizes the large intestinal environment, limiting pathogenic bacteria and their destructive by–products. Due to Burdock's beneficial influence over intestinal microflora, blood–lipid composition often improves. It is not uncommon for root preparations to lower LDL and VLDL (very low density lipoprotein) levels. The result will be incremental, but still of note.

Furthermore, due to Burdock's inulin content, it is well used for what is popularly called "leaky gut syndrome" – a title meant to describe a symptom picture of skin allergies, joint inflammation, fatigue, and colon instability dependent upon proliferation of harmful colon bacteria, their by–products, and heightened leukocyte activity. For this purpose, combine Burdock with Yucca. The combination tends to stabilize beneficial flora levels, while binding harmful endotoxins.

Burdock seed preparations, due to their lignan content, most likely have a mild estrogen receptor affinity. As estrogen antagonists, use the seed tincture or encapsulated seed powder as a preventative for estrogen–dependant prostrate and breast cancer.

The term alterative sums up Burdock's abilities the best. It is an older medical term, born of a time when allopathy was an equal brother to homeopathy and nautropathy, used to classify a substance, usually a plant, or to describe its property. Simply, it is a plant that positively changes or alters elimination, immunity, cellular metabolism, and detoxification, or other related factors that promote healing.

INDICATIONS

- Skin conditions, inflammatory, chronic
- Gout
- Acid–based kidney stones
- Antioxidant, cardiovascular
- LDL/VLDL, to lower
- Intestinal flora imbalance
- As an alternative

COLLECTION

Gather Burdock's mature first year roots. They will be prime to harvest from fall through winter. The roots of second year plants, if not half–rotted, will make an inferior medicine. Burdock seed is collected from the second–year plant. That is a simple matter. Removing the seeds from their encasement, will prove to be much more labor intensive. Both the root and seed of Burdock are commercially available.

PREPARATIONS

Use root capsules or the root cold infusion to capture Burdock's inulin content. For non–inulin applications the fluidextract of the root is the optimal preparation.

DOSAGE

- Root infusion, cold or standard: 4–8 oz. 2–3 times daily
- FPT/DPT of root (50% alcohol): 45–90 drops 2–3 times daily
- Fluidextract of root: 15–45 drops 2–3 times daily
- Capsule (00) (root): 2–3, 2–3 times daily
- DPT of seeds (50% alcohol): 15–45 drops 2–3 times daily
- Capsule (00) (seed): 2, 2–3 times daily

CAUTIONS
None known.

OTHER USES
In Japanese cuisine Burdock (Gobo) is cultivated and utilized as a root vegetable. Although medicinally not as potent, its polysaccharide content is significant. Gobo is well applied for its inulin properties.

BUTCHER'S BROOM
Liliaceae/Lily Family

Ruscus aculeatus
Sweet broom, Knee holly, Box holly

DESCRIPTION
As a low–growing, shrubby, evergreen perennial, Butcher's broom is a unique Lily family bush. Typically between 3'–5' in height the plant has bright green stems and tiny scale–like leaves. Flowers form on leaf–like stems, appearing as though originating from the center of each "leaf". The red ovoid fruit ripen in early autumn. Like closely related asparagus, Butcher's broom prolifically sprouts from root colonies.

DISTRIBUTION
A successful plant, Butcher's broom is found throughout the Mediterranean region, northern Africa, western Asia, and southern Europe, including the British Isles. Its ability to thrive in an array of soil types and microclimates affords the plant with the title of invasive weed in a number of regions. It is also planted widely as an ornamental.

CHEMISTRY

Saponins: ruscogenin, neoruscogenin, ruscin, desglucoruscin, desglucodesrhamnoruscin; flavonoids

MEDICINAL USES

Rich in old–world history and lore, Butcher's broom held an important place in European plant–based tradition. Favorably viewed by both English herbalists Gerard and Culpepper its use in period folk medicine was important.

Reinvented, today Butcher's broom is a plant of modern European phytotherapy. Currently its most direct use is in addressing CVD (chronic venous disorder), a poorly understood disturbance of the microcirculatory, affecting an array of venous tissue, associated capillary beds, and surrounding tissue/skin groups. Leg, varicosities, edema, and related ulceration, are the main symptoms of CVD.

Butcher's broom works to increase venous tone. The plant's tightening effect diminishes capillary bed/venous tissue distention, limiting protein/fibrin–leakage edema. Under Butcher's broom adrenergic influence even the valve–like venous junctures are augmented, resulting in improved leg circulation, ultimately lessening varicose disturbances.

Hemorrhoids, essentially varicosities affecting the anal region, are diminished by the plant as well. All the same mechanisms by which Butcher's broom is found therapeutic for the extremities, likewise affects other trunk areas.

Both internal and external application are well proven, generally well–tolerated, and complement each other nicely. Standardized products abound since the plant's formative years were spent in European phyto–pharmaceutical testing grounds.

Currently two steroidal saponins, ruscogenin and neoruscogenin, are considered responsible for Butcher's broom's effect on venous tissue (doubtlessly there are other constituents making an impact). Their vasoconstrictive qualities are evident in the results obtained by the plant's use.

INDICATIONS

♦ Venous laxity, lower extremity and trunk (external and internal)
♦ Varicosities (external and internal)
♦ Edema/Ulceration, venous involvement (external and internal)
♦ Hemorrhoids (external and internal)

COLLECTION

Although both leaves and roots contain saponins, the roots are decidedly more potent. Easily dug they rhizomatous and fleshy.

PREPARATIONS

Fresh and recently dried material will be of therapeutic value. Cut/sifted and powdered material with longer storage times will be of inferior quality. Standardized preparations have a well–proven track record. Both crude and standardized materials are commercially available.

DOSAGE

♦ FPT/DPT (60% alcohol): 30–60 drops 2–3 times daily
♦ Fluidextract: 15–30 drops 2–3 times daily
♦ Ointment/Oil: as needed

CAUTIONS

External preparations applied to ulcerated skin may prove to be irritating. In these cases use Calendula or another healing vulnerary. Occasionally some of the plant's saponin–derived acridity is transferred via the fresh plant tincture. Diluting in an adequate amount of water should diminish any transitory throat/esophageal discomfort.

OTHER USES

The plant's bundled twigs and branches were once used in broom making. Basket weavers also used the tough but flexible branches in their craft.

CALENDULA
Asteraceae/Sunflower Family

Calendula officinalis
Marigold, Garden marigold, Pot marigold

DESCRIPTION

A somewhat small, but showy annual, Calendula's most notable feature is its flowers. On occasion measuring 4" across, they are typically orange or yellow, but some variation is to be expected due to the presence of cultivars. The plant's foliage is hairy and pale green. Leaves are oblanceolate or spatulate and sessile or petioled.

DISTRIBUTION

A plant native to the Mediterranean region, Calendula now is found practically world–wide through its use as a bedding plant or in the herb garden. Throughout parts of the Northeast and western United States it is now considered naturalized due to its popular ornamental use and prolific seeding habits.

CHEMISTRY

Essential oils; flavonoids: kaempferol, quercetin, isoquercitrin, rutin; phenolic acids: chlorogenic, caffeic, coumaric, and vanillic; sterols; carotenoids: neoxanthin, violaxanthin, luteoxanthin, auroxanthin, flavoxanthin, mutatoxanthin, antheraxanthin, lutein, cryptoxanthins, carotenes; tannins; saponins; triterpene alcohols; triterpenoid fatty acid esters: lauryl, myristoyl, and palmitoyl; esters of faradiol; polysaccharides; a bitter principle; mucilage; resin.

MEDICINAL USES

Calendula is mainly used externally as a healer of tissue. The plant is well known in its application to ulcers and wounds. In either case it lessens inflammation and speeds healing of skin and tissue. Although not as strong, as a tissue stimulant the plant shares some qualities with Arnica. Locally Calendula has a mild effect on increasing white blood cells counts, which not only helps fight infections, but also increases tissue granulation and healing time. But most likely the plant's overall healing influence is due to its array of flavonoids and carotenoids. Not only are they profound antioxidants but they also serve as a sort of tissue nutritive. New, organized tissue will form more quickly, which makes the plant's application well suited to situations where the skin's epithelial layer has been removed or damaged. Applied to burns with or without Aloe, it will reduce scarring. Even continually applied alone or with St. Johns wort, Calendula is superb in lessening scar formations from wounds, surgery, and of special interest to women – post–operative cesarean–section scars. As a warm poultice, combined with Marshmallow, it shows success in bringing abscesses to a head. In these situations, after cleaning the area, apply Calendula ointment to the abscess's cavity.

The plant lessens varicosities and other laxities of venous tissue. Due to Calendula's vaso-constricting effect it is especially useful for lower leg/ankle issues in which poor fluid movement causes capillary bed engorgement, and often ulceration and infection.

As a douche or wash Calendula tea is soothing and healing to vaginal and cervical inflammations. Combined with Echinacea and Thuja it makes an excellent suppository for cervical dysplasia whether related or not to HPV (human papillomavirus).

Calendula made as an eyewash is well applied to minor conjunctivitis. Prickly poppy will be found more effective for bacterial involvement; Goldenseal for allergy induced ocular inflammations.

Although the plant is mainly considered an external medicine, the tea or tincture diluted in warm water makes an excellent preparation for healing oral, esophageal, and upper gastric ulcers and erosions. Like other topical approaches, surface area contact is necessary for the healing of involved mucus membranes. With 3 cups of tea daily, benefit should be noticed within a week.

INDICATIONS

- Ulcers/Wounds/Abscesses (external)
- Scar formation (external)
- Varicosities with associated ulceration (external)
- Capillary circulation, impaired (external)
- Vaginal/Cervical inflammation (external)
- Cervical dysplasia (external)
- Conjunctivitis (eyewash)
- Ulcers, oral, esophageal, gastric

COLLECTION
Deep orange flowers will be more potent due to higher carotenoid levels. With pruners snip the flowers from the plant. These are then allowed to dry or tinctured fresh.

PREPARATIONS/DOSAGE
- FPT/DPT (80% alcohol): 10–30 drops 2–3 times daily
- Fluidextract: 5–10 drops 2–3 times daily
- Eyewash: 3–4 times daily
- Ointment/Oil/Salve: as needed
- Douche/Sitz bath/Wash: as needed
- Suppository: 2–3 times daily

CAUTIONS
None known with proper use.

CANNABIS
Cannabaceae/Hemp Family

Cannabis sativa, C. indica, C. ruderalis
Hemp, Marijuana, Wild cannabis

DESCRIPTION
Cannabis's botanical classification is imperfect at best. What causes such a problem with the plant's taxonomy is the great length of time it has been domesticated, selected, and cross–breed.

Loosely Cannabis can be separated into three morphological and use types. The Cannabis sativa type is tall and loosely branched with narrow leaflets. It is mainly cultivated for fiber and seed uses; its cannabinoid content is diminutive. C. indica is compact and conical shaped with wider leaflets. This is the main drug variety, both for medical purposes and otherwise. The C. ruderalis type is short, branchless, and weedy. It is considered a wild version of C. indica or C. sativa.

Cannabis is a dioecious annual. Herbaceous in habit, the plant's leaves are serrated, palmately compounded, and composed of usually 5, 7, or 9 leaflets, but occasionally up to thirteen, reducing to sometimes only one at the upper growth tip. Lower leaves are typically opposite, whereas the upper leaves are alternate. Its angular stem may appear almost mint–like.

Both male and female flowers form from leaf axils; both are greenish. Males develop into long, branched, drooping panicles; female flowers are erect, clustered, and catkin–like. Cannabis's fruit, technically not a seed, is a compressed achene enclosed within an ovate bract. Flowers, leaves, and stems are all covered by a viscid pubescence.

DISTRIBUTION
Native to Central Asia, Cannabis is now cultivated world–wide for its fiber, seed, or medicinal/psychoactive use. In Afghanistan, doubtlessly one of the epicenters of the plant's indigenous range, large expanses are left to its cultivation.

CHEMISTRY
Cannabinoids: δ–9–tetrahydrocannabinol, δ–8–tetrahydrocannabinol, cannabinol, cannabidiol, cannabicycol, cannabichromene, cannabigerol.

Due to selective breeding cannabinoid (especially THC or δ–9–tetrahydrocannabinol) content has increased significantly – from the 1960's 1–3% to today's 6–13%. Both physical and cerebral influences are dependant on this group of compounds.

MEDICINAL USES
Although I had deliberated for a time on whether or not to include Cannabis in this work, ultimately I had little choice as it fits the criteria of the others: it is very popular (unfortunately though for the wrong reasons), and most relevantly, it is

a medicinal plant. Its legal status should be kept in mind, but ultimately responsibility for its effects, for good or bad, should be placed upon the adult user.

Cannabis use stretches back before recorded history, probably rivaling Corn and Myrrh in continual usefulness. It certainly ranks among a strata of plants known to influence culture and society, both ancient and modern.

In many painful conditions Cannabis is warranted. The urinary tract is one region where the anesthetic effects of the plant is profoundly felt. It will be found pain relieving to bladder, urethra, and even kidney centered distresses. The burning and discomfort of cystitis and urethritis are particularly soothed by Cannabis. It is more relieving to chronic and subacute inflammations than acute sensitivities. Even in low–grade kidney sensitivity/inflammation it will be of use. Consider it specific for the urinary irritation of interstitial cystitis and the chronic urinary symptoms of multiple sclerosis. Although the plant has little actual antibacterial influence its effects over the region should not be underestimated.

Compounding its pain relieving effect is its influence over smooth muscle constriction. Used during urinary stone passage, due to its reduction of spasm and constriction, Cannabis will be found opening to the area.

The plant has control over other spastic states/pains as well. Tremors, muscular stiffness, and seizure activity of all sorts will be modified to some degree. Epileptics and suffers of multiple sclerosis will especially benefit from the plant if not using conventional medicines.

Menstrual cramps as well as other uterine irritabilities, such as the pains of endometriosis, will be quieted. For men, seminal vesicle irritation is usually subdued as well. The cramping pain of diarrhea is specific for the plant, as is biliary and renal smooth muscle irritation. The hectic cough of chronic bronchitis is abated, and will be found particularly useful taken before bed.

Cannabis has influence over neuralgias of all types. Whether related to abrupt injury or slower progressing ailments, its effects are usually a welcomed relief. The pain of shingles and sciatic/lumbar/trigeminal impingement is well addressed.

Suffers of terminal illness, when pain and sensitivity are the norm will feel eased by the plant. Possibly its most important use, to lend relief to the afflicted who are dying, Cannabis will help dull the contortions of the body. Unlike the overt suppression of opiates, Cannabis allows a greater range of function.

An externally applied liniment will accent internal use of the tincture for these pain syndromes. Topical application for the pain and inflammation of arthritis and injury is an old and successful application.

As an appetite stimulant profound effects will be seen in individuals who suffer from anorexia connected to nervousness and anxiety. When normal appetite is suppressed due to cancer or chemotherapy–radiation, Cannabis will spark hunger sensations. Its ability at curbing nausea – a typical symptom of conventional cancer treatment – is well noted.

Intraocular pressure and related glaucoma is poorly remedied by Cannabis due to the plant's short per–dose duration of activity (2–3 hours). Plus, there currently exist conventional medications with little side effect.

Upon the mind the plant has interesting influences. If there is depression it generally is found uplifting; if anxious, then calming. Of course there are exceptions, some will find the plant deranging and others will be unaffected.

It is not my desire to repeat what can be found in countless drug culture manuals concerning Cannabis's cerebral influences. As far a the plant's label by some as a "sacrament" to be used daily, solely for its mind altering effects...at least have the honestly to know that you are not able to take the world, in all of its tragedy and comedy, sober.

INDICATIONS

♦   Urinary tract pain, irritation, and constric-

tion
- Menstrual cramps/Uterine irritability
- Gastrointestinal spasm
- Hectic cough of chronic bronchitis
- Pain, nerve tissue/smooth muscle (external and internal)
- Lack of appetite/anorexia

COLLECTION
The whole plant is active. Compared to the male flowers or leaf, female flowers will have higher concentrations of cannabinoids. Cannabis indica will be the strongest. C. sativa and C. ruderalis lesser so, but still useful medicines, though in today's Cannabis aficionado field numerous variants and hybrids exist, making pure selection nearly impossible.

Although the dried female flowering tops are standard in drug trade, as is Cannabis resin or hashish, in most states Cannabis is illegal to cultivate and to possess. About a dozen states have enacted "medical marijuana" and "personal use" laws, usually at conflict with federal law. In this country, farmers of low cannabinoid Cannabis sativa varieties (industrial hemp) for seed and fiber use, are plagued by legal contention, red tape, and stigma.

PREPARATIONS
Internal, liquid preparations are recommended, due to their effects being more tissue oriented. Smoked Cannabis has more profound, yet effervescent, cerebral effects.

DOSAGE
- FPT/DPT of flower and leaf (80% alcohol): 5–30 drops 1–3 times daily
- Liniment/Ointment: topically as needed

CAUTIONS
Used short–term for what the plant is indicated for should not cause a problem. Some users may find longer–term use addictive. The most obvious drawback to consistent use is Cannabis's pronounced cerebral influence. Permanent dulling effects on mental process seems to be obvi-

ous with long–time users...a.k.a. "pot head" and "stoner". It is fairly well documented that when used heavily as a recreational drug, particularly in adolescence, the plant can and often does lead to long–lasting neurobiological changes affecting function and behavior.

"Adult user" is stressed here; unless dealing with a cancer situation, due to the plant's cerebral effects and related illegal status, a minor will hardly benefit from Cannabis. There are many other plants that are successful replacements for Cannabis's secondary applications; see Therapeutic Index. Do not use while pregnant or while nursing.

The Law.

OTHER USES
Fiber, oil, and food.

CASCARA SAGRADA
Rhamnaceae/Buckthorn Family

Rhamnus purshiana
Sacred bark, Chittem bark

DESCRIPTION
Cascara sagrada is a small tree or large shrub reaching heights of 35'. Older trunk and branch bark is gray, whereas twigs and branches are red to brown. The elliptic, 2"–6" leaves are thin and have tapered bases. Leaf margins are entire or toothed, surfaces are smooth or slightly hairy with prominent veins. The plant's inconspicuous flowers form in small groupings; they each have 5 sepals and 5 petals. Fruit are black, 2/5" in diameter, and 3–seeded.

DISTRIBUTION
Cascara sagrada ranges through much of Northern California and is found as far north as Montana and British Columbia.

CHEMISTRY
Anthraquinones; flavonoids; tannins.

MEDICINAL USES

Cascara sagrada is a well known bowel stimulant, but unlike other anthraquinone–containing laxatives such as Aloe and Senna it is less apt to cause dependency. The tea is best used in mild to moderate chronic constipation, when stools are dry and difficult to pass. Taken before bed the plant works well with the body's natural rhythm by setting up a bowel movement for the morning. Used this way rarely does the plant cause griping, or a watery stool. Although Cascara sagrada can be used long–term, intestinal health is best regulated through proper diet and fluid intake.

The plant's secondary influences also work to remedy constipation: Cascara sagrada is a bitter tonic, stimulating upper gastrointestinal response. It is also a biliary stimulant. These attributes, in concert with its activity over the large intestine make the plant a key therapy for upper, mid, an lower gastrointestinal deficiencies.

One lesser known activity of Cascara sagrada is its arthritis lessening effect. It is not as strong in pain relief as Creosote bush or Turmeric, but when applied properly, some find the plant remarkable. Suffers of rheumatoid– or osteo– arthritis whose pain is dependant on constipation, often find Cascara sagrada quite relieving. It is no secret how the plant works in these situations. Through stimulation of the large intestine and the liver, tissue wastes are eliminated more efficiently, hence a reduction in inflammatory potential occurs. With the exception of acute pain from injury, most inflammatory conditions, including allergies (if chronic constipation is part of the picture) will respond positively to the plant.

INDICATIONS

♦ Constipation, chronic
♦ Liver deficiency
♦ Arthritis with constipation

COLLECTION

Select a secondary branch with thin and unfissured bark. With a knife, or sometimes hands are adequate, strip the bark from the branch.

PREPARATIONS

Mainly a concern for the individual personally collecting and using Cascara sagrada, the bark should be aged before using. Two methods can be used. Once dried, set aside for 6 months or place the bark in an oven or a dehydrator, set at 120 degrees, for 8–12 hours. The first method is more reliable, the latter should be used mainly if the bark is needed immediately. Either method reduces the harshness of the green/freshly dried bark.

DOSAGE

♦ DPT (30% alcohol): 1–2 teaspoons 1–2 times daily
♦ Fluidextract: 10–30 drops 1–2 times daily
♦ Bark decoction/Cold infusion: 2–6 oz. 1–2 times daily

CAUTIONS

Due to potential uterine stimulation by the plant's anthraquinones, do not use during pregnancy. A laxative effect will be seen in nursing babies if used by the mother. Cascara sagrada is fine for children – reduce the dosage accordingly by weight.

CATNIP

Lamiaceae/Mint Family

Nepeta cataria
Catmint

DESCRIPTION

Catnip is a short–lived, herbaceous perennial with erect or semi–erect branching stems. Although not nearly as pubescent as Horehound, Catnip too has a white to grayish pubescent coating, particularly on its upper portion. Leaves are green above and grayish–hairy below. They are deltoid to ovate with crenate to serrate margins. The flowers form in spikes or cymes, with each corolla being 2–parted and white with purple spots. Catnip's small seeds, or nutlets, are ovoid, brown, and somewhat flattened.

DISTRIBUTION

Native to Europe, Catnip is now naturalized extensively throughout temperate North America. Look to semi–shady, disturbed areas.

CHEMISTRY

Main volatiles: nepetalactone, citronellol, geraniol, citral, germacrene, d caryophyllene, spathulenol.

MEDICINAL USES

There are no surprises when evaluating Catnip's therapeutic influence over the body. Part sedative, part diaphoretic, and part carminative, the plant is useful for mild complains, particularly those of children.

Use the infusion as a mild calming agent, particularly in cases in which there is mental/ emotional agitation that disturbs digestion. Catnip has marked carminative properties, so its use in gastrointestinal pain and fullness from gas and bloating will be found of benefit, especially if worry and anxiety are factors. The plant has a marked anesthetic effect on the stomach lining, as do many Mint family plants, making the tea or tincture useful for both nausea and vomiting. If alcohol use is the culprit a duel therapy of Milk thistle taken before the drinking episode, and Catnip the day after, will be effective in reducing alcohol toxicities and any residual stomach upset.

For colicky babies, several tablespoons of warm tea is an old remedy. Not only will the herb curb cramping and flatulence but it will also sooth the infant's troubled state of mind. For this purpose, it combines well with Fennel. As an old stand–by, it is effective and pleasant tasting. Like Wood betony a cup of Catnip tea is useful in relieving childhood headaches, particularly if there is associated worry and agitation.

For women whose period, through stress and worry, becomes late and troublesome, Catnip will lessen abdominal discomfort. It is not a menstrual stimulant such as Pennyroyal or Wormwood but a quieter of surrounding muscle coats. In all aspects Catnip's strength is in its gentleness. It does not influence abruptly, but subtly nudges.

Lastly for fevers, hot Catnip tea is a mild diaphoretic, similar to Spearmint in effect. If drunk cool, the tea is less diaphoretic, but more tonic in nature, and better applied to previously mentioned gastrointestinal and anxiety complaints.

INDICATIONS

- Gas pains and bloating
- Nausea/Vomiting
- Colic
- Menstruation, late, with anxiety
- Fever, mild

COLLECTION

Gather the upper half of the Catnip, flowering or not. After drying garble the leaves and or flowers from the stems. Discard the stems as they have little value.

PREPARATIONS

Tincture preparations are inferior but they are included here due to their popularity as an ingredient in stomachic combinations, i.e. Catnip and Fennel.

DOSAGE

- Herb infusion: 4–8 oz. 2–3 times daily
- FPT/DPT (50% alcohol): 30–60 drops 2–3 times daily

CAUTIONS

None known.

CAYENNE PEPPER
Solanaceae/Nightshade Family

Capsicum frutescens
Red pepper, Bird pepper, Chili pepper, African pepper, Ají, American cayenne, African cayenne, Guinea pepper

DESCRIPTION

Cayenne pepper describes both a particular plant[8] (Capsicum frutescens) and a certain grade of Capsicum powder. The plant, and historically the main source of the herbal medicine, is native to Central/South America. The plant's name is derived from Cayenne, the capitol of French Guinea, where the plant is found in abundance.

Described here is the main perennial species – C. frutescens. But chances are if the plant produces, small–tapering, orange–red, and very hot fruit, it has been, or at one time will be called, "Cayenne pepper". It is more of a description applied loosely throughout the spice–medicinal herb sectors, and less of a concrete plant or item.

Cayenne pepper or Capsicum frutescens when found in its native temperatures is a short–lived perennial. From 3'–5' in size, it is a fast–growing evergreen shrub. Leaves are ovate to ovate–lanceolate and can be up to 4⅔" long by 1¾" wide. Greenish to yellowish–white flowers occur in node groupings. The elongated–tapering, red to reddish–orange fruit can be up to several inches in length. The placenta and attached seeds (coating) contain the highest amounts of spiciness (capsaicinoids).

DISTRIBUTION

Since the plant has been cultivated for thousands of years its specific place of origin is difficult to ascertain, but some suggest the Panama region of Central America. Today the plant is found pan–tropically, extensively naturalized and cultivated throughout the world.

CHEMISTRY

Capsaicinoids: capsaicin, dihydrocapsaicin; carotenoids: α–carotene, β–carotene, cryptoflavin, zeaxanthin, β–cryptoxanthin, 9–cis–capsanthin; ascorbic acid.

MEDICINAL USES

Cayenne pepper has a rich history of western medicinal use, but it is only one variety that is

useful. Don't be fooled by the "it must be Cayenne pepper" line of thought. Essentially, if the pepper is hot it will work.

Most hot–chili peppers have been categorized by their spiciness. The Scoville scale, used by the spice industry for nearly 100 years, measures each pepper's pungency in terms of heat units. Cayenne ranks between 30,000–50,000 heat units, habanero, between 100,000–500,000 units, common bell pepper has a ranking of 0–1 unit. All pepper's heat is dependant upon the amount of contained capsaicin, which alone has a ranking of 16,000,000 units. This capsaicinoid is found primarily within the fruit's inner white fibrous material, which holds the seeds (hot peppers can be made much more mild by scraping this layer from the opened fruit).

Cayenne's therapeutic effect is dependant upon capsaicin. This compound has a fascinating influence on contacted tissue groups – so much so that early descriptions of Cayenne as a simple circulatory stimulant need to be reevaluated.

Cayenne has a unique bi–polar effect. Upon initial exposure there is intense peripheral and central nerve ending excitation – depolarization and discharge – resulting in burning pain and/or warmth and tissue stimulation.

With continued reapplication these influenced afferent neurons become unresponsive, not only to Cayenne, but also to pain signals from other injuries – sprains, arthritis, ulcerations, etc. This is also why individuals who have consistently ingested Cayenne, or other culinary chilies, typically have a much greater "burn tolerance". In a sense, pain receptors have been "burned out". This effect is only temporary; continual exposure is needed to keep nerve endings unresponsive.

Initially, Cayenne augments gut secretions and musculature activity. Here it is best applied to weak, asecretory digestion, commonly seen in the aged, sick, and metabolically oppressed. After continued application its stimulatory powers become less, and are replaced by an analgesic effect. Suffers of chronic upper gastrointestinal

---

8   Exceptions include a number of variants of Capsicum annuum and C. baccatum – also considered "Cayenne".

ulceration normally see a reduction in pain and inflammation with its use.

If the situation applies, small amounts combine well with bitters and/or aromatics. Cayenne's indication is similar to most other bitter–aromatic combinations. The main difference though is a regional circulatory deficiency, noticeable by pale and dry oral mucosa, often including the tongue. Use it to stimulate the appetite, digestion, and gastrointestinal movement – especially if there is pain.

For sore throats, head colds, and sinusitis several drops of the tincture added to warm water and used as a gargle will prove effective. Again, it is best if the affected mucosa is pale and dry, and the condition is somewhat chronic, but regardless, some good will come of it. With regular gargling, tonsillitis will be hedged towards betterment. Using the tincture as a liniment, it can also be externally painted on the affected area.

For the common cold when there are chills and an accompanying low fever, the plant will serve to speed the body's recovery. Similar to immune stimulants, Cayenne's excitation of circulatory energies amplify the body's response to bacterial/viral invaders, hence bringing about resolution in a more timely manner.

As a purely constitutional medicine, Cayenne fits a certain subset of individuals. Cold extremities, particularly after a drop in ambient temperature, weak pulse, pale skin, and weakened digestion, are just some indications that point to Cayenne's use. Older persons, through the inevitable aging process, when loss of circulatory energy is usually a certain fact, will benefit from the plant's influence.

Externally, the powder made into a plaster will be found warming and analgesic – a specific for chilblains. Unlike Mustard, Cayenne will not cause tissue redness or blistering of the skin. It is not rubefacient but a nerve ending desensitizer. Applied to arthritic pain, chronic sport's injuries, lower back pain, and even pelvic discomfort due to reproductive pain, the plant will be found relieving. Applied to the bronchial region, it will subdue the pains of pleurisy. The tincture or liniment rubbed into the temples, forehead, or nape of the neck, relieves headaches, and may serve as a migraine abortive. Raynaud's sufferers respond to external applications. Nueragias of all types are quieted to varying degrees. Essentially if there is tissue or nerve pain, usually Cayenne will help.

The powder is a decent clotting agent, and can be used topically for cuts and such that do not require stitches. It is only recommended as a snuff for nosebleeds for the most sadomasochistic of individuals. It is effective, but at a price.

The plant's antibacterial and antifungal qualities are not monumental, but should be noted. It works well if there is a double involvement of nerve–tissue pain and a corresponding infection.

INDICATIONS

♦ Digestion, weak, asecretory
♦ Sore throat/Tonsillitis (gargle)
♦ Sinusitis (gargle)
♦ Common cold with fever and chills
♦ Weak circulation in the aged and sick
♦ Arthritic pain/Sport's injuries, chronic (external)
♦ Headache (external)
♦ Pleuritic pain (external)
♦ Nueragias (external)
♦ Cuts/Scrapes (external)

COLLECTION

Simply gather the fruit when ripe; dry well spaced.

PREPARATIONS

Cayenne is commercially available. I recommend purchasing the whole dried fruit and powdering it as needed for tinctures and plasters. If this is unavailable the powder can be purchased in various strengths, or "heat" levels. The capsules taken internally can be a decent preparation, but may cause gastrointestinal/anal burning. Reduce dosage, and gradually work to a preferred dose. The tincture can be diluted in water.

DOSAGE

- ♦ DPT (80% alcohol): 2–10 drops 1–3 times daily
- ♦ Capsule (0): 1–2, 1–3 times daily
- ♦ Plaster/Liniment/Ointment: as needed

CAUTIONS

Mucus membranes: ocular tissues, sinuses, and gastrointestinal tissues will be much more sensitive than external dermal layers. After initial application if there is excessive burning reduce the dose. The area should feel warmed and stimulated...not on fire. If using externally make sure to wash hands thoroughly after application. Contact with the eyes (or genital area) without doing so will be distressing!

Normal use poses little concern, but used in large amounts, long–term, it is unclear if capsaicin is carcinogenic or anticarcinogenic. Certainly it has an effect on inflammatory mediators, at times being amplifying, at others, sedating.

Internally Cayenne does have a mild anti-platelet effect. This quality poses no problem in healthy individuals, but it may cause clotting time inconsistencies if taking pharmaceutical blood–thinners. Full doses are not recommended during pregnancy.

OTHER USES

Like other chilies Cayenne can be used as a condiment.

CHAMOMILE

Asteraceae/Sunflower Family

Matricaria recutita (Matricaria chamomilla, Chamomilla recutita)
German chamomile, Manzanilla

DESCRIPTION

Chamomile is a small branching annual, usually no more than 2′ in height. The plant's leaf morphology is variable – lower leaves tend to be tripinnate, the upper ones bipinnate or simply pinnate. Numerous flower stems arise from each branch's growth tip, upon which small conical flowers develop. Surrounding ray flowers are initially spreading, then at maturity reflexed. Achenes are 3–5 ribbed.

DISTRIBUTION

The plant is native to central Europe and western Asia. Cultivated extensively, particularly in Germany and Hungary, it is a common herb garden companion plant. It is certainly grown in this country, as well as others.

CHEMISTRY

Sesquiterpene lactones: eudesmanolides, germacranolides, guaianolides, α–bisabolol, bisabololoxides a and b, farnesene, chamazulene; flavonoids: apigenin, chrysin.

MEDICINAL USES

Chamomile is known particularly as a child's remedy, not for its lack of potency, but because it is so well tolerated. As a soothing tea it is best used for stomach and intestinal irritation, particularly associated with nervousness and anxiety. Its ability at relieving nervous dyspepsia and colic verges on remarkable. The gastrointestinal upset and general irritability that sometimes accompanies infants when teething is soothed by Chamomile.

It is an excellent tea for ulcerative conditions of the stomach and small intestine. One of its better applications is in quieting pre–ulcer inflammation. Chronic gastritis as well as matured ulcers will heal more quickly under its use. Spastic conditions of the colon, particularly if there is accompanying inflammation will also respond positively to the plant.

As a sedative, the tea will relieve mild insomnia if taken before bed. Mental unease from overwork and stress tends to be quieted as well. Often women respond more reliably to Chamomile's influence than men: whether hormonally connected or not it is particularly useful for emotional hypersensitivities. Use Chamomile when nervous system irritation, triggered by emotional or mental stress, causes muscular or nerve sensitivity. For these purposes Chamomile combines well with Passionflower. Chrysin having influence over GABA receptor sites is only one flavonoid shared by both.

The hot tea is useful in promoting menstruation when suppressed by stress, cold temperatures, or wintertime respiratory infections. Chamomile is not an emmenagogue per se, but serves to correct imbalances that may lead to suppressed menses. Occasionally menstrual cramps are lessened by the hot tea as well. It is a mild remedy for uterine irritability towards the end of pregnancy.

As a mild diaphoretic used during feverish states, the hot tea is capable for both children and adults. Although not as vigorous as Peppermint, Elder, or Yarrow, Chamomile is best for fevers arising from sickness due to stress and overwork.

Topically, Chamomile ointment or oil is an excellent antiinflammatory. In nearly all skin conditions if there is redness and irritation, external application will be found healing. Eczema and allergic dermatitis are particularly soothed by its application. In fact consider both external and internal use of the plant a gentle yet effective remedy for allergic outbreak and sensitivity. If predisposed to topical inflammation due to animal hair, dander, or other environmental allergens keep stock of Chamomile for it will prove useful.

Wounds, skin ulcers, and bedsores will show improvement under the plant's influence. Inflammation will be reduced, healing will be quickened, and the situation's overall improvement will make Chamomile an efficient remedy. Lastly as a simple mouthwash used 3–4 times a day Chamomile is excellent in healing oral ulceration, due to allergy, habitual Tobacco use, and even aphthous stomatitis (canker sores).

INDICATIONS
♦ Irritation, gastrointestinal
♦ Dyspepsia, due to anxiety
♦ Colic
♦ Gastrointestinal upset, due to teething
♦ Ulcers, peptic
♦ Gastritis
♦ Spastic colon
♦ Insomnia/Anxiety/Mental unease
♦ Amenorrhea/Dysmenorrhea
♦ Fever, mild
♦ Eczema/Allergic dermatitis (external)
♦ Wounds/Skin and mouth ulcers/Bed sores (external)

COLLECTION
The flower heads are gathered with pruners or by hand.

PREPARATIONS
All sorts of proprietary preparations are available. Internally, the simple flower head infusion will be the most reliable way to utilize the plant's therapeutics. Most external preparations are of use, with the ointment being most widely used. Chamomile essential oil is commercially available; use diluted or undiluted for external application. Internally, the essential oil/spirit, due to the missing flavonoid component, will be less effective than whole plant preparations.

DOSAGE
♦ Flower infusion: 4–8 oz. as needed
♦ External preparations: as needed

CAUTIONS
Safe for children and use during pregnancy, Chamomile is one of the most wildly used herb teas today. Some individuals highly allergic to Sunflower family plant pollen (Ragweed, Goldenrod) may have a reaction to Chamomile.

CHASTE TREE
Verbenaceae/Vervain Family

Vitex agnus–castus
Monk's pepper, Indian spice, Safe tree

DESCRIPTION
Chaste tree is a large, deciduous bush or small

tree capable of obtaining heights of 20'–25'. The plant's 5–7 lance shaped leaflets are palmately arranged and are supported on long leaf stems. Each leaflet is dark green above and much lighter beneath. Like other Vervain family plants the leaves are oppositely arranged along ridged upper stems. The spike–like racemes form at branch ends. Individual flowers can be a variety of colors – lavender, blue, and white are typical. Each is tubular with 5 fused petals, which curl under at the flower's opening. The fruit are surrounded by a hardened layer and resemble peppercorns. They are green when young but dry to a purplish–grey. When crushed their smell is distinctly aromatic and spicy.

DISTRIBUTION

Originally a plant of the Mediterranean region of southern Europe, northern Africa, and western Asia, Chaste tree is now found throughout warmer parts of the United States. The plant is extensively naturalized through the Southeast and is found as a thriving ornamental in warmer southwestern regions.

CHEMISTRY

Iridoid glycosides: agnuside, aucubin, agnucastoside a, b, and, c, mussaenosidic acid; flavonoids: casticin, orientin, isovitexin, luteolin, artemetin, isorhamnetin; diterpenes: vitexilactone, vitexlactam, rotundifuran; phenylbutanone glucoside: myzodendrone; α–pinene, β–pinene, limonene, cineole, sabinene.

MEDICINAL USES

Chaste tree is best used by women who suffer from premenstrual breast tenderness and heavy menstrual bleeding associated with longer than 28–day menstrual cycles. The plant is doubly indicated if lifestyle stress and moderate to heavy caffeine use is present. While inhibiting excess prolactin levels Chaste tree supports proper corpus luteum function and therefore progesterone level. The plant is effective in rectifying anovulatory cycles, corresponding infertility, secondary amenorrhea, uterine fibroids, and excessive

menstrual bleeding dependent upon excessive cellular proliferation of the endometrium – all essentially issues of progesterone deficiency.

Because of Chaste tree's alignment with the Vervain family the plant tends to be a mild sedative, even outside of its diminishing effect on stress mediated prolactin release. This makes Chaste tree useful in premenstrual discomforts with associated anxiety, mood swings, and irritability. The plant is equally indicated in beginning stages of menopause. It combines well with Motherwort in reducing hot flashes and associated irritability.

Chaste tree is of use in reestablishing coherent menstrual cycles after prolonged estrogen–based contraception. Moreover, an important distinction between Chaste tree and oral or topical pharmaceutical–grade progesterone use is necessary: progesterone, as it naturally occurs, is a reproductive hormone that is dependent upon a healthy corpus luteum and proper levels of FSH (follicle stimulating hormone) and LH (luteinizing hormone). Chaste tree supports correct corpus luteum function and therefore is pro–progesterone. Oral or topical use of progesterone does little for the corpus luteum but only for tissues that respond to that hormone. The use of progesterone for PMS or associated corpus luteum deficiency issues is like putting a new stereo in an old truck; great tunes but still the same truck.

Traditionally Chaste tree, as its name implies, has been used as an anaphrodisiac. I personally have seen several men use Chaste tree to curb libido because of their wives unavailability. One man became somewhat frightened after observing practically all penile sensation had left him. After discontinuing Chaste tree normal functioning returned after 2–3 weeks. Lastly Chaste tree has been found to increase milk production in lactating women.

INDICATIONS

♦ Premenstrual discomforts with breast tenderness, agitation, and anxiety
♦ Heavy menstruation

♦ Anovulatory cycles
♦ Uterine fibroids, subserous
♦ Perimenopause
♦ Insufficient lactation

COLLECTION

Strip the mature fruit from the branch ends. Dry normally.

PREPARATIONS/DOSAGE

♦ DPT (60% alcohol): 30–40 drops 2–3 times daily
♦ Fluidextract: 10–25 drops 2–3 times daily
♦ Capsule (00): 2–3, 2–3 times daily

It is important to note that the effect of Chaste tree may not be perceived immediately. Often several months of use is needed to notice the plant's benefit.

CAUTIONS

Do not use during pregnancy.

CINNAMON

Lauraceae/Laurel Family

Cinnamomum verum (Cinnamomum zeylanicum)
Ceylon cinnamon, True cinnamon

Cinnamomum loureiroi (Cinnamomum loureirii)
Saigon cinnamon, Vietnamese cinnamon

Cinnamomum cassia
Cassia

DESCRIPTION

In the wild Cinnamomum is a bushy evergreen tree reaching heights of 20'–50'. Many of its numerous branches tend to grow horizontally or even droop. The 4"–7" long, generally 3–veined leaves are entire, ovate to ovate–oblong, and shiny green. The spreading cream–colored flower clusters form from branch ends and have a disagreeable smell.

DISTRIBUTION

Cinnamomum is a widely distributed genus. It is represented by over 300 species throughout the Tropics and Subtropics of North, South, and Central America, Australia, Southeast Asia, and the South Pacific.

CHEMISTRY

Main volatile and oleoresin compounds for Cinnamomum verum: e–cinnamaldehyde, α–copaene, α–amorphene, δ–cadinene, terpinen–4–ol, β–caryophyllene, coumarin, α–muurolene, β–bisabolene, cadina–1(2), 4–diene, ortho–methoxy cinnamaldehyde, cubenol, 1–heptadecene, 1–nonadecene, tetracosane, octacosane, nonacosane.

MEDICINAL USES

Out of a whole collection of Cinnamomums, the species listed here are only several that are commercially known as Cinnamon. The plant is firstly known as an aromatic stomachic, meaning it is well applied to dyspepsia, nausea, and gas pains. Like most spice herbs it acts as a carminative. It is soothing to an upset stomach, and if given sweetened, children usually are fond of the tea.

The intestinal tract is also favorably influenced by Cinnamon. It is specifically indicated as an intestinal astringent. Preparations are best used in cases of diarrhea if there is accompanying spasm. The plant works well to curb the nausea and diarrhea of food poisoning. An added benefit here is its influence over a number of bacterial strains that are problematic in these situations. Cinnamon's volatile oils are distinctly antibacterial, making the tea or tincture suitable for an array of related gastrointestinal issues.

The plant is a decent hemostatic. The spirit or tincture, is able to check passage hemorrhaging in a number of different regions. For the gastrointestinal tract, Cinnamon is best used to check the bleeding of gastric and duodenal ulcers. Caution should be used in its application to the intestinal ulceration of crones disease. Cinnamon's aromatics are membrane stimulants, so the plant's effect on involved tissues may be irritating. Use small amounts tentatively.

Passive hemorrhaging from uterine fibroids is lessened with Cinnamon. Minor tissue trauma, resulting in uterine bleeding after childbirth will diminish with the plant as well. Also mid-cycle spotting and heavy or lengthy periods will reduce under its influence. In these cases Cinnamon exerts its effect not by any hormonal influence, but by its combination of aromatics and tannins. In tandem they serve as vasoconstrictors. Cinnamon is well combined with Canadian fleabane for all of these mentioned hemostatic applications.

More recently Cinnamon has shown to improve blood glucose levels in fasting diabetics by about 20%. Its hypoglycemic effect appears related to its ability at increasing insulin sensitivity. Combined with soluble fiber/pectin, diet, and exercise the tincture or infusion taken 2–3 times daily is a sensible enough approach. If dependant upon elevated blood sugar levels, cholesterol and triglyceride levels also tend to improve.

INDICATIONS
♦ Nausea/Dyspepsia/Gas pains
♦ Diarrhea with spasm
♦ Bacterial infection, gastrointestinal
♦ Food poisoning
♦ Passive hemorrhaging
♦ Hyperglycemia

COLLECTION
Farmed Cinnamon trees are generally never allowed to reach mature sizes. Through the frequent coppicing of the shoots, a single tree may produce for many years. The bark is separated from the core wood of the coppiced shoots, and formed into "quills". Initially the bark is whitish, but then through drying turns a characteristic yellowish–brown. Sri Lanka is the largest grower–exporter of True cinnamon or Cinnamomum verum.

PREPARATIONS/DOSAGE
♦ DPT (60% alcohol, 10% glycerin): 30–60 drops 2–3 times daily
♦ Bark infusion: 4–6 oz. 2–3 times daily
♦ Spirit: 10–30 drops 2–3 times daily

CAUTIONS
Do not use the essential oil/spirit internally during pregnancy. Excessive amounts may cause digestive upset.

OTHER USES
Cinnamon is best known as a spice and flavoring. Like nearly any other medicinal plant high in aromatics it is antibacterial and antioxidant. Known intuitively to keep perishables from spoiling, surely this fact accentuated its use as a food spice.

Cinnamomum camphorata was initially the only source of camphor. Today though is it mostly synthesized.

CLOVE
Myrtaceae/Myrtle Family

Syzygium aromaticum (Eugenia aromaticum, E. caryophyllata)
Caryophyllus

DESCRIPTION
Clove is a small, evergreen, pyramidally–shaped tree. Its bark is smooth and gray. Leaves are green and shiny, obovate, oppositely arranged, and 4" long by 2" wide. Its distinct midrib is surrounded by many parallel veins. If bruised or broken most parts of the tree are distinctly fragrant. The compact, cylindrical flowers form in clusters at branch ends.

DISTRIBUTION
Native to a few of the Maluku Islands[9] in Indonesia, Clove thrives along with Mace and Nutmeg in this tropical region of the Pacific. Cultiva-

9 This island group is also known as the Spice Islands, a region at one time dominated by colonial powers, particularly the Dutch. At the height of their grip the Dutch eliminated great stands of the tree in neighboring areas as to ensure their control of this valuable commodity.

tion occurs today in similar latitudes: Zanzibar, greater Indonesia, Madagascar, India, Pakistan, Sri Lanka, and Brazil.

CHEMISTRY

Ellagitannins: syzyginins a and b; main volatiles: eugenol, trans–caryophyllene, α–humulene, eugenol acetate.

MEDICINAL USES

The effectiveness of Clove as a carminative, stimulant, anesthetic, and antiseptic is almost wholly derived from the bud's volatile oil content. Clove is distinctly aromatic and to most is familiar, arousing memories of autumn spiced teas, or Christmas–time potpourris.

Internally use Clove for nausea and indigestion with gas pain originating from the stomach or the intestines. For nausea and vomiting, particularly when the original offending material has been regurgitated, and the activity is now dependant upon reflex, the plant will be helpful. Use it for the nausea and vomiting of food poisoning. Not only is it a useful carminative but also it will be found directly inhibiting to wide array of food–borne pathogens. Clove added to disagreeable tasting tinctures and teas often makes the body's reaction more favorable.

Like many other volatile aromatics, Clove is stimulating to gastric secretion. This is accomplished by the plant's dilatory influence on stomach lining vasculature. Unlike bitter tonics that have little effect on local blood dynamics, Clove provides more blood, therefore gastric activity to the area.

As for Clove's anesthetic effect, it is most well known to temporarily relieve dental pain. It should be applied directly to the offending tooth. Make sure to limit contact with the gum, as the undiluted essential oil will cause irritation.

The spirit made with the essential oil can be used topically as a muscle rub. The pain of various sport–type injuries will be dulled by its application. Skin conditions that are prone to itch, such as chronic eczema, will be soothed by the essential oil made into an ointment. All essential oil based preparations are distinctly antibacterial and antifungal. They can be applied to infected cuts and such, speeding recovery. As an antifungal agent, it is inhibiting to a wide array of infections. It is particularly well applied to Candida albicans involvements.

Use Clove for reducing the outbreak of the herpes group of viruses (HSV, chicken pox/shingles, etc.). Combined internal (tincture, tea, or capsules) and external (diluted essential oil) application will be most effective. For this purpose it combines well with Mugwort or Wormwood tea.

In Unani and Ayurvedic systems Clove is used as a male aphrodisiac. Recent studies suggests that Clove in fact does have influence, but in a biphasic way. Normal to conservative dosing with the tea, tincture, or capsules appears to augment androgen levels. Larger doses have an inverse effect, lessening reproductive parameters.

Lastly, like most spice plants, Clove has significant antioxidant properties. Generally considered to be on–par with vitamin E, this quality will benefit individuals when using the plant for its more direct uses.

INDICATIONS

- Nausea/Indigestion with gas pains
- Nausea/Vomiting from food poisoning
- Dental pain (external)
- Sports injuries (external)
- Cuts, as a disinfectant (external)
- Fungal infections (external)
- Herpes group (external and internal)
- As an aphrodisiac
- As an antioxidant

COLLECTION

The unexpanded flower buds are gathered after turning green to a bright red. After drying, the bud is separated from the pedicel/peduncle (stem). Both buds and stems enter the market, buds priced higher than stems. Often stems are an adulterant in Clove bud powder. They are also used as a base material in Clove essential oil extraction.

PREPARATIONS

A number of forms can be used therapeutically. By far the most common is the essential oil. For internal use it is to be prepared as a spirit. For topical use, depending on the situation, use the ointment, spirit, or diluted/undiluted essential oil. For Clove's anesthetic effect on dental pain, use the essential oil undiluted, carefully though to avoid the gums.

DOSAGE

♦ DPT (70% alcohol): 10–20 drops 2–3 times daily
♦ Spirit: 10–20 drops 2–3 times daily
♦ Capsule (00): 1–2, 2–3 times daily
♦ Liniment: topically as needed
♦ Essential oil: topically as needed

CAUTIONS

Excessive internal use may cause gastrointestinal, renal, or hepatic irritation. As a tea flavoring during pregnancy its use is fine. Stronger tincture/spirt preparations are not recommended due to their higher concentration of volatiles.

It appears Clove (particularly eugenol) inhibits platelet aggregation. This is no concern for healthy individuals; but for individuals taking blood–thinning pharmaceuticals, there may be potentiation issues.

OTHER USES

Of course as a spice; Clove is also a main ingredient in "Chai"[10].

COFFEE

Rubiaceae/Madder Family

Coffea arabica
Arabica coffee, Mountain coffee

---

10 In the near east Chai is a nearly universal word for "tea", usually green or black tea, and has nothing to do with the popular Clove–Ginger–Cinnamon combinations in vogue today.

DESCRIPTION

Coffea arabica grows to be a large bush or small tree. Though usually between 25'–35' high when left in its wild state, it is often kept at 6'–12' in order to facilitate harvesting. The plant's wavy–green, glossy leaves are leathery, opposite, and 2"–5" long by 1½"–3" broad. White flowers form in axillary clusters. About the size of a cherry, Coffee berries (actually a drupe) are red to purplish when ripe. Each contains 2 seeds.

DISTRIBUTION

Indigenous to Ethiopia and Yemen, Coffea arabica is cultivated from Mexico to South America and in eastern Africa.

CHEMISTRY

Purine alkaloids: caffeine, theobromine, and theophylline; sterols: cycloartenol, 24–methylenecyloartanol, cycloeucalenol, obtusifoliol, citrostadienol, 24–methy– lenelophenol, stigmasterol, sitosterol, campesterol, stigmastanol, campestanol; chlorogenic acids.

MEDICINAL USES

Several species of Coffee are popular in commerce today. Along with Coffea arabica, which has the longest documented use as an energizing beverage, there is C. robusta and C. liberica. Actually the latter two species have slightly higher caffeine contents. They all can be used interchangeably.

As one of the most popular herbal supplements taken today, Coffee deserves its own monograph. Like Tea, Yerba Maté, Kola, and Guaraná, Coffee's principal alkaloid and stimulating agent is caffeine. Like other caffeine containing plants if used properly Coffee is therapeutic. Unfortunately though, it has been much maligned, mostly by the puritanical fraction (relating to diet anyway) well established in today's alternative medicine landscape.

As an energizing beverage Coffee is decidedly effective. Autonomic (sympathetic branch) and central nervous system stimulation is certainly pronounced under the plant's influence

– blood pressure, heart rate, and respiration are all amplified to some degree. Its effect increases muscular contractility and mental prowess, being useful for both the laborer[11] and the thinker.

There is of course a limit to which Coffee, or caffeine, will continue to stimulate the body. Only to be pushed so far, fatigue and sleep will eventually take hold; it is no match for the body's need to rest and replenish itself.

Coffee's secondary attributes, which make the plant distinct from other caffeine sources, are its stimulatory influences on the gastrointestinal tract and liver. It is a mild bitter stimulant, moderately increasing gastric secretion, preparing the stomach for food. Peristalsis is promoted along the intestines as is bile secretion within the liver. Besides Coffee's traditional use as a morning stimulant, helping to dissipate the visages of sleep, certainly its bowel stimulation is as nearly well known. Habitual Coffee drinkers often rely upon the beverage in order to have the first bowel movement of the day. Take it away, and not only is the brain in a fog, but intestinal movement is slowed to a crawl.

A strong cup of coffee is a useful cerebral vasoconstrictor. Use it to lessen the pain of headaches when red eyes, flushed face, and a throbbing quality are the main symptoms. Migraine headaches often respond well to the plant, especially if vasodilators such as Clematis and Anemone have been tried as preventatives with no results.

The Coffee enema, greatly popularized by the Gerson therapy's approach to the treatment of cancer, is in fact a decent, yet unorthodox, way of receiving Coffee's stimulation.

INDICATIONS

♦ As a stimulant, sympathetic/central nervous system

♦ Fatigue, physical/mental
♦ Indigestion, poor secretion
♦ Mild constipation
♦ Headache and migraine, as a vasoconstrictor

COLLECTION

Coffee fruit is picked when fully mature. The outer pulp–layer and seed membrane are then removed through various methods. The "bean" is then roasted, and here coffee acquires its characteristic aroma and taste.

PREPARATIONS

Standard water percolation, when a filter is used, will produce a standard dose of caffeine and some secondary hepatic/biliary effects. "Cowboy" or "Camp" coffee, when whole beans, or grounds are simply boiled, will produce a beverage which contains caffeine but also one that has a higher lipid fraction. Liver, gallbladder, and intestinal effects will be strong. Also "Cowboy" coffee has been shown to raise cholesterol levels, making its extended use problematic.

DOSAGE

♦ Water percolation: 4–8 oz. 1–3 times daily
♦ Fluidextract (25% alcohol, 10% glycerin): 30–60 drops 1–3 times daily

CAUTIONS

Abnormally high blood pressure is a common result of excessive caffeine intake. One cup of coffee a day usually does not pose a problem; however one pot may. Particular to excessive Coffee use is gastritis, loose stools, and liver tenderness. Nervousness and muscular weakness are a number of nervous system side effects.

Headaches, lethargy, and disordered digestion, including constipation are a number of occurrences seen when Coffee as a regular staple is omitted from a daily diet. Take anything long enough and its physiologic effects become interlaced and graduated with the body's. Remove that article, and withdraw symptoms are common and should be expected.

---

11   It is a common practice, during the forced road marches of infantry training, to use the standard issue freeze–dried Coffee crystals as a dip of sorts. Placed between the jaw and check it is allowed to slowly dissolve, releasing caffeine to in turn stimulate the heart, lungs, and skeletal muscles, increasing performance under demanding conditions.

COMFREY
Boraginaceae/Borage Family

Symphytum officinale
Knitbone, Boneset

DESCRIPTION

Comfrey is a coarse, large–leaved, bristly perennial. Leaves are 2"–11" long. Lower leaves are larger and petiole borne; upper leaves are smaller and are occasionally sessile. As a summer flowerer the typical Borage family coiled inflorescence is distinctive. The calyx is deeply lobed and bristly like the rest of the plant. The corolla is generally red to purple. The small seeds or nutlets that follow are black and shiny.

DISTRIBUTION

Comfrey is a European native. Here in the temperate United States, if it is not planted in the garden, it is an escapee, mainly found in disturbed areas. Occasionally where it was once planted as an ornamental, it is found in remnant stands.

CHEMISTRY

Triterpenoid saponins; phytosterols; pyrrolizidine alkaloids: intermedine, lycopsamine, symlandine, symphytine, echimidine; allantoin.

MEDICINAL USES

As with most medicinal plants used today, if objective scientific research is applied, their traditional uses are substantiated or at least clarified. In Comfrey's case, due to a configuration of events, the research that today is used to site Comfrey as a toxic plant was and still is misapplied. The short story, that an array of PAs (pyrrolizidine alkaloids) found within Comfrey are harmful agents and a number of hepatoxic cases have been linked to the plant's usage should be looked at more closely.

1. Not all PAs are created equal. Depending on the family–genus–species, some PA–containing plants are completely non–toxic (Echinacea) or are overt poisons (many Senecio species). These differences are due to the type of contained PA. The American garden variety of Comfrey falls more to the non–toxic side of the continuum, whereas Russian varieties contain higher percentages of the more toxic PA, senecionine.

2. The few cases of hepatotoxicity that were "reported" for Comfrey use in the late 80s/early 90s mainly involved individuals who had preexisting liver–centered illnesses, and/or who were users of hepatotoxic drugs. At least one individual ingested an extraordinary amount of the herb daily (10 cups of tea/"handful(s)" of tablets daily) – a huge dosage for *any* plant.

3. Comfrey toxicity is mainly theoretical and is essentially based only upon animal studies. Purified PA fractions (not Comfrey) were feed to rats, who then developed hepatotoxic reactions. High administered PA to body weight ratio, and the fact that not all animals process PAs the same, factor into the alarmist result. Pigs, cows, chickens, and horses are less sensitive to PAs than rats, rabbits, goats, and sheep.

4. Where do humans fit in? The fact is we don't really know, but most likely the situation with Comfrey is not a dire as some would suggest. Some perspective is needed. How many individuals die each year of liver–related pharmaceutical/over–the–counter poisonings? Hundreds, if not thousands. How many individuals have succumbed to the *rational* use of *only* Comfrey, with no pharmaceutical/prior disease history...zero!

5. Comfrey's overall usage history is so empty of toxicity report, it is strange that an apparent concentration of cases developed when they did. With some speculation it is not far–fetched to suggest that the few individuals supposedly affected by "Comfrey toxicity" were stricken, despite, not because of Comfrey[12].

12 I find it remarkable, yet typical that an individual can be on an organ transplant list, taking a slew of pharmaceuticals, drinking alcohol to excess just to dull the misery of the situation AND taking an herbal remedy. If the indi-

Both Comfrey root and leaf can be used externally to speed healing of ulcers, wounds, and cuts. The compound allantoin found in abundance in Comfrey speeds the breakdown and liquidation of defunct tissue, pus, and wound secretions, while stimulating tissue granulation. It is of great use in chronic wound management. A poultice made with the fresh plant is optimal, if need be the dried plant can also be used. Salves and ointments are secondary, but still will make a difference.

"Maggot therapy" – surgically applied maggots to poorly healing, infected wounds, is a new twist on an ancient practice. It has a small but staunch following. Maggots work to speed the healing of wounds due to their feeding on infected and necrotic tissue, but most importantly their excretions contain allantoin. So if a handful of maggots are not available use Comfrey.

Although not as serious as wound management, external applications are excellent in healing anal fissures. After each bowel movement make sure to gently clean the area, then apply the salve. Reapplication is important, especially before bed.

As an internal vulnerary, leaf and root preparations should be used, although if skittish after reading the PA segment, use leaf material only – it has a much lower alkaloid content. Comfrey can be used for any type of structural damage, from that of broken bones and fractures, to soft and connective tissue injuries. The plant speeds healing, holding an almost legendary reputation.

Due to Comfrey's mucilaginous qualities, its demulcent activity has a noted effect on a number of organ systems. The tea makes a soothing cough reliever, particularly if from irritated throat tissue. Lastly for urinary tract irritation, the plant will be found of benefit. Both bladder and kidney pain, from any number of likely causes, will be lessened due to Comfrey's soothing effect on inflamed tissue.

vidual dies due to precarious health, guess what is blamed for that person's death...you betcha...the herb.

INDICATIONS

♦ Ulcers/Wounds/Cuts (external and internal)
♦ Anal fissures (external and internal)
♦ Broken bones/Fractures
♦ Connective/Soft tissue damage
♦ Ulcers, gastric
♦ Cough from irritation
♦ Urinary tract irritation

COLLECTION

The whole plant should be collected. Be sure to dry the roots well; they are very mucilaginous. The use of a dehydrator will help.

PREPARATIONS

"Pyrrolizidine alkaloid free" Comfrey is commercially available, usually in tincture and capsule form. If purchasing non–processed Comfrey or growing the plant for internal use make sure it is from American stock.

DOSAGE

♦ Herb infusion: 4–6 oz. 2–3 times daily
♦ Root decoction: 2–4 oz. 2–3 times daily
♦ FPT/DPT of herb/root (50% alcohol): 20–40 drops 2–3 times daily
♦ Fresh root/herb poultice: as needed
♦ Oil/Salve/Ointment (root): as needed

CAUTIONS

Aside from potential toxicities already explained, none. Regardless, to err on the side of caution it is not recommended during pregnancy or while nursing.

CORN SILK

Poaceae/Grass Family

Zea mays
Corn, Indian corn, Maize

DESCRIPTION

Being monoecious Corn has separate male and female flowers on the same plant. Male flowers above are arranged in terminal racemes. Enveloped in a thin wrapping of leaves (later in development known as the husk), female flowers form beneath leaf sheaths. Each kernel or germ has an attached long style terminating outside of the husk. Collectively the styles are know as Corn silk, from which each kernel potentially is fertilized. Once pollinated the silk dries quickly. Depending on variety, once ripe, kennels are of an array of colors; white, yellow, purple, black, and even molted combinations are common.

Some consider Corn to be the most significant domesticated grain crop today. Veiled by the mists of time its shaping through simple cross–breeding practices started nearly ten–thousand years ago. From what plant or plants did modern–day Corn originate is a matter of debate, but it looks fairly certain that another species of Zea, Teosinte, is involved. Also ancient pre–domesticated Corn appeared not too differently than some Grama grass varieties today. Regardless of Corn's ancient ancestors its transformation has been guided by human hands to the extent that it can not successfully propagate without manually planted seeds.

DISTRIBUTION
Although native to the Americas, the place where initial domestication occurred is vague. Presently southern Mexico is agreed upon by researchers and historians as the area of origin. Quickly spreading throughout the Americas, especially the southwestern region of the United States, Corn held a significant place in American Indian culture.

CHEMISTRY
Anthocyanins; flavonoids; phenols.

MEDICINAL USES
Corn silk tea is specific for the urinary tract. Not many other herbs can rival its focused soothing influence over the area. Use liberal amounts of the tea for most any type of inflammation/irritation/pain centered around the kidneys, bladder, urethra, or ureters. For painful urination, be it from tissue irritation or outright infection, Corn silk will give relief. For active infections, the addition of an antimicrobial herb will provide stronger effects.

When dealing with chronic or acute nephritis Corn silk's soothing qualities are well noted. The herb is not as specific as Goldenrod as a "nephron tightener", but what Corn silk lacks in Goldenrod's specifics, it makes up in generalities. Through reducing kidney tissue inflammation the organ's filtering process improves lessening albumin in the urine.

The herb's most prominent use though is to encourage urinary deposit breakdown. 2–3 cups a day, given time, will facilitate the litholysis of even the most stubborn of kidney stones. Corn silk will also reduce the pain and irritation, and facilitate healing of involved tissues after the deposit's passage. Like Marshmallow, Corn silk is mild tasting and child–safe.

INDICATIONS
♦ Painful urination
♦ Cystitis/Urethritis
♦ Nephritis, acute and chronic
♦ Lithiasis
♦ Pain and irritation of urinary deposits

COLLECTION
The silk can be gathered prior to or after pollination. Collect the silk in one hand while cutting the strands at the top of the ear with the other. Dry well–spaced. Corn silk is also commercial available.

PREPARATIONS/DOSAGE
♦ Silk infusion: 4–8 oz. 2–3 times daily
♦ Fluidextract (40% alcohol): 30–60 drops 2–3 times daily

CAUTIONS
None known.

OTHER USES
Various culinary, industrial, and research oriented uses; from glue to straw hats, most parts of

Zea mays are put to use.

CRANBERRY
Ericaceae/Heath Family

Vaccinium macrocarpon
American cranberry

DESCRIPTION
Of a trailing, low–growing habit, Cranberry is a robust, evergreen[13] perennial with glabrous–elliptic leaves. Commonly rooting at runner nodes, small upright stems rise above the root/runner mass and in the late spring/early summer produce long, narrow, recurved flowers. Fruit are red and large for the genus.

DISTRIBUTION
A North American species, Cranberry is native to eastern Canada, northeastern Unite States, south to isolated pockets within Tennessee, finally west to the Great Lakes region. Now though due to commercial production the plant has escaped its tame environs and is well established in temperate regions of the Pacific Northwest. Bogs and related wetlands are the plant's ideal habitat.

CHEMISTRY
Proanthocyanidins: epicatechin, catechin, epigallocatechin; anthocyanidins: cyanidin, peonidin; flavonol glycosides: myricetin, quercetin, kaempferol; main volatiles: ethyl acetate, octanol, α–terpineol, benzoic acid; ascorbic acid.

MEDICINAL USES
There is no question that Cranberry works to curb urinary tract infections. Used this way for nearly 100 years, it is truly a successful American folk remedy. A special recognition should be reserved for the plant due to its use even among individuals who don't believe clearly proven medicinals such as Garlic or Echinacea ("first tier"

herbals) are beneficial.

Cranberry works to curb urinary tract infections through two avenues. First, it is a mild urine acidifier. Its effect here is probably not that appreciable due to only a very small pH change seen in the urine after taking the plant. Secondly, Cranberry's flavonoid (particularly proanthocyanidins) fraction is broadly inhibiting to E. coli's attachment to the endoepithelial tissue that lines the urinary tract. Exposure to Cranberry actually changes the organism's shape and functionality, making it easily passed with urine from the body. The combination of these two activities makes Cranberry an effective, yet simple remedy.

The most practical application for Cranberry is daily juice intake for suffers of chronic, reoccurring UTIs (urinary tract infection). Due to anatomical differences women typically are more susceptible to these infections than men. The juice or whole fruit will also be of great benefit to the elderly and the disabled, who are likewise troubled.

Most Heath family plants exert similar effects. From Uva–ursi and Manzanita, to Pipsissewa and Pyrola, they all will be useful, to varying degrees for alkaline urinary tract infections. To receive the fullest benefit from any of these plants, including Cranberry, it is paramount to reduce simple carbohydrates from the daily diet. Be them from refined sugar or flour, or even fruit, it makes little difference; all will increase urinary pH[14], making the involved tissue more susceptible to bacterial colonization.

Another factor if troubled by UTIs is that of hygiene. The large intestine's content is the main source for E. coli in these situations. Women are particularly prone to UTIs due to a particularly short urethra and its close proximity to the anus. After bowel movements, wipe from front to back; bathe or wash daily – simple considerations that make a difference.

Cranberry is a significant source of antioxidant flavonoids: proanthocyanidins, anthocya-

---

13 Usually evergreen in the Southeast, leaves turn reddish–brown during the dormant season of more northern latitudes.

14 Excessive calcium, magnesium, and potassium from food or supplementation can also raise urinary pH.

nins, etc. Generally health promoting, use as a food with medicinal overtones.

INDICATIONS

♦ Urinary tract infections, alkaline urine

COLLECTION

Pick the fruit when ripe; dark red varieties will be found stronger than the others.

PREPARATIONS

Barring personal collection, Cranberry preparations are widely available in both natural food stores and regular markets. Pure, unsweetened, from concentrate or not, Cranberry juice is preferable. The fresh or frozen fruit can also be eaten.

DOSAGE

♦ Juice: 3–4 oz. 2–3 times daily
♦ Fresh or frozen fruit: 1–2 oz. 2–3 times daily

CAUTIONS

None known.

OTHER USES

Jam, juice, sauces, etc.

CREOSOTE BUSH

Zygophyllaceae/Caltrop Family

Larrea tridentata (Larrea divaricata var. tridentata, Covillea tridentata)
Chaparral, Greasewood, Little stinker, Hediondilla, Gobernadora

DESCRIPTION

At maturity Creosote bush is approximately 8'–10' tall by the same dimension wide. Flexible, ash–colored stems rise vertically, or nearly so, from the ground. When growing on desert flats it has a distinctive funnel–like appearance with the top section of the plant having the widest radius. Most of the leaves are collected in groupings among the upper branches. The leaflets are fused in pairs and resemble a "packman". The younger leaves are particularly resinous and shiny; with age, their luster diminishes. The yellow petals of the flower have a particular way of twisting perpendicularly to the reproductive center, making the arrangement fan–like. When mature the small fuzzy seed capsules separate into individual wedges, called mericarps.

Beyond normal seed germination, Creosote bush has a relatively unique way of reproducing. The plant is very adept at cloning. If the root crown of Creosote bush is imagined as a circle, clones are created on the circumference, increasing the root crown's diameter. After a time the center roots die of old age, leaving numerous, physically independent, genetically identical clones spread out in a localized area. Eventually as this process continues plants spread outward like ripples in water created from a dropped stone. Some extremely old plants have been dated in southern California to be approximately 12,000 years old. The ages of these ancient plants were determined by calculating the known outward growth rates with the furthest distance genetically identical clones were apart from each other.

DISTRIBUTION

Creosote bush can be found throughout the Sonoran, Mojave, and Chihuahuan Deserts. Huge expanses are found in valley bottoms and basins. It more sparsely occupies slopes and rocky hillsides.

CHEMISTRY

Lignans: nordihydroguaiaretic acid, dihydroguaiaretic acid, isoguaiacin, norisoguaiacin; flavonoids: apigenin, gossypetin, herbacetin, kaempferol, luteolin, morin, myricetin, quercetin; saponins: larreagenin a, larreic acid, erythrodiol; monoterpenes: α–pinene, limonene, camphene, linalool, borneol, camphor, bornyl acetate; sesquiterpenes: α–curcumene, calamine, β–santalene, edulane, α–bergamotene, cuparene, β–eudesmol, farnesol, α–agarofuran.

MEDICINAL USES

If there is one plant that is the medicinal hallmark of the southwestern deserts, it is Creosote bush. Combining traditional perspectives from White, American Indian, and Mexican usage, together with science–based evidence, it is no wonder that the plant is considered a panacea. Looking at Creosote bush's main spheres of influence, that of a unique antiinflammatory, antioxidant, and antimicrobial agent, we are more able to define and understand the plant's therapeutic use.

Creosote bush is sedating to pro–inflammatory mediators. Leukotriene and leukocyte activity, histamine and prostaglandin release are all diminished. This makes Creosote bush useful in lessening rheumatoid arthritis pain and soreness. For the above problem it combines well with Yucca. Many also find relief by soaking in a Creosote bush bath. Likewise, in asthmatic conditions the plant reduces bronchial airway stuffiness through diminishing the "heat" of the autoimmune process. For other systemic autoimmune hypersensitivies, Creosote bush is often found helpful, as it is also profoundly antioxidant in nature. Topically it has been used with success in resolving psoriasis and eczema, particularly in combination with deeper liver therapies – removing dietary and environmental allergens are also important steps.

Creosote bush inhibits several prominent viruses that are troubling in these times of social excesses. HPV (Human papillomavirus), the cause of genital warts and cervical dysplasia, is sensitive to Creosote bush's NDGA (nordihydroguaiaretic acid) content as is HSV (herpes simplex virus) types 1 and 2. A douche of Creosote bush tea applied twice daily or a suppository used before bed are both effective approaches for either virus affecting vaginal and/or cervical tissues. Otherwise, topical use of the oil or salve is efficacious. Cold sores respond very well to external salve application.

Studies are not consistent in regard to the plant's antimicrobial/antifungal activity but observable results have been positive, particularly topical application of Creosote bush to infected cuts and skin punctures. The salve is also a "must–have" when living in venomous spider/cone–nose insect territories. Continually applied Creosote bush is remarkable in reducing the deleterious effects of these varmints.

Although internal use of the plant as a cancer therapy is controversial at best, external preparations are useful in resolving a particular form of premalignant squamous cell carcinoma, called actinic keratosis. These reddened and sometimes scaly patches arise on sun–damaged skin. A topical pharmaceutical preparation of NDGA, called Actinex, is currently used in the treatment of the condition. By dry weight Creosote bush contains 2–10% of NDGA – whole herb preparations are adequate and chances of adverse skin responses are limited.

INDICATIONS

♦   Rheumatoid arthritis (external and internal)
♦   Asthma
♦   Psoriasis/Eczema (external)
♦   HPV (external)
♦   HSV–1 and –2 (external)
♦   Cuts/Abrasions (external)
♦   Venomous and non–venomous insect bites (external)
♦   Actinic keratosis (external)

COLLECTION

Collect when new leaf growth is apparent. Using your thumb and forefinger strip the leaves that form in clumps towards the outer–most branch ends. The leaves are easily pulled from their branches; if the flowers and seeds are collected this also is fine. The resin that builds up on your hands does not come off even with the most vigorous scrubbing. Applying a high proof alcohol will help in removal.

PREPARATIONS/DOSAGE

♦   DPT (75% alcohol): 20–40 drops 1–3 times daily
♦   Leaf infusion (standard or cold): 2–4 oz. 1–3 times daily (1 teaspoon of herb to 1 cup of water)

- Ointment/Oil/Salve: as needed
- Douche: 1–2 times daily

CAUTIONS

Do not use Creosote bush while pregnant or nursing. Use of the plant is also not recommended if there is existing liver impairment or inflammation. Do not use Creosote bush with other drug therapies that may effect the liver, be they over–the–counter or prescription.

There were a number of cases, particularly in the early nineties that implicated Creosote bush in triggering liver inflammation. Most cases were self–resolving after discontinuing Creosote bush. The two individuals who required liver transplants took the plant for over a year and either drank regularly an undisclosed amount of alcohol or took a cocktail of pharmaceutical and over–the–counter drugs. In summation Creosote bush is therapeutic if used properly by healthy individuals. Nevertheless, when used as a cure–all for long periods, Creosote bush can be problematic. There are no cautions for the plant's external use.

DANDELION

Asteraceae/Sunflower Family

Taraxacum officinale (Leontodon taraxacum)
Chicoria

DESCRIPTION

Dandelion is a small perennial arising from a single or branched taproot. Both the leaves and flowers originate from the plant's root crown. Lacking branches, the dark green leaves are between 2"–12" long and are deeply lobed. Yellow flower heads arise on hollow stems, which can be 1'–2' long. The puff–like seed clusters are wind dispersed. Each achene is attached to a parachute–like grouping of silky hairs making dispersal easy. If damaged, the entire plant exudes a milky sap. Dandelion in low elevation, arid locales tends to be diminutive in size and weaker in strength compared to its high moun-

tain and cold country relatives.

DISTRIBUTION

Dandelion is found throughout most of the country. This European native is extremely robust and versatile, making the best of what it is given. Lawns, gardens, grassy parks, and roadsides are common places for the plant.

CHEMISTRY

Sesquiterpene lactones: eudesmanolides, germacranolides, guaianolides; phenyl–propanoids; phenolic acids: caffeic acid, chlorogenic acid; flavonoids: apigenin, luteolin, chrysoeriol; coumarins: scopoletin, aesculetin, cinnamic acid esters (monocaffeyltartaric acid, chlorogenic acid, chicoric acid), hydroxycinnamic acid; triterpenes; β–amyrin, taraxol, taraxerol; carotenoids: lutein; phytosterols: sitosterol, stigmasterol, taraxasterol; polysaccharide: inulin.

MEDICINAL USES

Dandelion's use as a gastric and hepatic/biliary stimulant is straight–forward. The tea or tincture taken before meals is a reliable bitter tonic. It increases digestive prowess by stimulating an array of gastric secretions. Use the plant if prone to indigestion and combine it with Peppermint or Ginger if there is a tendency for bloating. Dandelion is stimulating to bile production by the liver and release by the gallbladder, therefore small intestinal fat digestion is augmented. The plant tends to be more cooling to the liver than other hepatic stimulants such as Barberry, so its use in liver inflammations, like hepatitis C, is well–fitted. In fact alone or combined with Milk thistle, Dandelion reduces liver sensitivity, upper body tightness, and itchy eyes and skin associated with subacute liver inflammation. Moreover, a cup of roasted or plain Dandelion root tea before breakfast is an effective way of thinning bile so gall stones tend not to develop. 1–2 cups a day over several months will diminish established gall stones from overly concentrated bile.

Dandelion, particularly the leaf, is diuretic. It is indicated in resolving uric acid kidney stones and acts systemically in eliminating uric acid deposits responsible for gout.

Dandelion has a substantial inulin content within its roots. Due to the body's inability to digest this complex carbohydrate, inulin enters the colon intact promoting beneficial microflora growth, particularly of bifidobacteria. This in turn stabilizes the large intestinal environment, limiting pathogenic bacteria and their destructive by–products. Use Dandelion in the nefarious "leaky gut syndrome" – a title meant to describe a symptom picture of skin allergies, joint inflammation, fatigue, and colon instability dependent upon proliferation of harmful colon bacteria, their by–products, and heightened leukocyte activity. For this purpose, combine Dandelion with Yucca. The combination tends to stabilize beneficial flora levels, while binding harmful endotoxins.

Writing about Dandelion and its virtues Doctor Geo F. Collier stated in an 1843 issue of The Lancet: "The great objection to its use will be that it costs nothing, and may be made by everyone, without pharmaceutical mystery or expense." (Some things just never change).

INDICATIONS
♦ Indigestion
♦ Liver/Biliary congestion
♦ Poor fat digestion
♦ Uric acid kidney stones/Gout
♦ Poor intestinal health

COLLECTION
Gather Dandelion leaf when verdant and hydrated during the spring and summer. The roots of the plant can be dug all year, but are strongest during colder seasons, particularly in the fall when they contain up to 40% inulin. Dry the leaves normally. Split the taproots length–wise before drying.

PREPARATIONS
The root powder in capsules or the root cold infusion is the best way to receive the plant's inulin content.

DOSAGE
♦ Root decoction: 2–6 oz. 2–3 times daily
♦ Leaf infusion: 4–8 oz. 2–3 times daily
♦ FPT/DPT of root (40% alcohol): 60–90 drops 2–3 times daily
♦ Fluidextract of root: 20–40 drops 2–3 times daily
♦ Capsule of root (oo): 2–3, 2–3 times daily

CAUTIONS
Do not use if there is a biliary blockage.

OTHER USES
Although slightly bitter, the young leaves are used as a potherb. Fresh or lightly sauteed add them to salads or other cooked greens.

ECHINACEA
Asteraceae/Sunflower Family

Echinacea angustifolia
Narrowleaved purple coneflower, Coneflower

Echinacea pallida
Pale echinacea

Echinacea purpurea
Purple coneflower, Missouri snakeroot

DESCRIPTION
Echinacea angustifolia is an herbaceous perennial. The entire plant is covered by a layer of stiff hair, making it rough to the touch. The plant's leaves are lanceolate to oblong and are borne on short petioles; upper leaves are smaller and are sessile. All species of Echinacea have distinct involucral heads with a common combination of disk and ray flowers. E. angustifolia's flowers are light pink to purple; at ¾"–1½" long its ray flowers are showy. The plant's seeds are distinctly 4–angled.

Like Echinacea angustifolia, E. pallida is also a hairy herbaceous perennial. Its leaves are oblong to lanceolate with the upper ones smaller and sessile. Ray flowers are 1½"–3½" long and are purplish to white.

Echinacea purpurea is the largest of the group profiled here. It can reach heights of 3'– 4', with leaves occasionally as large as 7¾" long by 5⅘" wide. They are serrated with contracted bases; mature leaves have petioles which can be up to 10" in length. Heads are typical and are composed of involucral bracts. Ray flowers are 1"–3¼" long, and are reddish–purple to pink.

DISTRIBUTION

All Echinaceas are prairie plants. E. angustifolia is found throughout the Great Plains. From central Minnesota it extends through most of the plain states to northwestern Indiana. E. pallida is found from southwestern Indiana, south through eastern Kansas to northeastern Oklahoma. E. purpurea is found from northeastern Texas and Oklahoma east to Georgia, and north to Ohio and Michigan.

CHEMISTRY

For Echinacea purpurea: caffeic acid derivatives: caftaric acid, chlorogenic acid, caffeic acid, cynarin, echinacoside, cichoric acid; alkamides (isobutylamides); polysaccharides; arabinogalactan–proteins.

MEDICINAL USES

If there is one plant in the history of western herbal medicine that could be appointed front–runner, it would be Echinacea. Once a favorite of 19th century Eclectics and Thomsonians, the plant still holds sway over 21st century herbal therapeutics. In the case of Echinacea, unlike other herbs that are trendy in application, the reason for its long–lasting position is simply its effectiveness. The fact that Echinacea stimulates positive responses in so many different conditions makes its application vast. In the past, before the advent of microbiology, the activity of this herb was viewed with something approaching awe; it just could not be explained simply as a stimulant, or as a vulnerary, or even as an alter-ative, although its action, at times, had these and other qualities. We now know that Echinacea, being an immune stimulant, affects a wide array of situations because immunological depression and infections can take on such prosaic manifestations.

Use Echinacea when immunological weakness is apparent, presenting itself as chronic sore throats, colds, and sinus infections. It is well used both as a preemptive, and as a situational when counteracting common wintertime viruses. As a mouthwash and gargle, used for laryngitis and pharyngitis, the plant's effect, although peculiar in sensation, is healing. It can either be used as a once–a–day preventative, or as a daily regiment in these throat conditions that are slow to resolve. A more serious condition, strep throat, which often leads to tonsillitis, can be especially helped by the gargled tea or tincture mixed in a little water. Combined equally with Yerba mansa or Goldenseal, it will provide even more profound relief. For sinusitis, prepare Echinacea as a nasal spray or wash, and use several times a day.

Chronic skin conditions that are dependant upon "bad blood" will show marked improvement through Echinacea's amplifying of white blood cells. Poorly healing skin, slow wound resolution, and boil development, particularly in response to stressful episodes, are key for the plant's application. Both topical and internal use are indicated. Abscesses can be either brought to a head or resolved internally by both topical and internal application. An Echinacea poultice made with a base of Marshmallow powder, combined with a stimulant such as Ginger, will prove efficacious in its effects. Application should also be made to infected wounds and ulcers, and aptly if there is surrounding tissue necrosis. Apply liberally especially if there is septicemia, and of course internal use is as important, particularly in such a potentially serious condition.

It is worth mentioning here that this is the gray area that herbal and conventional medicines share – serious conditions that herbs may perform well in, but that conventional medicine typically excels in. The brave, faithful, or at least the desperate will find Echinacea, I believe, no failure. In the past we had no option, it was either take the bitter herb, or suffer; and sometimes we suffered even if we did take what was known to work. Today healing sometimes is too easy, especially in the realm of microbial infections. Antibiotics, with all of their side effects, and resistance issues, typically work. So to the ones who want to try it the old way, who risk a little more, I doff my hat.

Unlike straight forward expectorants or antitussives, many of which through their volatile oil content inoculate lung space, or mucus membrane stimulants such as Goldenseal or Yerba mansa, which alter surface tissues making them more resistant to offending bacteria or viruses, Echinacea works more deeply to stimulate innate immunity. The plant stimulates the body's resistance through a number of related, yet different avenues. It is as if when Echinacea's compounds enter the systemic circulation, surrounding cells, be them free–floating leukocytes or stationary tissue cells, their presence is interpreted as an insult; but not strong enough to send the body into revolt. Macrophages, neutrophils, and lymphocytes are stimulated by Echinacea's polysaccharides and glycoproteins. They become more active in the presence of the plant due to their interpretation of these polymeric compounds. By acting as a pseudo–pathogen Echinacea gives off a certain scent that the body then responds to. It is a rues, a trick really, for no damage is done, only an increase in the body's defensive capacity takes place.

Several bioactive component groups are involved in Echinacea's influence of the immune system. The polysaccharides within the plant stimulate macrophages to produce increased amounts of interleukin–1 and –6, and tumor necrosis factor–α. The prowess of resident macrophages within alveolar tissue of the lungs is increased. The effect on the liver's defensive line (kupffer cells) also is amplified. Overall Echinacea stimulates innate immunity but has little affect directly on T and B–lymphocytes and NK (natural killer) cells of acquired immunity.

The alkylamides inhibit 5–lipoxygenase and cyclooxygenase, two pivotal enzymes involved in prostaglandin production. Because some prostaglandins are thought to be involved in NK cell suppression, Echinacea works indirectly to augment levels of these immunologic cells. Less well defined, cichoric acid also has been shown to have immunomodulatory effects.

Echinacea pallida has the highest echinacoside content out of the three plants discussed here, making its antihyaluronidase activity also the strongest. Even though E. angustifolia has smaller amounts (E. purpurea has none), it is still of service. Both plants inhibit hyaluronidase, a ubiquitous cellular enzyme that specifically contributes to the inflammatory process of tissue injury. They are protective and stimulatory of extracellular matrix, collagen, and ultimately properly formed tissue. Use these two varieties of Echinacea, internally and externally for their wound healing abilities. Pain, redness, and swelling will diminish from Echinacea's antiinflammatory properties. Chronic inflammations, such as tendonitis or bursitis, improve under the plant's use as well.

As a venomous snakebite remedy Echinacea is one of herbalism's favorites. The beginnings of its use here, is credited to the American Indians who lived around the plant. Following this, the plant was in the forefront as a frontier medicine for snake bites. Before the advent of antivenoms, Echinacea rued supreme in this application. The root poultice used externally intermingled with liberal use of the tea or tincture taken internally is the surest way to proceed. It is thought that Echinacea's antihyaluronidase activity must have some beneficial effect on the situation as most snake venoms contain varying amounts of hyaluronidase.

As with many other medicinal plant uses modern medicine has rendered some of them obsolete...maybe this is one of them. I have had no chance to treat rattlesnake bite in my private practice. Naturally the emergency room is the best place to begin, but if I were placed in a leveled position, in which treatments with conventional medicines were not available, I would reach first for Echinacea. The plant does deserve a look back in conjunction with antivenom treatments or when conventional treatments are failing.

Echinacea has good inhibitory effects on HSV (herpes simplex virus), both oral and genital (both acyclovir–resistant and sustainable strains). Internal and external use will also prove beneficial to chicken pox and shingles infections.

INDICATIONS

- Laryngitis/Pharyngitis/Tonsillitis/Strep throat
- Upper and lower respiratory tract infections
- Sinusitis
- Poorly healing skin
- Boils/Abscesses (external and internal)
- Septicemia
- Immune suppression, general
- Chronic tissue injuries
- Tendonitis/Bursitis
- Snakebites, venomous (external and internal)
- HSV–1 and –2 (external and internal)
- Shingles/Chicken pox (external and internal)

COLLECTION

As there is not much prairie that has been untouched by development, farmland, or pasture conversion, depending on local plant quantities, some regional collection may need to be halted. In various states, Echinacea is listed as a threatened plant. In others, it is found abundantly.

Of course cultivation is an option, as it is easily grown from seed. Not all, but the majority of the world's supply comes from the cultivated plant.

PREPARATIONS

The entire plant can be used, although roots, flowers, and the immature seed heads will be strongest. Due to the plant's isobutylamide content, a unique metallic–numbing sensation is quickly felt when the plant is chewed. Echina-

cea's medicinal potency is not solely determined by this peculiar sensation, but it does give some indication.

DOSAGE

- FPT/DPT (70% alcohol): 30–90 drops 2–3 times daily; in acute situations, every 1–2 hours
- Fluidextract: 10–30 drops 2–3 times daily
- Infusion (cold or standard): 4–8 oz. 2–3 times daily
- Fresh or dry plant poultice: apply and change several times a day
- Mouthwash/Gargle/Nasal spray: 4–5 times a day

Like Valium being derived from Valerian, the myth that Echinacea should only be taken for two weeks at a time is told and re–told in countless health–food store settings. It is fine taken for longer.

That said, there will be a natural action/reaction when any plant or drug is used. In the case of Echinacea, immediately after the plant is discontinued, affected white blood cell counts typically dip, then shortly return to normal. This is homeostasis at work; we are pulled in one direction, only to be pulled in the other before achieving the middle ground again.

CAUTIONS

Considering the plant's effectiveness and strength, individuals have very little to be concerned with in regards to side effects. As with any plant in the Sunflower family, sensitive individuals may respond allergiclly to medicinal use of the flower heads. I have never observed Echinacea being problematic in autoimmune conditions, such as asthma or rheumatoid arthritis, but it is theoretically possible given the activity of the plant. Echinacea should not be used if taking immune suppressant pharmaceuticals.

ELDER
Caprifoliaceae/Honeysuckle Family

Sambucus nigra
Elderberry, Black elder, European elder

DESCRIPTION

Usually no more than 30' tall, Elder is a fast–growing, small deciduous tree. Leaves are arranged in an odd–pinnate pattern; one leaflet terminates a bunch of 3–9 (usually 5). Each is 2"–5" long and 1"–2" wide. The cream to white, small 5–petaled flowers form in flat–topped clusters, referred to as corymbs. When ripe the blackish–purple fruit droop in clusters; each are about the size of a small pea.

DISTRIBUTION

A tree with a significant range throughout much of Europe, Elder is also indigenous to parts of Africa and Asia. It is successful in a variety of habitats and soil types.

CHEMISTRY

For Sambucus canadensis, a closely allied blue–fruited Elder: triterpenes: α–amyrin palmitate, balanophorin, oleanolic acid; flavonoids: cyanidin, cyanin, quercetin, rutin; monoterpene: morroniside; steroids: campesterol, β–sitosterol, stigmasterol; sambucine.

MEDICINAL USES

Elder is chiefly diaphoretic, making its application to fevers, particularly if they are low to moderate in temperature, warranted. If the skin is hot and dry Elder will reliably promote sweating. With Elder or any diaphoretic, timing and preparation are important factors. The tea needs to be hot and should be drunk during the latter part of the day and before bed. Body temperate tends to naturally rise throughout the day and into the evening, so using the therapy in accordance with the body's innate rhythm only makes sense. Keeping the body warm with a hot bath and/or blankets will also promote sweating. Once the fever breaks, usually in the middle of the night, it is important to change perspiration soaked clothes and bedding. Depending on the severity of the infection, this cycle may repeat itself several times before finally resolving. Diaphoretic therapies work with the bodies innate intelligence by augmenting a genetically coded process. In essence elevated body temperate, or fever, serves to stimulate immune system activity. Fever is not an illness, but a natural infection–fighting defense. Modern conventional approaches typically strive to suppress a temperate through Tylenol, etc., truly opposing the body's proven infection–fighting approach.

Children will certainly benefit from Elder, and other diaphoretics such as Spearmint and Ginger. Fevers dependant upon wintertime viral infections: common cold, sinusitis, bronchitis, and even the flu, will be dealt with efficaciously. If the fever resolves the infection has as well. Depending on secondary symptoms Elder will combine well with Echinacea, Wild indigo, or other immune stimulants.

There are times when diaphoretic approaches to an infection are inadequate. In these times, when fevers are dangerously high, or when other threatening symptoms delineate a severe infection, the usefulness of pharmaceuticals out weights their drawbacks.

The tea drunk cold is diuretic, especially if there is no elevated temperature. External preparations are distinctly antimicrobial and antifungal. Elder is usefully applied to these situations particularly if the affected tissues are edematous, slow to heal, and tend to ulcerate.

Elder has been found to inhibit varieties of Salmonella and Shigella dysenteriae, so its application to gastroenteritis coincides with traditional use for the plant in Guatemala. The leaf and flower tea are somewhat similar in effect to now popular Elder fruit or Elderberry preparations, which relatively speaking are recent in application.

INDICATIONS

♦ Fevers, dry, low to moderate temperature, with lung centered viruses

- Fluid retention
- Wounds, edematous, ulcerated, slow to heal, with or without bacterial or fungal involvement (external)

COLLECTION

Prune the last foot or so from flowering branch ends or collect the flowers and leaves separately. The fruit clusters can be collected in bunches and then separated from their respective small stems.

PREPARATIONS

The flowers are simple enough to dry; the leaves though can be problematic. If they are not dried quickly they often mildew, turn black, and become unusable. Dry quickly in a warm and arid environment or use a dehydrator.

DOSAGE

- Leaf/Flower infusion: 2–4 oz. 2–3 times daily, though often less of the leaf tea is needed as it can be more stimulating

CAUTIONS

Like any vasodialating herb, Elder can potentially increase body temperature very briefly before promoting diaphoresis. Be mindful of this when using it in higher febrile states.

OTHER USES

Any fruit of blue–black Elder types are sweet and edible raw. Jams, jellies, and wines are made from them.

ELEUTHERO

Araliaceae/Ginseng Family

Eleutherococcus senticosus (Acanthopanax senticosus, Hedera senticosa)
Siberian ginseng, Devil's shrub, Touch–me–not, Wild pepper, Taiga root

DESCRIPTION

A robust deciduous shrub, at maturity the plant can reach heights of 6'–10'. Its classic Ginseng family leaf arrangement is conspicuous: 5–7 toothed leaflets arranged in a palmate pattern. Eleuthero's spiny stems are distinct. Blue–black fruit develop from its inconspicuous ball–like flower clusters.

DISTRIBUTION

Mainly a boreal forest plant of the Far East, Eleuthero thrives in the cold winters and moderate summers of the Taiga. Its native region encompasses parts of Korea, Japan, northern China, southeastern Russia, and a number of ex–Soviet states, including Siberia.

CHEMISTRY

Triterpenoid saponins; flavonoids; polysaccharides; lignans; sterols; coumarins; phenylpropanoids.

MEDICINAL USES

Behind the Iron Curtain, during the height of the Cold War, Soviet scientists spent a substantial amount of time researching the therapeutic benefits of Eleuthero. Developed as a cheap and abundant analog to Panax ginseng, State–run programs were developed to supply professional–level athletes and the working class with an herbal supplement designed to increase performance and productivity. Certainly Eleuthero increased work–place productivity, mainly by reducing the days missed due to sickness, but an olympic herbal edge? That still remains to be seen. Compared to what today's professional athletes and sport's figures take, that Cold War–era supplementation seems so tame.

Eleuthero and its more "muscular" relatives, Panax and American ginseng, at their cores are stress response modulators. That they work is known; how these plants work still baffles researchers to this day. Yes, we know catecholamine/cortisol responses are modified. In some situations under the influences of these plants certain tissue groups demand less input, enabling resources in an over–stretched environment to be received elsewhere. And inversely in some situations Ginseng family plants tend to be excitants, increasing the body's demand for energy and building blocks.

Regardless of what is known or not of the plant's mechanics we can always go back to the traditional indications, which fortunately for us hold true whether or not we understand the minutia. Whichever plant is in the spotlight, sight must not be lost of what the plant does (gleaned through direct observation), for how the plant is suppose to work. Ideally they should be one and same, but often they are not.

If American and Panax ginseng are the main dishes than Eleuthero is the aroma – an adaptogenic essence. Not as gross in effect as the others, it will be found more subtle and gradual in influence. All three plants are tonics, but consider this one the most gentle.

For the debilitated, weakened, aged, and those of lowered vitality, Siberian ginseng will provide a sense of strength and stability. Even if normally robust, but weakened from illness, the plant will decrease recovery time. Recuperative factors such as immunity, tissue oxygenation, and cellular metabolism will be augmented.

Like others of the family, the plant will not be found reliable in its sport's enhancing attributes, especially by competitive level athletes, whose tuned physical responses are, or are close to, optimal. Strangely though for normally fit individuals who are under an inordinate amount of chronic–type stress: war zone conditions for a GI, severe grief/anxiety, or over–work, Eleuthero will stabilize the catecholamine/cortisol environment, providing a physiological break from the insult.

Eleuthero is a membrane stabilizer having good influence over the liver, nervous system, and blood. As a hepatic antioxidant, individuals will appreciate its cooling effects on hepatocyte inflammation, usually occurring in response to viral exposure or environmental toxicities. Lipid peroxidation is retarded, lessening atherosclerotic plaque formation, making tonic use of this plant a long–term cardiovascular therapy.

"Ginseng abuse syndrome" is rarely seen with Eleuthero, making it safe for hypertensive individuals. Eleuthero's more gentle qualities make the plant ideal for individuals who don't need the extra stimulation.

INDICATIONS

◆ Lowered vitality, from age, illness, or stress
◆ Stress, chronic, from grief, anxiety, or over-work
◆ Cellular inflammation, hepatic, neuronal, or cardiovascular
◆ Antioxidant, general

COLLECTION

Roots are typically dug in the fall. Like many other perennial bushes the root bark and less woody rhizomes are more active than the inner wood of the tap root. Unfortunately commercial grade Eleuthero root contains woody and non–woody parts. Quality and potency problems are likely due to this fact.

PREPARATIONS/DOSAGE

◆ DPT (60% alcohol): 60–90 drops 2–3 times daily
◆ Fluidextract: 20–40 drops 2–3 times daily
◆ Cold infusion: 4–6 oz. 2–3 times daily

CAUTIONS

However unlikely, "ginseng abuse syndrome" is possible with Eleuthero, otherwise it is a generally benign plant.

EPHEDRA

Ephedraceae/Joint–Fir Family

Ephedra sinica
Ma huang

DESCRIPTION

A small shrub, no more than 2'–3' in height, Ephedra is mainly composed of semi–woody vertical stems and branchlets. Leaves are inconspicuous and scale–like forming at segment bases. Male and female flowers develop on separate plants.

Male pollen cones are found in whorls at stem nodes; female seed cones are terminal or axillary and are red and fleshy when mature. Seeds are two, brown to grayish–brown.

DISTRIBUTION

Ephedra is indigenous to Mongolia and China; plains and mountain slopes.

CHEMISTRY

Six main alkaloids: ephedrine, pseudoephedrine, methyl ephedrine, methyl pseudoephedrine, norephedrine, norpseudoephedrine; an array of flavonoids.

MEDICINAL USES

The Ephedra monograph is as fitting a place as any for the "take responsibility for your own actions" tangent. There is currently an official ban[15] of Ephedra sales by the FDA. Why, you might ask? Because Ephedra contains a number of sympathomimetic alkaloids: they tend to increase body–wide adrenergic responses, the most noted – blood pressure. When Ephedra is used in *excess*[16] the plant has some negative side–effects (renal vasoconstriction and cardiac stimulation), which have been a component in over a dozen cardiovascular–related deaths throughout the past 15 years.

The reader must understand herbs are not just play things to be used like a flavor of the week, but are pharmacologically active substances. Granted, many are benign enough, but some are drug–like in their effects. Ephedra is such a plant. And used when there is a prior cardiovascular weakness or condition only reflects on the ignorance of the user and the sales-manship of the supplement company. Used as a sport's supplement: add a cardiac stimulant to an already stressed heart, no problem! As a diet aid: I haven't eaten for a whole week and with this herb I feel great!

My apologies for the sarcasm, but I have no sympathy for the knucklehead who knows the herb is a stimulant, but who takes enough to have a heart attack. Ephedra is known on the street; it is common knowledge. Safe usage and warning information is prevalent.

Is it right that the FDA stepped in and banned Ephedra? Should we all suffer a lack through the stupidity of a few? It is a judgment of our intelligence that we let these regulating bodies make decisions for us.

As a medicinal plant, because, not despite its nervous system effects, Ephedra is a superb bronchial dilator. Used symptomatically in spasmodic bronchial constriction, typically accompanying an (humid) asthmatic episode, the tea or tincture is quick acting. The lungs become less constricted, breathing improves lessening sensations of heaviness and oppression.

Allergy and hayfever responses affecting the upper respiratory tract – throat, sinuses, etc. – are reduced as well. Sinus discharge is dried and nasal breathing improves. Using Ephedra as a decongestant (or diaphoretic) when sick is not a wise usage of the plant. The body is already stressed or compromised to some degree. Energy reserves are needed in the healing/virus–fighting process, not in nervous system stimulation.

Ephedra is not a healing tonic. It has no long–term virtue. Used short–term, symptomatically it is useful in a limited fashion.

INDICATIONS
♦ Congestion, bronchial/nasal

COLLECTION

The plant's stems are collected usually without male/female cones. It is then dried and cut for various grades. The bulk of Ephedra comes from inner Mongolia.

---

15 Interestingly there is no ban of over–the–counter pseudoephedrine (cold medications/diet aids). It is found in much higher concentrations in these products than in its crude source, Ephedra.

16 A supplement used to increase metabolism or "energy levels" – code name for diet aid or sport's supplement – will almost always be used in excess because the mind set of these individuals is not rational. It also must be noted that the vast majority of Ephedra supplements contain added concentrates or isolates of ephedrine, increasing the chance of toxic reaction.

PREPARATIONS/DOSAGE

♦   Stem infusion: 2–4 oz. 1–2 times daily
♦   DPT (50% alcohol): 20–40 drops 1–2 times daily

CAUTIONS

Do not use if suffering from renal or heart disease, diabetes or hypertension – basically if you are sick or unwell do not use Ephedra, except as indicated above. Do not use if nursing or pregnant. Watch for insomnia, anxiety, hypertension, heart palpitations, headache, and blurred vision with larger doses.

OTHER USES

Makers of illegal "crystal–meth" or methamphetamines are using pharmaceutical grade ephedrine or pseudoephedrine found in over–the–counter cold "medicines" as a base, and not Ephedra.

EUCALYPTUS

Myrtaceae/Myrtle Family

Eucalyptus globulus
Blue gum, Gum tree

DESCRIPTION

Eucalyptus is a large, stately tree. It is a rapid grower and can reach heights of 130 '. The trunk typically has persisting strips of shedding bark. Its long branches are exceptionally smooth. Leaves are long, bluish–gray, lanceolate to sickle–shaped, and if crushed are aromatic. It is an easy variety to recognize due to its large, solitary flowers and fruit.

DISTRIBUTION

The tree is common to coastal areas throughout California. It is native to Australia.

CHEMISTRY

β–amyrin, erythrodiol, uvaol, acetyloleanolic, acetylbetulinic, acetylursolic, betulinic, and ursolic acids.

MEDICINAL USES

Firstly, Eucalyptus is a suburb antiseptic. The plant's array of antimicrobial volatile oils are effective against a whole contingent of pathogens. The essential oil is the strongest preparation, and can be applied undiluted or diluted with olive oil. The poultice, fomentation, or wash, although less potent, also are of use, and should be used if there is any sensitivity to the essential oil. Its topical use is well suited for infected and inflamed wounds, cuts, and similar injuries. Eucalyptus will benefit old ulcers and bed sores that have become infected. A douche made from the tea is useful in treating chronic vaginitis, particularly if there is discharge.

As a chest rub, the essential oil is excellent at stimulating bronchial secretions. It combines well with internal use for chronic bronchitis with a dry cough and difficultly produced discolored phlegm. Like other herbal medications such as Ligusticum or Lomatium, which contain antiseptic aromatics, Eucalyptus also inoculates the pneumatic environment. Take the plant if there is need for a stimulating expectorant with antimicrobial properties. It is particularly useful in chronic lung conditions when there is general weakness, such as in the aged, or in the midst of a chronic episode of bronchitis. Inversely Eucalyptus has a restraining effect on excessive respiratory discharge and associated cough, particularly if arising from a weakened state of health. Again the key lung state that the plant is best suited to positively affect is debility. Not only are tea and tincture preparations useful, but the inhaled aromatic–containing steam should not be overlooked. Used alone or combined with White sage the inhaled steam method is excellent at treating common sore throats, and the more serious, strep throat. Inhale the herb infused steam 3–4 times a day. Especially for strep throat, it combines well with internal immune/lymphatic stimulating herbs, such as Echinacea, Red root, or Wild indigo.

Cystitis, urethritis, ureteritis, especially with

mucus discharge, are indicators for Eucalyptus's application. One caution here: if there is an active infection the plant can be irritating to the kidneys. To minimize the plant's kidney irritating potential combine it with Corn silk or Marshmallow.

Eucalyptus tea, taken 4–6 oz. at a sitting, is soothing to the stomach. Through its carminative activity it relieves gas and indigestion caused from stomach content fermentation. If gastritis or dyspepsia is the result of abnormal stomach bacteria, such as in the case of mild food poisoning, Eucalyptus should prove relieving. Related belching, coated tongue, and foul mouth taste should equally improve shortly with its use.

INDICATIONS

- Wounds/Cuts/Abrasions, as a disinfectant (external)
- Ulcers/Bed sores, as a disinfectant and to stimulate healing (external)
- Vaginitis (external)
- Bronchitis, chronic, with dry cough
- Sore throat/Strep throat
- Cystitis/Urethritis/Ureteritis
- Dyspepsia/Gastritis, from fermentation
- Food poisoning

COLLECTION

Simply clip the newer leaves from the tree. Dry normally.

PREPARATIONS/DOSAGE

- FPT/DPT (60% alcohol): 20–40 drops 2–3 times daily
- Leaf infusion: 4–6 oz. 2–3 times daily
- Spirit: 10–20 drops 2–3 times daily
- Essential oil: topically as needed
- Douche: 2 times daily

CAUTIONS

Due to Eucalyptus's renal stimulation do not use in kidney disease or inflammation.

OTHER USES

It is a common practice for the essential oil to be used in saunas or steam rooms for its decongesting qualities.

FENNEL

Apiaceae (Umbelliferae)/Carrot Family

Foeniculum vulgare
Fennel seed

DESCRIPTION

A biennial or short–lived perennial, Fennel stands 3'–5' in height. Both leaf and stem are numerously divided – leaves so much so that they appear feather–like. Lower and mid stems are significantly inflated. The small yellow flowers develop in large umbel clusters; they are terminal and compounded. The tannish–brown seeds are ¼" long and ribbed.

DISTRIBUTION

Indigenous to extensive parts of Europe and Asia, Fennel ranges far and wide. It is advantageous and does well in moist and disturbed soils. In the United States, as in other regions, it is cultivated in the garden and exists as a successful escapee.

CHEMISTRY

Aromatics for Fennel seed: α–thujone, α–pinene, camphene, sabinene, myrcene, α–phellandrene, p–cymene, limonene, cineole, β–ocimene, γ–terpinene, fenchone, camphor, terpinen–4–ol, methyl chavicol, cis–anethole, anisaldehyde, trans–anethole, germacrene d, tetradecanoic acid, hexadecanoic acid, tetradecane, 1,2 benzenedicarboxylic acid, dioctyl ester, pentadecane, 1–hexadecanol, hexacosane, 1–octadecanol, 7–octadecanone.

MEDICINAL USES

Fennel is a simple Carrot family carminative. Its agreeable nature and pleasant taste make it a useful medicine for children; in fact it is an old standby for colicy babies. Combined with Catnip, the two plants make an excellent formula designed to diminish the gastrointestinal spasm and gas of colic – a teaspoon of each is usually all that is needed. A strong cup of tea is a sure remedy for dyspepsia with nausea. Young and old alike will benefit from the plant's soothing qualities.

For lactating mothers who are having difficulties producing sufficient quantities of milk, often Fennel tea is just what is needed. If stress or nervousness is a factor, besides removing the stressor (often not possible), combine Fennel with a sedative like Passionflower. Although not as strong as some other menstrual stimulants, a strong cup of Fennel tea often stimulates menses. An added benefit here is the plant's tendency of reducing menstrual cramps.

INDICATIONS

♦ Colic
♦ Gastrointestinal spasm and gas
♦ Dyspepsia with nausea
♦ Insufficient lactation
♦ Amenorrhea/Dysmenorrhea

COLLECTION

There are over a dozen Foeniculum vulgare varieties on the market today. Although Germany is best known for its quality grade, Fennel is grown nearly world–wide. Some varieties are more flavorful and aromatic than others. When purchasing Fennel be sure that it is aromatic and tastes spicy–sweet. Occasionally Fennel is adulterated with Bitter fennel or Foeniculum piperitum, identifiable by the smaller seed size and slightly bitter taste.

If collecting your own, the seed cluster umbels can easily be snipped from the plant. Place them in a paper bag to dry fully; after which the seed is easily separated from the stem material. Fennel is easily grown in the garden – a wide range of cultivars are available.

PREPARATIONS/DOSAGE

♦ Seed infusion: 4–8 oz. 2–3 times daily
♦ FPT/DPT (50% alcohol): 30–60 drops 2–3 times daily

CAUTIONS

An infrequent cup of tea during pregnancy is fine, though Ginger or Spearmint is better used for the nausea of morning sickness.

OTHER USES

As a seasoning or food spice Fennel's Licorice–like flavor is well known.

GARLIC
Liliaceae/Lily Family

Allium sativum
Ajo

DESCRIPTION

Garlic stands between 1½′–3¼′ tall. The above ground portion arises from a thick–sectioned, membrane–coated bulb. Its flat, sheath–like leaves develop from the plant's scape. Flowers form in an umbel–like arrangement. Garlic's 6–segmented perianth is whitish–green; stamens over–reach the perianth segments.

DISTRIBUTION

Generally cultivated, Garlic is also found as an escapee in fields and meadows.

CHEMISTRY

Organosulfur compounds: γ–glutamylcysteine, s–allyl cysteine, alliin, allicin, ajoene; a number of seleno–compounds; flavonols: apigenin, isorhamnetin, kaempferol, luteolin, quercetin, myricetin; inulin.

MEDICINAL USES

Garlic is one of our most potent kitchen medicines. Historically significant, common, easily grown, and most importantly medicinal, Garlic deservedly commands a ranking position among a number of useful spice herbs. When looking over Garlic's attributes instead of asking, "what does Garlic do?" it is better asked "what does Garlic not do?". It is a broadly–acting folk medicine used world–wide.

The plant's effect on the cardiovascular system is well proven. Its most reliable application is toward elevated LDL (low density lipoprotein) and VLDL (very low density lipoprotein) levels. A moderate reduction in these circulating cholesterols is typically seen in 2–4 weeks of supplementation (½–1 gm. of clove daily). Although long–term use is needed to see significant results, arteriosclerotic plaques will reduce under Garlic's influence. It is suggested that Garlic's effect here is through its stimulation of hepatic cholesterol's conversion to bile salts or simply its reduction due to the plant's inhibition of liver cholesterol biosynthesis.

Garlic's most significant use as a cardiovascular medicine is its application towards a tendency. If cardiovascular issues run in the family or an array of sub–symptoms point to future troubles, use Garlic as a preventive. The plant's ability at reducing plasma concentrations of homocysteine [17]is noteworthy.

Any serious approach to cancer prevention should include either Garlic from dietary sources or its supplementation. Through clinical trails it clearly has shown anticarcinogenic activity. Many types of tumors have shown inhibition under its influence. Garlic appears to affect metastases in several ways. Being antioxidant, enhancing a number of detoxification pathways, and having a direct influence over mutagenic cells, all play a part in Garlic's effect of cancer.

The plant's antimicrobial activity is vast. Results will clearly been seen with both internal and external applications. From fungal and viral infections to bacterial infections, Garlic will make a difference. If the situation is especially severe often the plant is combined with conventional pharmaceuticals. Chances are if it is an unwanted organism, Garlic will have some affect. Even Giardia and Entamoeba strains, the culprits of traveler's diarrhea and giardiasis are inhibited by Garlic.

17 Circulating levels of homocysteine have become an important indicator of future cardiovascular disease, particularly occlusive problems and ischemic heart disease in diabetics.

A piece of freshly sliced clove can be placed directly on topical infections. This approach is one of the most reliable for wart removal – keep the slice on the wart 24/7, change everyday. Typically within 7–10 days the wart will fall off on its own. With topical use, particularly on sensitive skin, some tissue irritation may result – really unavoidable with this type of concentrated application.

Candida or bacterial derived vaginitis responds well to a clove suppository. Care should be taken not to nick or bruise the clove after removing its outer paper–like covering. After placement the clove should be left for 8–12 hours at a time. Many women find this technique more practical if used before bed. A fresh clove should be used daily. If tissue sensitivity or irritation develops discontinue and try a douche of Barberry or Oregongrape.

For vaginal/cervical (HPV) human papillomavirus infection, combined application of the clove suppository with internal use is a suburb treatment. Its antiviral use for any of the herpes group of infections will likely speed resolution.

As an age–old remedy for childhood ear infections, place a drop of two of tincture, fresh juice, or herbal oil directly in the offending ear. This can be repeated several times a day. Results will be noted in a day or so. Lastly, Garlic–breath is finally good for something: a wide range of oral–periodontal bacteria are inhibited or killed by the plant's *strong* aromatics.

INDICATIONS

♦ LDL/VLDL levels, elevated
♦ Cardiovascular disease, as a preventative
♦ Cancer, as a preventative and adjunct therapy
♦ Infection, bacterial, fungal, viral (external and internal)
♦ HPV infection
♦ Herpes virus group
♦ Childhood earache/infection

COLLECTION

In temperate climates Garlic is typically harvested throughout the summer months when its leaves begin to brown. Whole, intact bulbs store well for an intermediate period of time. Make sure to keep dried, powdered Garlic in a sealed container in order to preserve its volatile content.

PREPARATIONS

Fresh is the best. Lightly sauteed comes in second. Fresh and dry plant tinctures are serviceable, as are the encapsulated powder and the oil, prepared through the alcohol intermediate preparation. Proprietary products – aged extracts, odorless, or standardized for certain constituent levels – are more uncertain.

A fine way of utilizing Garlic is through juicing a couple of cloves. After mixing the juice with other vegetable juices or teas, drink. This done two or three times a day will provide a strong systemic effect.

DOSAGE

♦ Fresh clove: 1–2, 1–2 times daily
♦ Fresh clove: topically as needed and as a suppository
♦ FPT/DPT (65% alcohol): ½–1 teaspoon 2–3 times daily
♦ Oil: as needed

CAUTIONS

Garlic does provide a mild blood–thinning or antiplatelet effect. Usually this influence is beneficial, especially for individuals under stress with cardiovascular disease tendencies. It is of no concern for healthy individuals. Even if taking conventional blood–thinning pharmaceuticals (warfarin) in combination with Garlic there should be little reason for concern (although some monitoring with mega–doses is wise). Garlic's volatiles from a freshly crushed clove can irritate sensitive skin and mucus membranes.

OTHER USES

Onion has many of the same health benefits of Garlic, only to a lessen extent. Consider it Garlic's little brother. Both have significant amounts of inulin/fructooligosaccharides. Entering the colon intact, these complex carbohydrates promote beneficial flora growth, particularly of bifidobacteria. This in turn stabilizes the large intestinal environment, limiting pathogenic bacteria and their destructive by–products.

GINGER
Zingiberaceae/Ginger Family

Zingiber officinale
Jamaican ginger, African ginger, etc.

DESCRIPTION

Ginger is a 2'–3' tall perennial. During its growing season the plant's deciduous stems rise vertically with leaves alternately forming from sheath–like areas. They are 6"–8" long, about an inch wide, sessile, acute, and linear–lanceolate. Flower stalks arise from stem sides, are ½'–1' tall, and terminate in a bract–like cluster of greenish–yellow, purple (with yellow spots) flowers. Ginger's fruit is an oblong capsule.

DISTRIBUTION

Although originally native to Tropical Asia, Ginger is extensively cultivated throughout tropical regions in both hemispheres; China, India, Indonesia, and Nigeria are the top producers.

CHEMISTRY

Diarylheptanoids; vanilloids: gingerol, paradol; shogaols; zingerone; sesquiterpene hydrocarbons: zingiberene, curcumene, farnesene, bisabolene, β–sesquiphellandrene; monoterpenoid hydrocarbons: cineole, linalool, borneol, neral, geraniol.

MEDICINAL USES

Ginger tea drunk while hot, or the tincture added to hot water is a reliable diaphoretic to be used when feverish. The plant will surely as any other diaphoretic cause sweating when the skin is dry and core body temperature is elevated. Its effect, is largely dependant upon an array of aromatics. Taken at the onset of a general cold, particularly if chills accompany the episode, is a popular and effective way of countering wintertime distresses. Its warming properties and familiar taste tend to bring ease to the situation.

For the gastrointestinal tract Ginger is an effective medicine. The tea, tincture, essential oil, or even good quality powdered root taken in capsule form are all useful.

As a carminative, Ginger reduces nausea, gastrointestinal spasm, and gas associated with most cases of diarrhea. It is an excellent tonic–therapy for individuals whose stomach or bowels are weak from constitutional factors. Besides Ginger's carminative effects the root does contain several natural proteases, making it useful in resolving indigestion and stasis, especially from protein induced dyspepsia.

Along with the general nausea from disagreeable food or day–after alcohol hangover, Ginger is an effective remedy for the stomach upset of motion sickness. Here take a dose or two of Ginger before the troublesome movement, then every hour or two as needed. Legendary among sailors for sea sickness (motion sickness on water), still to this day Ginger is held in high esteem for such matters. It also will be found very helpful in curbing the nausea, food aversion, and taste changes that result from conventional radiation/chemotherapy treatments. Lastly the tea is well known to reduce the nausea and vomiting of morning sickness. A cup or two in the morning is usually all that is needed.

Combined with Oregongrape or Simaruba family plants, Ginger is indicated in most cases of food poisoning when intestinal spasm or borborygmus is evident. The aged will find Ginger's secretory stimulant properties of benefit, particularly the plant's ability to increase salivation. Chewing on a piece of fresh Ginger, or the tincture held in the mouth is a sure way to trigger salivary gland secretion.

Women suffering from menstrual cramps with an attending sense of coldness will find Ginger's spasmolytic properties pain relieving. A poultice can be used over the lower abdomen in tandem with the internal tea or tincture. Although not as strong as a Mustard plaster, if skin irritation or redness is perceived make sure to remove the poultice.

As a medicine for arterial inflammation Ginger looks promising. Although a fairly new application for the plant, it is surmised that preparations serve as cardiovascular antiinflammatories, regulating AA (arachidonic acid) metabolites. Although proportionally not as strong as aspirin, Ginger inhibits AA–induced platelet release and aggregation. Serum cholesterols also show reduction, as does their excessive production by the liver.

Ginger's ability at relieving chronic tissue/ joint pain and associated inflammation needs no proving. Again through altering a number of AA pathway parameters, Ginger is appropriate for the chronic pain and inflammation of rheumatoid conditions, poorly healed sport–mechanical type injuries, and other situations when warmth and tissue stimulation feels therapeutic.

Within the realm of spice herbs, Ginger has little rival as a cancer preventative. A substantial amount of research has been conducted on the plant's ability at inhibiting carcinogenesis. Results are largely positive due to Ginger's ability to stimulate apoptosis–regulated cell death. This body–wide protective mechanism selects unhealthy or diseased cells from healthy ones, then initiates that cell's destruction. When this function is operating ideally cancerous cells are never allowed to thrive and subsequently spread to other regions of the body. Ginger's antioxidant and antiinflammatory properties also play a part in its chemoprotective role, as does its anti–angiogenic influence over developing tumors.

Among others types, several breast cancer lines and liver and gastrointestinal cancers (in vitro) have been inhibited with Ginger. It may not be miraculous in eradicating carcinoma, but it is certainly worthy as a preventative. For these broad antimutagenic purposes equal portions of Ginger and Turmeric serve as an excellent combination.

INDICATIONS

- Fever, dry skin
- Common cold, with chills
- Nausea, general
- Nausea, from motion/sea sickness
- Nausea, food aversion, and taste changes from radiation/chemotherapy
- Nausea and vomiting of morning sickness
- Gastrointestinal spasm and gas
- As a salivary stimulant
- Dysmenorrhea (external and internal)
- Inflammation, cardiovascular
- Inflammation/Pain due to rheumatoid conditions and chronic injury
- Cancer, preventative

COLLECTION

Before Ginger's rhizomes become tough and fibrous – 9–10 months after planting – they are easily dug being not far from the soil's surface.

PREPARATIONS

Both fresh and dry preparations will be effective. Although gingerol and shogaol ratios do change somewhat through the drying process, the end result, regardless of form is still therapeutically similar.

For the broadest range of Ginger's therapeutics whole plant forms should be used – teas, tinctures, or powdered root. The essential oil, containing only volatile elements, will be best used for its stomachic and diaphoretic properties. For this take 20–30 drops of Ginger spirit as needed. 2–3 drops of essential oil can also be dropped directly onto a sugar cube and allowed to dissolve in the mouth.

Although not a "correct" tea preparation per se, 1–2 teaspoons of fresh root is allowed to steep in hot water. Add lemon and sweeten to taste. It is an excellent cold and flu tea.

DOSAGE

- Root infusion: 2–4 oz. 2–3 times daily
- FPT/DPT (70% alcohol): 20–50 drops 2–3 times daily
- Fluidextract: 5–15 drops 2–3 times daily
- Spirit: 20–30 drops 2–3 times daily
- Poultice: as needed

CAUTIONS

Do not use the essential oil or spirit during pregnancy: this applies to any essential oil with its concentrated array of aromatics.

OTHER USES

Ginger as a spice, candied or crystallized, and Ginger soda are all popular consumer forms. Ginger ale made with real Ginger will curb nausea, but if serious therapeutic effects are needed use the purer medicinal forms.

GINKGO

Ginkgoaceae/Ginkgo Family

Ginkgo biloba
Maidenhair tree

DESCRIPTION

An extraordinary tree reaching heights of 60'–120', Ginkgo has somewhat of a horizontally oriented crown and deep anchoring roots. A medium green throughout the spring and summer, the leaves turn a distinct bright yellow during autumn, then shortly after fall to the ground. Leaves are fan–shaped with prominent radiating veins. They are 2"–6" long and occasionally bifurcate or partially split.

Being dioecious, male and female reproductive parts exist on separate tress. Males produce pollinating cones; females, small stems in which a set of ovules or "eggs" develop if pollinated. The fruit are 1" long by about ¾" of an inch wide, greenish–yellow to tan, and have a distinctive rancid butter smell.

DISTRIBUTION

A relic of an ancient time, the genus thrived in both the northern and southern hemispheres during the permian, laurasia, jurassic, and cretaceous periods. Today, Ginkgo biloba occurs naturally only in Zhejiang province, China, but even this is questioned by some authorities. It is suggested that like other ancient ginkgo trees they too were planted by people long ago. Some planted specimens are speculated to be nearly 3000 years old.

Long cultivated in China, then Korea, and Japan, they are associated with Buddhism and Confucianism. Trees planted at temple sites are responsible for Ginkgo's wider discovery and popularity today. First planted in the United States approximately 200 years ago, they are now a common ornamental.

CHEMISTRY

Flavonoid glycosides: quercetin, kaempferol, isorhamnetin; terpene lactones: ginkgolides a, b, and c, bilobalide; ginkgolic acids.

MEDICINAL USES

Ginkgo's application to circulatory disorders is vast due to the plant's kindly influence over this system. Its vasodilatory properties affect medium and small interior arteries and capillary beds. Peripheral and cerebral circulation is most profoundly influenced, as can be seen by the problems Ginkgo most successfully remedies.

Suffers of peripheral vascular disease and associated intermittent claudication will benefit from the plant's use. Walking distance, leg pain, and overall symptom picture improves with Ginkgo. Raynaud's disease (and syndrome), a vasoconstrictive condition affecting the extremities, also shows improvement under the plant's use. For this it combines well with a vasodialating nervous system sedative such as Skullcap.

Ginkgo will also produce favorable results applied to varicose conditions. Ulceration due to poor venous circulation, as well as hemorrhoids, will improve under the plant's influence.

Ginkgo specifically antagonizes PAF (platelet activating factor). The plant's influence over this compound, which is largely responsible for platelet grouping and some inflammatory responses involving an array of white blood cells, is inhibitory. Therefore Ginkgo has significance in limiting dietary or environmental allergic re-

actions. Even asthmatic bronchial constriction, if white blood and mast cell release are the chief causes, will be reduced.

Ginkgo has an interesting tissue protective effect. As a tissue prophylactic, when exposed to ischemia/hypoxia, both cerebral and myocardial areas suffer less damage under Ginkgo's influence. This has significance for anyone who has a history of stroke or heart attack, and related vasospasm or clot formation. By normalizing cellular ATP, glucose, and oxygen parameters, Ginkgo increases the affected tissue's stress tolerance. Ginkgo inhibits clot formation, through its effect on PAF, and also through its inhibition of the proteolytic enzyme, thrombin.

It is for good reason the plant is considered a remedy for many elderly complaints. Its influence over cerebral tissues and associated age-related mental deterioration is noteworthy. As mentioned earlier, Ginkgo increases cerebral blood flow, particularly to the white matter of the brain. Secondly, cerebral glucose utilization becomes more efficient. Both of these attributes have a marked effect on learning, memory, and congintion.

There are a number of symptoms that indicate cerebral insufficiency. They often are associated with early stage Alzheimer's disease, dementia (degenerative and vascular), and history of stroke. Ginkgo clearly improves the following related symptoms: confusion, lack of concentration, failing memory, absentmindedness, tiredness, depression, and anxiety. Even a number of non-cognitive symptoms improve with the plant's use, particularly, tinnitus, hearing loss, diminished eye sight, vertigo, dizziness, and headaches. These system-wide improvements are due to increased blood supply/glucose utilization in deficient areas. Depending on the situation's severity, Ginkgo has been shown to at least stave off further cerebral deterioration.

One memorable effect of Ginkgo was its restart of hair growth on a 70 year-old man's bald scalp – most likely due to improved capillary blood movement, affecting hair follicle nourishment. His wife was more excited than he was.

Enforcing the majority of Ginkgo's circulatory effects is its antioxidant influence. Typical of other botanicals containing antioxidant flavonoids, Ginkgo is a potent free radical scavenger. Its inhibitory effect on lipid/lipoprotein oxidation and hydrogen peroxide mediated damage to red blood cells will be found of use to nearly anyone suffering from an inflammatory condition. For neuropathy and related eyesight issues, most diabetics will respond favorable to a Gingko–Bilberry combination.

INDICATIONS
♦   Peripheral vascular disease
♦   Raynaud's disease/syndrome
♦   Varicose conditions, and related ulceration
♦   Hemorrhoids
♦   Allergic reaction, general
♦   Asthma, to reduce inflammation
♦   Stroke and heart attack prophylactic/recovery
♦   Blood clot formation
♦   Cerebral insufficiency
♦   Alzheimer's disease/Dementia
♦   Neuropathy

COLLECTION
If whole–plant leaf preparations are to be used, gather spring and early summer green leaves, as these are medicinally more potent than yellow–fall foliage (sometimes marketed as "Golden ginkgo"). Use dry.

PREPARATIONS
In Ginkgo's case, standardization has proven reliable and efficacious. The process removes much of the pant's mildly toxic ginkgolic acid content[18]. Use the standardized extract if trying to correct a problem; use crude preparations if in need of a low–dose maintenance.

DOSAGE
♦   Standardized extract: 100–300 mg. daily, taken in divided doses

---

18   A number of studies point to this group of compounds as allergens; not a poison, but possibly an irritant.

♦   DPT (60% alcohol): 30–60 drops 2–3 times daily
♦   Leaf infusion: 2–4 oz. 2–3 times daily

CAUTIONS
Theoretically Gingko should not be mixed with blood thinning pharmaceuticals, but a number of interaction studies (in humans) have been conducted with no concluding evidence to suggest potentiation or problem.

GINSENG
Araliaceae/Ginseng Family

Panax ginseng
Ren shen, Wild ginseng, Chinese ginseng, Korean ginseng

DESCRIPTION
Arising from an aromatic fleshy tap root, Ginseng produces a single stem, 1'–2½' feet in height. The rounded stems end in whorls of 5–8 palmate leaves. Each leaf is composed of 3–5 serrated leaflets. They are oblanceolate and dull to shiny green. The mature fruit form in drupes and are pea–sized and red.

DISTRIBUTION
Native to northeastern China, Korea, and eastern ex–Soviet Union, Ginseng at one time flourished in mixed–conifer mountain forests. Nearly identical in needs to American ginseng, it prefers rich soils and dappled shade.

CHEMISTRY
Triterpenoid saponins: ginsenosides (panaxatriols, panaxadiols), oleanolic acid; polysaccharides; phenolic acids: salicylic acid, p–hydroxybenzoic acid, vanillic acid, genistic acid, cis–p–coumaric acid, protocatechuic acid, syringic acid, cis–ferulic acid, trans–p–coumaric acid, gallic acid, trans–ferulic acid, trans–caffeic acid.

MEDICINAL USES
Classifiers had it right when they used Panax to

name the genus. Derived from the Greek word panacea, it is understandable that it was considered a cure–all; so many physical and mental parameters are affected by the plant. At the heart of Ginseng's "adaptogenic" influence is its modifying activity over the hypothalamus–pituitary–adrenal axis, or at least the tissue groups that respond to these glands. From immunity to endurance, from sex drive to mood, Ginseng has influence. Both the central and peripheral nervous systems are affected. Ultimately Ginseng is one of our most profound constitutional medicines, able to alleviate situations of deficiency, whether from the weakness of old–age or innate tendency.

Ginsenosides, a class of saponins, are considered Ginseng's main affecting agents. There probably is no other group of compounds known within the world of herbal medicine that are attributed with such an array of influences. They are essentially at the core of the plant's activity; but Ginseng's saponins are not the whole of the plant, possibly the heart, but not its entirety.

As an adaptogen, Ginseng (and others in the Ginseng family) exerts a sparing action on the adrenal medulla. In times of short–term, and especially long–term stress, it reduces stress–induced catecholamine secretion. Whether it is from a local influence, or mediated via the hypothalamus/anterior pituitary, Ginseng's specific mechanism of action is still open to debate. One thing is certain though, therapeutic changes are achieved through the plant's use.

Acting both as hormone and neurotransmitter, catecholamines are secreted in large quantities in useful fight or flight reactions, and also in response to (or as a cause of) numerous chronic ailments. It is less known that nearly every chronic disease or ailment is dependant upon a continued/chronic stress–response of some sort for its continuation, or at least its severity. Continued over–secretion of catecholamines eventually leads to that tissue's or organ's over reaction and eventual exhaustion and/or breakdown. Ginseng reduces the amplitude of our body's reaction to internal and external stress by lessening long–term stress–induced catecholamine secretion.

This influence of Ginseng is the main reason why so many qualities are ascribed to the plant. Cardiovascular, gastrointestinal, nervous system, metabolic, and even psychiatric conditions such as anxiety and depression are beneficially affected by Ginseng. The more stress is a factor, be it physical or mental, the more apt the condition will respond to the plant. Use Ginseng when the problem seems inescapable, and that inescapable quality takes on a life of its own.

In the weak and aged, as a promoter of physical stamina and endurance, Ginseng has little rival. Very different from the xanthine–caffeine group of plants, Ginseng is not a stimulant per se, but used as a tonic, over time it will increase work capacity. Although less reliable in its effects, athletes and workers whose performance is limited by exertion will see improvement under its use. Little will be seen by individuals preforming short–intense activities, such as weight–lifting, but for activities which involve long–term exertion, Ginseng will be performance enhancing.

Used as a strengthener Ginseng will probably not appreciably affect an individual who is healthy and robust. This is one reason why studies measuring the performance enhancing effects of the plant show contrasting results. Simply put, if an individual's system is already adept at managing stress responses or is efficient at a particular exercise, Ginseng has no gap to fill – ancient Chinese immortals aside, Ginseng will make no one super human.

Traditional wisdom suggests that the plant be used when innate vitality is waning. In these individuals it will seem life enhancing and restoring. Immune system activity responds, as the user is often plagued less by minor bacterial and viral infections and generally feels healthier through its use. Fatigue and tiredness, symptoms of so many chronic metabolic and immunologic syndromes, will diminish; to what degree depends on the severity of the situation. It is not that Ginseng only addresses the symptoms here, but the individual's core deficiency, which must exist for these problems to develop, is addressed.

Relatedly when sleep is disturbed from similar syndromes of dysfunction – fatigue during the day, restlessness during the night – Ginseng often provides a deeper, more restful sleep.

Stress–induced male libido/potency problems are remedied by Ginseng. As an aphrodisiac, erectile response is normalized. Quality and quantity of sperm increases. It is important to know that Ginseng is not drug or "viagra"–like in its effect. As a long–term tonic results will be seen, but when evidence is expected immediately, the user will be disappointed. One probable explanation of Ginseng's effect on male erectile tissue is its nitric oxide linked relaxation of the corpus cavernosum. Vasodilation of penile tissue allows for an increase in rigidity, girth, etc.

For women as well, when a harried, career–minded lifestyle is cause of sexual disinterest, try Ginseng. Even related fertility problems may be influenced. If the situation permits it, foster a sense of relaxation and maternal instinct. This alone will affect the reproductive environment profoundly.

Research has shown Ginseng as an effective cancer preventative. A capable protectant against a myriad of specific malignancies the plant modulates both cellular and humoral immunity as well as inhibiting carcinogenesis through a variety of mechanisms. The plant's ginsenosides, as well as its antioxidant phenolics, equally play parts. Patients with active malignancies, particularly who are weakened and feel set upon by radiation and chemotherapy treatments, will feel strengthen by Ginseng.

Aside from the activity of ginsenosides, the pant's phenolics are potent influences as well. This group of compounds is largely responsible for Ginseng's antioxidant behavior. And here the differences in preparation become apparent: the steaming process, making ginseng "red", substantially increases its phenolic content, therefore its antioxidant attributes. Inversely this steaming process reduces total ginsenoside content, but increases less polar ginsenosides, which doubtlessly is responsible for other therapeutic differences between the two preparations.

Ginseng is a useful cerebral–spinal stabilizer. It is surmised that under the plant's influence cellular membranes are kept better intact due to its marked antioxidant properties. Among other neuroprotective mechanisms, neuronal–specific apoptosis (programed cell death) appears modified by the plant, particularly if heightened as a result of ischemia or stroke. Ginseng is specifically indicated if there is a history of stroke–related dementia, memory loss, or disorientation. In fact nearly all age–related cognition/cerebrovascular problems will improve under the plant's influence. Even students, having need of increased mental concentration and retention will benefit from supplementation. For this use, Ginseng combines particularly well with Guaraná.

Not a specific medicine for the liver, such as Barberry, which serves as an overt chologogue, Ginseng's cellular protectant qualities nonetheless are well applied to this vital organ. Seen here, as in cerebral centers, it protects against hepatic oxidative injury. Its effects are smartly applied to the long–term hepatic stress of hepatitis C or virtually any condition if there is liver inflammation. For these purposes it combines well with Shiitake or Reishi mushroom.

Lipid metabolism is amplified. Typically Ginseng lowers LDL levels and raises HDL levels, overall producing a more healthy blood–cholesterol profile. Relatedly Ginseng fits suffers of "syndrome x", a metabolic tendency disposing the individual to high cholesterol/blood glucose/blood pressure levels. Although there are better herbs which will more profoundly affect these parameters, Ginseng is a medicine for the underling tendency.

Other regions or tissues groups are equally affected by Ginseng. Red blood cell membranes show stabilization under the plant's influence, leading to less injury derived hemolysis; this being of interest to athletes whose performance is due to the blood's oxygen carrying ability.

Ginseng is weakly estrogenic, ginsenosides having some affinity to estrogen receptor sites. Some women going through menopause may see some amelioration in discomforts, but all in all there are better herbs for such issues, i.e. Black cohosh or Chaste tree. Normal amounts typically will not have any adverse effect on the reproductive system.

INDICATIONS
- As an adaptogen
- Weakness of old–age/Reduced vitality
- Stress, especially long–term
- Fatigue/Tiredness from immunologic/metabolic dysfunctions
- Libido, diminished
- Male erectile problems
- Cancer, as a preventative
- Fatigue/Weakness from conventional cancer treatments
- Memory–loss/Dementia, especially age related or from ischemia or stroke
- As a hepatic antioxidant
- Blood cholesterol/Blood glucose, elevated
- Red blood cell stabilization

COLLECTION
Extensively cultivated in China and Korea, Ginseng represents a plant that has transitioned from a wildcrafted medicine to one that is a strictly controlled crop. Ginseng growing/export is a large and successful industry (as medicinal plants are concerned).

Truly wild Ginseng is virtually extinct in forests of China and Korea – its status is much worse than that of wild American Ginseng. Due to inaccessibility, the Russian federation stands are slightly more stable, but still are at potential threat from poachers fueled by fantastic market prices.

PREPARATIONS
Ginseng root comes in two base forms: the unprocessed dried root, or White ginseng (uncured), and the steamed fresh root (then dried), or Red ginseng (cured). Normally dried the root is cream to tan in color. After steaming the root becomes dark red, almost translucent, rust colored.

Both forms share a majority of therapeutic properties. Some constituent differences are due to a particular conversion triggered by the curing (steaming) process. Cured Ginseng's antioxidant activity is distinctly higher, making its uses towards cancer, liver–lipid disturbances, and cerebral stabilization slightly more pronounced. Use uncured Ginseng for the plant's well known adaptogenic properties. Realize though, using one or the other is fine tuning its application. If all you have is one particular form its use will be fine for whatever application.

Due to whole root quantities being unable to keep up with demand, there have been a number of interesting attempts to fill this lack. The most successful, using suspension cultures, is the cultivation of Ginseng's finer rootlets, or advantageous roots. An immense amount of root mass in able to be grown in a relatively short period of time. Ginsenoside content is superior in this often over looked part of Ginseng. Compared to 5 year–old whole roots, 5 year–old rootlets contain nearly 3 times the amount of ginsenosides! Even 1 year–old rootlets, ounce–per–ounce, contain more ginsenosides than the main body of a 5 year–old root. These finer rootlets are harvested, dried, powdered, and used in many Ginseng demands when the actual whole root is not needed – extracts, tablets, powders, etc. Among Ginseng parts and preparations it is a sleeper; in this case the slight is more powerful than the showy.

Unfortunately throughout Ginseng's history, adulteration, as with many higher–priced herbals, has been/is a reality. Fortunately though this deceit is usually well–controlled, at least by reputable bulk herb retail/wholesalers who routinely test authenticity. Encapsulated or tablet form Ginseng, which nearly every supplement maker has alone or in combination, is entirely another matter. Reputable brands generally will not pose an issue; generic or discount brands are more problematic. Either way, to be safe, purchase the whole root or bulk powder from a trustworthy source.

The roots are poorly water soluble, making alcoholic and powdered preparations choice. Of course chewing and swallowing a small section of dried root is a perfectly fine method and in some ways surpasses the other more "advanced" modes in simplicity and directness.

Both Ginseng leaf and berry are medicinal as well. The dried leaf is primarily used as tea material, i.e. tea bags. The berry, although a more powerful medicine for hyperglycemia and equally "syndrome x" suffers, is not a popular article of commerce.

DOSAGE

♦ Capsule (00): 1–2, 1–3 times daily
♦ DPT (70% alcohol): 15–30 drops 1–3 times daily
♦ Dried whole root: 1–3 small pieces daily

CAUTIONS

Within normal dosing ranges Ginseng has few cautions. "Ginseng abuse syndrome" as it is labeled, is the occasional result of taking too much Ginseng, especially red or cured Ginseng. Elevated blood pressure, restlessness, and insomnia are common symptoms. That higher doses of Ginseng affect the body this way is not unusual considering the bi–phasic quality of the plant.

GOLDENSEAL

Ranunculaceae/Buttercup Family

Hydrastis canadensis
Yellow root, Yellow puccoon

DESCRIPTION

Goldenseal is a small herbaceous woodland perennial. During the spring a simple 6" to 1' long stem arises from the plant's root. Usually two unequal leaves form; they are pubescent, 5–7 lobed, and serrated. From the base of the upper leaf a single flower, lacking petals, but having prominent greenish–white sepals, develops. The flower does not linger; shortly the fruit forms. Though non–edible, it appears Raspberry–like, crimson, and composed of numerous carpels.

DISTRIBUTION

Like American ginseng and Black cohosh, Goldenseal is native to temperate forests of the eastern part of the country. It prefers moist, rich, and acidic soils. Adequate canopy coverage by hardwood trees is important for Goldenseal, as it grows poorly in direct sunlight, preferring dappled shade. Found in twenty seven states it ranges from Quebec and Ontario to Arkansas and Georgia. In nearly every state it is considered either threatened or endangered.

CHEMISTRY

Isoquinoline alkaloids: hydrastine, hydrastinine, canadine (tetrahydroberberine), canadaline, iso–corypalmine, berberine; flavonoids; volatiles.

MEDICINAL USES

Even though Goldenseal is one of the most popular herbs used today, along with Echinacea the plant's influence is still not properly understood. I suppose if Goldenseal was used appropriately there would not be such a scarcity of wild populations. It is a prime example of a medicinal substance that is over utilized, poorly understood, and much exploited. What it is used for and what it is good for are two very different things. Unfortunately Goldenseal (along with Echinacea) is considered "good" for nearly everything. If the user of Goldenseal understands one thing about the plant's application, it will be hard to stray from proper use: apply it to chronic mucus membranes conditions.

Goldenseal is a mucus membrane tonic. Its stimulatory power is best applied to situations where affected tissue lacks sufficient vitality to overcome lingering disturbances. Chronic head colds, sinusitis, and rhinitis will be helped by the internal tincture and/or a nasal wash. Unresolving pharyngitis, where the affected membranes do not respond to strictly antimicrobial approaches, will benefit from Goldenseal. For all of these issues, as with most others that Goldenseal addresses, look for unchecked mucus discharge accompanying the regional problem. Certainly the gargled tincture will not hurt, but the plant's application to tonsillitis is unreliable. Combined with Eucalyptus or White sage as a gargle, and internal Wild indigo and Red root, it will prove more reliable. The nasal wash for post–nasal drip will curb mucus development, therefore reducing associated nausea, cough, and throat clearing.

As a bitter tonic Goldenseal, has little rival. When digestion is weak, there is low–grade irritation of the area producing a coated tongue, the plant will be found beneficial. Chronic gastritis, even if it is of alcohol abuse, is nicely soothed by it as well. Long–standing ulceration of the stomach, small, or even the large intestine, will be furthered towards resolution. Attention to the state of ulceration is an important consideration here. Use it only if the ulcer is subacute or chronic. If the ulceration is acute, try Marshmallow or Slippery elm.

Gastrointestinal irritation following bacterial associated food poisoning is another indication for the plant's use. If there is copious mucus, lingering nausea, and diarrhea after the main bout, it will be found soothing. As a restoring tonic for sufferers of biliary/intestinal disarray from prolonged illness, alcohol abuse, or constitutional weakness, Goldenseal should hold a main spot in any therapy geared towards recovery. Care should be taken not to use the plant in acute inflammatory complaints, as the situation may worsen due to Goldenseal's stimulatory nature.

As a tissue strengthener for the rectal area, both internal and external use will be of benefit if there is risk of prolapse. With or without associated hemorrhoids the applied ointment or retained enema will do good. Anal fissures, rectal ulcers, or any acute inflammation of associated tissue will likely be aggravated by full strength topical applications. Weak ointments or half–strength enemas will do good though; internal use is also indicated in these situations.

Abnormal vaginal and uterine secretions are checked by Goldenseal. Whether discharge is from a functional hormonal imbalance or an external problem such as a vaginal flora disruption or an overt microbial/fungal infection, a douche or sitz bath will prove useful. If there is active inflammation, take care not to make the solution too strong, otherwise some irritation may develop.

Just as Goldenseal checks excessive mucus discharge in chronic conditions, it has some power over circulatory problems of a similar nature. Passive hemorrhage of the gastrointestinal tract often is checked efficiently, be it from ulceration or erosion of mucus membrane surfaces, often associated with diarrhea or dysentery. Passive hemorrhaging of the bronchial, renal, or uterine regions, are reduced less reliably.

As an eyewash Goldenseal will be found soothing and superior to many complicated mixtures for inflamed outer–ocular disorders. In cases of conjunctivitis, if there is copious discharge, Goldenseal's antibacterial and astringent qualities will be found useful. Eye redness and irritation from allergies and exposure will be equally soothed.

Factoring into many of Goldenseal's effects is the plant's inhibitory action over a myriad of bacterial, fungal, and parasitic strains. Both berberine and hydrastine are implicated in these activities. It is important to note that Goldenseal preforms poorly if used solely as an antibacterial herb. This single–minded approach, using Goldenseal for only its antibacterial qualities is the main reason why it is in nearly every brand's formula for wintertime colds to jock itch. For straight–forward bacterial/fungal infections use Oregongrape, Barberry, or even Coptis; they will prove just as effective.

Goldenseal is often listed as an immune stimulant. This simply is not true. This false label maintains its presence due to the plant's inclusion in a majority of "shotgun" Echinacea–based formulas.

The greatest disservice to the plant is its mythical reputation as a "cleanser" for drug testing. Every weekend partier who normally wouldn't eat a salad, knows of the supposed effect Goldenseal has on Cannabis detection through urinalysis. Fact: Goldenseal having any effect on the matter is an herban legend. What does have influence though is drinking 3–4 gallons of water a day prior to the drug test – that is of course if the individual makes it to the drug test. Drinking that much water in such a short time period is a major stress on the kidneys and will almost certainly skew electrolyte balance possibly prompting a hospital visit.

INDICATIONS
♦ Head cold/Sinusitis/Pharyngitis, chronic
♦ Dyspepsia/Gastritis, chronic
♦ Gastrointestinal ulceration, chronic
♦ Passive hemorrhage of gastrointestinal tract
♦ Diarrhea/Dysentery, as a follow–up
♦ Hemorrhoids/Anal fissure/Rectal ulcer (external and internal)
♦ Leucorrhoea/Vaginitis (external and internal)
♦ Conjunctivitis (eyewash)

COLLECTION
After gaining popularity by Eclectic introduction, Goldenseal has been over collected since the latter part of the 19th century in an attempt to fulfill market demand. Currently wild populations still continue to decline, even though collection of the wild plant has been outlawed in many states[19]. Certainly habitat loss due to urbanization plays a part as well.

Although obvious but needing to be stated, wild Goldenseal should not be collected. Like American ginseng, Lady slipper, and Unicorn root, Goldenseal needs to be left alone[20], or even helped to recover. You as the consumer can make a difference in Goldenseal's future. Purchasing only cultivated roots (or use other botanicals) does have an effect by sending a message to the grower and the poacher. Cultivation is tedious but generally successful.

19 Goldenseal was placed on the CITES (Convention on International Trade In Endangered Species) list in 1997.
20 This is one of the darker sides of the herbal medicine field. The endangerment of a plant due to its benefit to us is a complicated and unfortunate issue. Profiteers, marketers, the unaware public, and ignorant professions dispensing the plant are all at fault. Goldenseal, or any other medicinal plant, is just not that good to warrant its extinction. There are many other botanicals, or combinations thereof, that equal or even surpass Goldenseal ability.

PREPARATIONS
There are alternatives[21] to Goldenseal. Combine a berberine containing herb such as Oregongrape or Barberry with either Bayberry or Yerba mansa (Anemopsis californica). Using equal portions of each mimic Goldenseal part in chemical make-up, and part in astringent stimulation.

Both root and leaf are medicinally active with the leaf being about ⅓ to ½ as potent as the root. Unlike the root, the leaf makes a decent tea. Unless noted the following dosages are for the root.

DOSAGE
♦ FPT/DPT (60% alcohol): 30–60 drops 2–3 times daily
♦ Fluidextract: 10–20 drops 2–3 times daily
♦ Capsule (00): 2–3, 2–3 times daily
♦ Leaf infusion: 2–4 oz. 2–3 times daily

CAUTIONS
Goldenseal, although safe in normal doses, in principle is not a plant to take during pregnancy or while nursing. Excessive doses can lead to nausea, gastrointestinal irritation, and possible hepatic/renal irritation.

OTHER USES
It was once used as a dye plant by the Cherokee.

GOTA KOLA
Apiaceae (Umbelliferae)/Carrot Family

Centella asiatica (Hydrocotyle asiatica)
Indian pennywort, Brahmi, Pegaga

DESCRIPTION
A small annual tending to be under foot due to its diminutive size, Gota kola forms a loose spreading, low cover. Leaves are semicircular, reniform, net–veined, with shallow lobes. Each is supported on a long, weak, 4"–8" long petiole.

21 Rarely in clinical practice do I use Goldenseal, preferring alternate combinations.

The small, pink to light green flowers form in umbels; seed capsules are ridged and pumpkin-like.

DISTRIBUTION

Originally a wetland plant of India and similarly terrained Asia, Gota kola, centuries ago, spread throughout the South Pacific, Madagascar, Africa, Turkey, and many points in between. Even in parts of the southeastern United States there is Centella erecta, a variety that is considered nearly identical in all aspects (except genetically); almost certainly the American variety descends from C. asiatica. Look to wetland edges and moist and sunny areas. Possibly our variety can be used in a similar fashion.

CHEMISTRY

Triterpene saponins: asiaticoside, asiaticodiglycoside, madecassoside; ursane saponins: asiatic acid, brahmic acid, isobrahmic acid, madecassic acid, betulinic acid; flavonoids: quercetin, catechin, rutin; mono- and sesquiterpenes: campesterol, stigmasterol, sitosterol, α-pinene, β-pinene, myrcene, γ-terpinene, bornyl acetate, α-copaene, β-elemene, β-caryophyllene, trans-p-farnesene, germacrene-d, bicycloelemene; pectins; terminolic acid, vanillic acid, succinic acid.

MEDICINAL USES

Gota kola comes to us from Ayurveda, the traditional system of healing practiced in India. Here in the West, where we usually forgo talk of chakras and humors, the plant is mainly employed for skin, cognitive, and stress complaints. The plant has enjoyed a fairly recent resurgence in western herbal medicine. Although it has been a well known plant medicine in the west since the 1990s, it was written of as far back as 1857 by the Lancet: "This is the name of a new drug which has lately been much used in France in the treatment of cutaneous afflictions." and "It exercises a particular virtue over various cutaneous afflictions, particularly those of long standing and dependent on the presence of syphilitic or scrofulous taint. It has been administered with success in cases of leprosy[22] and elephantiasis."

Topically, more so if combined with internal use, Gota kola has a marked effect on tissue healing. The ointment applied to poorly healing wounds and ulcerations, bedsores, and burns is usually successful and very well tolerated. The plant's mechanisms are not fully known but we do know both fibroblasts are affected and collagen synthesis is augmented. Interestingly the plant appears not to have an effect on VEGF (vascular endothelial growth factor) produced from keratinocytes. This nuance along with its reducing effects on tissue inflammation and keratinocyte hyperproliferation coincides with the plant's positive influence of psoriasis.

Apply the plant to leg and foot ulcers of both advanced diabetes and CVD (chronic venous disorder). Needless to say internal therapies here are paramount in regaining some sort of equilibrium but topical approaches are a good starting point.

As a significant antioxidant, Gota kola is best applied to two areas: cognition and the heart. Its influences of memory, spatial awareness, and mood seem to go beyond those of a plant simply affecting free radicals and the like. Shortly after taking the plant a peaceful and focused calm arises. Thoughts become less jumbled, names become easier to recall, and power of concentration increases.

For the elderly with pre-dementia or beginning stage Alzheimer's disease, Gota kola is well applied. Its calming and focusing qualities will improve mental/emotional outlook and function. It has been suggested that Gota kola slows the neurodegenerative processes which underlie these behavioral disorders. Surface membranes of cerebral neuronal tissue are kept better intact. The antioxidative powers of catalase and SOD (superoxide dismutase) are amplified, which remove harmful oxygen-based inter- and extra-

22 Today Leprosy or Hansen's disease is largely manageable with antibiotic therapies. Gota kola probably will help with the tissue alteration that occurs from the responsible bacterium: Mycobacterium leprae, but a cure? Go with the antibiotics.

cellular by–products. Here it combines well with Ginseng or Ginkgo.

Modern–day research appears to confirm what Ayurvedic doctors have known for centuries: Gota kola given to mentally retarded children will calm and increase their ability. Given to epileptics, seizure frequency and intensity will diminish. It's not a cure, but as something natural, with virtually no side effect, it should at least be called a kindly therapy when applied to most disturbances based on neuro–cerebral impairment.

An emerging area of Gota kola influence is the cardiovascular system. The heart, particularly myocardial tissues are protected by the plant's saponins and related derivatives. Like its effect on neuronal tissues, catalase, SOD, glutathione peroxidase, and glutathione–s–transferase, all radical scavenging enzymes, are keep better intact and are amplified. Cellular damage through oxidative stress is reduce through the plant's usage. This has direct bearing on individuals who fit the "heart attack" or myocardial infraction profile. Not a prophylactic, but a buffer; if a heart attack does happen the resulting necrosis and cellular damaged will not be as extreme. If angioplasty or open heart surgery is unavoidable take Gota kola for two weeks prior to the operation, and while healing afterwards; it will reduce related tissue damage. Of course it is better not to have a heart attack, or heart surgery. Only using Gota kola for cardiovascular centered complaints, without changing stress/lifestyle/dietary conditions, most likely will not have a lasting effect.

INDICATIONS
- Wounds/Ulcerations/Bedsores/Burns (external and internal)
- Psoriasis (external and internal)
- As a cerebral/cardiovascular antioxidant

COLLECTION
Common picking grounds: third–world–country ditches with collecting water, wetland margins, etc. can be somewhat precarious when it comes to bacteria/chemicals/and other unhealthful substances. There is a decent amount coming from Hawaiian production. Not important with all herbs, but in Gota kola's case, look for organic.

Often the whole plant is collected, leaf, stem and spreading rhizome, but just the leaf and stem are as common in commerce. Either combination will work.

PREPARATIONS
Standardization for Gota kola is in vogue today. Remember though, for a long time people have been successfully utilizing the plant without the present–day pharmaceutical–like trend. Crude preparations, if made from quality material will be fine. The best preparation is to eat the plant fresh. If that is not possible, then the tea from the recent herb, or the fresh or dry plant tincture are all active.

DOSAGE
- Fresh herb: small handful 2–3 times daily
- FPT/DPT (50% alcohol): 30–60 drops 2–3 times daily
- Herb infusion: 4–8 oz. 2–3 times daily
- Ointment: as needed

CAUTIONS
None known.

OTHER USES
In various eastern cuisines, it serves as refreshing side dish. It can be eaten alone or added to salads. It is not known whether it increases longevity or power, but mythologically Gota kola is linked to Taoist masters and Indian kings.

GRINDELIA
Asteraceae/Sunflower Family

Grindelia squarrosa
Gumweed, Curlycup gumweed

Grindelia nuda var. aphanactis (Grindelia aphanactis)
Curlytop gumweed

DESCRIPTION

As a biannual or short lived perennial Grindelia squarrosa stands between 1′–3′ in height. Older plants are typically multi–stemmed; younger ones may only have one main stem, but both have many–branched tops. Leaf blades are usually toothed (but on occasion they are entire) and are oblong to oblanceolate. They are about 2–4 times longer than broad. Flower heads are sticky with resin and are composed of sizeable involucres with spreading or recurved phyllaries. Each flower head matures with 25–40 ray flowers. Similar in appearance, the flower heads of G. aphanactis are composed of disk florets.

DISTRIBUTION

Roadsides, disturbed soils, and open grassy areas are places to find Grindelia squarrosa. Found throughout three–fourths of the country, its range is extensive. From California it ranges to Texas, north to Wyoming and further into Canada, finally east to mid and northeastern states. It is absent from most of Southeast.

G. nuda var. aphanactis is mainly found throughout the southwestern region of the country. From California it ranges to Texas and north to Utah and Colorado.

CHEMISTRY

Essential oil content for related Grindelia robusta: α–pinene, camphene, β–pinene, p–cimene, limonene, γ–terpinene, cis–pinen–2–ol, p–cymene, terpinolene, α–campholenal, nopinone, camphor, trans–pinocarveol, pinocarvone, isoborneol, borneol, p–cymen–8–ol, terpinen–4–ol, myrtenal, methyl chavicol, myrtenol, verbenone, trans–carveol, cis–carveol, carvone, perilla aldehyde, (e)–anethole, bornyl acetate, δ–elemene, α–cubebene, α–copaene, α–humulene, γ–muurolene, germacrene d, β–selinene, bornyl isovalerate, γ–cadinene, δ–cadinene, germacrene–b, spathulenol, humulene–oxide, t–cadinol, β–eudesmol, calamenol.

MEDICINAL USES

As long as it is sticky and aromatic virtually any species of Grindelia can be used medicinally. A number of species were official, and at one point in time California's G. camporum was considered the main source plant.

Grindelia is useful in a number of chronic to sub–acute bronchial conditions. Indicators for the plant are: sense of constriction, rawness of the pectoral membranes, and dry cough. Its most prosaic use is its application to chronic bronchitis characterized by a non–productive, dry cough. Through the plant's aromatics, bronchial membranes are moistened, assisting expectoration. Of equal benefit is the antimicrobial nature of these oils, which help in fighting any infection that may reside in the area. The plant does have a dual quality though. Like Sage in the way it modifies secretions, Grindelia in weakened individuals, particularly the aged, will check bronchorrhoea. For a number of plants that are found stimulating to the body, it is not uncommon for opposite symptoms within a condition, in different people, to be remedied. It may appear paradoxical, but the strengthened tissues or organ dictates the path to health. In some that may mean increased secretion, in others, less.

For those who suffer from asthma, or at least asthmatic–like breathing as a constitutional tendency, Grindelia will be helpful. The same indicators previously mentioned for the plant's use apply here: constriction, labored breathing, and dry cough or membranes. In these people Grindelia will be found opening to the lungs. Breathing will be eased. Used solely or combined with Ligusticum, emphysema sufferers will also take note of the change in tissue oxygenation.

Smoked alone, or with Lobelia and/or Datura, Grindelia has a quick symptomatic effect on the spasmodic constriction of an asthma attack. It will be found opening and relieving to constriction. Not a healing approach, but one that will give results in an acute situation.

Seen with many aromatic expectorants the kidneys, bladder, and urethra are all influenced by Grindelia's antimicrobial volatiles. The tincture or fluidextract can be used for long–standing, chronic infections, as well as non–resolving irritation, with or without mucus discharge.

Grindelia's best kept secret is in its healing activity on the rash of poison ivy. A century and a half ago a lotion, made by diluting the fluidextract with water, or the fresh plant poultice was once considered one of the best plant medicines for the condition. Today it still preforms. Jewelweed can keep its place as king of the East in treating this troubling rash, but for the West, where rhus dermatitis can be just as troubling in mountain regions, use Grindelia.

Apply the ointment to old, poorly healing ulcers, or to any skin condition where repair of the epithelium is necessary. Chronic eczema also responds well to the plant.

INDICATIONS
- ◆ Bronchitis with a dry cough
- ◆ Asthma, with bronchial irritation
- ◆ Emphysema
- ◆ Urinary tract infection/irritation, chronic
- ◆ Poison ivy rash (external)
- ◆ Chronic skin ulcers (external)
- ◆ Chronic eczema (external)

COLLECTION
Gather the flowers and leaves by simply grasping them between your fingers; then pull. The immature flower heads can be collected alone if abundant. Their resin content tends to be higher. After collecting for several minutes your hands should be sticky with resin.

PREPARATIONS/DOSAGE
- ◆ FPT/DPT (70% alcohol): 20–50 drops 2–3 times daily
- ◆ Fluidextract: 15–30 drops 2–3 times daily
- ◆ Ointment or poultice: externally as needed

CAUTIONS
Possible bronchial and renal irritation with over use; do not use during pregnancy.

GUARANÁ
Sapindaceae/Soapberry Family

Paullinia cupana var. sorbilis (Paullinia cupana)
Brazilian cocoa

DESCRIPTION
Guaraná is a bushy climber. Shrub–like to vine–like, the plant's large, alternating, green leaves are borne on long petioles. A number of leaflets comprise each leaf; they are arranged in an odd–pinnate composition. Each is 5"–6" long and 2"–3" across. Flowers are cream to light yellow and form in axillary panicles. The grape–sized fruit are ovoid. Each contains 1–3 black, aril–covered seeds.

DISTRIBUTION
Guaraná is found in Brazil, primarily in the Amazon basin. It is cultivated in the same region.

CHEMISTRY
Tannins: catechin, epicatechin, epicatechin gallate; methylxanthine derivatives: caffeine, theophylline, theobromine; saponins.

MEDICINAL USES
Similar in use to Kola nut, Guaraná is yet another caffeine–methylxanthine containing plant. Methylxanthines, especially caffeine, represent 2.5–5% of the plant's dried weight (substantially higher than Coffee), so it is understandable that it is mainly used as a general metabolic stimulant. Under the plant's influence the force and rate of the heart is increased; respiration is amplified, as is muscular contractility and mental alertness. It can certainly be used as a sport–type supplement as well as a mental study aid.

For intermediate stretches of time Guaraná increases physical and mental performance. It is not uncommon for the plant's stimulation to last four to six hours, longer than the stimulation of Coffee–based caffeine. It will be found more steady, with muted highs and lows. This phenomenon is largely due to methylxanthine–tannin–lipid based complexes, which the body breaks down more slowly than the caffeine–based complexes of Coffee. The differences in solubility between Guaraná and Coffee are evident when making a simple infusion/decoction: Coffee produces a uniformly saturated tea; Guaraná, a milky solution, with some sediment, underscoring its non–polar compounds.

Interestingly Guaraná's performance increasing effects can not be attributed to its caffeine content alone. The plant's stimulant, tonic–like action is better tolerated and certainly more health–promoting than caffeine used singularly. This is possibly due to the plant's antioxidant tannin content. That said, tannins as antioxidants are popular these days (see Tea). In moderate quantities they are health promoting as free radical scavengers, etc. but in large amounts they chronically disrupt gastrointestinal membranes, making these sensitive tissues prone to dysfunction.

Due to the plant's caffeine content it is also a cerebral vasoconstrictor. It gives some relief when used in inflammatory–type headaches/ migraines with pulsating pain and red–irritated eyes.

If appetite is weak, Guaraná is not recommend due to its suppressant qualities. It will curb the appetite and increases lipolysis sufficiently enough to encourage weight loss, but it carries the same risks as other caffeine containing diet aids. Due to its tannin content and adrenergic synergism rapid intestinal movement and diarrhea is often abated.

A possible limiting factor in Guaraná's use, besides the obvious problems from excess caffeine intake, is its high tannin content. Take enough of the plant to curb diarrhea and over–stimulation of the central nervous system becomes as issue. Take the plant for the caffeine stimulation and some may find it constipating due to the high tannin content. Oh, well.

INDICATIONS
- As a cardiovascular, muscular, mental stimulant
- Vasoconstrictor for headaches/migraines
- Diarrhea

COLLECTION
The seeds are shelled, washed, and roasted.

PREPARATIONS
Guaraná is commercially available in bulk powder and occasionally whole seed form. Capsules, tablets, tinctures, and an array of combination products are commonly found in retail establishments.

DOSAGE
- DPT (65% alcohol, 10% glycerin): 30–90 drops, 1–3 times daily
- Fluidextract: 20–30 drops 1–3 times daily
- Capsule (00): 2–3, 1–3 times daily

CAUTIONS
Cardiovascular disease; hypertension.

OTHER USES
Guaraná, in the form of extracts, syrups, and distillates, is extensively employed as a stimulating/ flavoring agent by the soft drink sector.

HAWTHORN
Rosaceae/Rose Family

Crataegus laevigata (Crataegus oxyacantha, C. oxyacanthoides)
Midland hawthorn

Crataegus monogyna
Common hawthorn, English hawthorn

DESCRIPTION
No more than 12′ in height, deciduous and spiny, this small tree has moderately serrated and prominently lobed leaves. Flowers are whitish to pink and showy – they cluster in tightly packed corymbs. The large red fruit are ¼″ or more in diameter and contain 2–3 seeds.

Crataegus monogyna is slightly larger in stature. Leaf lobes are pronounced. Flowers are

1–styled; fruit is 1–seeded.

Hybrids between Crataegus species are common. The genus has always been problematic as true species identification with some specimens is nearly impossible.

DISTRIBUTION

For Crataegus laevigata: native to western and central Europe. C. monogyna's range is somewhat more expansive. It is found from western Europe to northern Africa to western Asia. Both species are extensively planted as ornamentals and borders throughout Europe and temperate North America. Throughout the Northeast C. monogyna can be found in a feral state around road sides, field margins, and other disturbed areas.

CHEMISTRY

Flavonoids: hyperoside, vitexin; procyanidins.

MEDICINAL USES

As a heart medicine there is no other herb with such a positive, yet gentle influence than Hawthorn. Discoveries through research are consistent with traditional application, which is a nice confirmation since not all herbs have that luxury.

The plant affects the entire cardiovascular system, but particularly the coronary artery and the muscle fibers of the heart. Coronary artery blood flow is increased. This activity augments heart tissue nutrition and oxygenation, particularly if the heart, due to cardiovascular disease, is devitalized. Another influence the plant has on vascular dynamics is its effect on blood movement. Similar to Garlic, peripheral vascular resistance is decreased. Blood literally passes by vascular walls with less drag. Small vessel networks of the heart are actually revascularized if damaged from tissue ischemia or infraction.

Partly due to Hawthorn's flavonoid portion, its overall effect is cardioprotective. When there is blood/oxygen deficiency the plant will increase cell death tolerance while improving myocardial performance. Hawthorn affords a definite

amount of cell membrane preservation and protection from overall damage.

The plant's influence on the heart beat is positively inotropic, meaning it increases the force of the heart's contraction. While doing this Hawthorn paradoxically decreases the organ's workload. Hawthorn usually steadies the rate as well, proving worthy in most arrhythmia disturbances, or erratic action of the heart. As far as rate is affected, if the heart is under exaggerated sympathetic influence (outside of exercise/overt physical exertion), usually it is slowed; if stressed from disease or hypertension, beats per minute will drop to a more healthy level.

Hawthorn's specific application to cardiovascular maladies is impressive. Almost no derangement is uninfluenced by it, possibly with the exception of bradycardic situations, but even here case by case analysis may deem some treatable with Hawthorn. The reason the plant affects so many heart issues is because virtually every problem can be helped if the organ is strengthened and performs more efficiently. Yet cardiac glycosides too (Digitalis) do this, but unlike Hawthorn with its ability of increasing activity with little or no corresponding stress, they often increase blood pressure. Hawthorn strengthens yet does not over stimulant.

Due to Hawthorn's increase in blood delivery to the heart, and its influence on the myocardium, incidence of angina pectoris and associated shortness of breath, discomfort, and chest oppression are reduced. I have observed significant results with both mitral and aortic valvular regurgitations. The plant's effect is not so much on the malformed valve, but on improving the heart's ability of compensation. It is impressive to see an individual's cardiac output scored at a stage III before Hawthorn, then stage II while drinking 24 oz. of tea daily, with no adjunctive pharmaceutical treatment[23]. Of course Hawthorn has limits. I have observed the plant having little effect on severe valvular situations and on SA/

23 Pharmaceutical beta blockers, ACE inhibitors, and calcium channel blockers may improve the symptomatic picture if suffering from heart disease, but none of them actually increase life span.

AV node disturbances.

High blood pressure is often reduced (10–20%), be the problem essential hypertension as a symptom from arteriosclerosis or valvular/structural problems. Both systolic and diastolic readings are influenced. Pulse rates during Hawthorn supplementation usually fall approximately 10% as well. These indicators point to reduced workload. Exercise tolerance and anaerobic threshold increases, indicating the heart is able to do more with less stress on the myocardium.

Hawthorn combines well with cardiac glyco-side containing plants, i.e. Convallaria, Cactus, or Digitalis. In fact due to Hawthorn's moderating influence usually less is needed for a therapeutic effect.

Some secondary problems associated with cardiovascular disease, or just plain and simple old hearts, are benefited by Hawthorn: pulmonary edema and edema of the extremities. However, often stronger heart–affecting medicines are need here. Chronic indigestion related to heart weakness is also relieved to varying degrees.

Whether suffering from atherosclerosis, or wanting to prevent the condition, Hawthorn is one of the best herbal remedies we have. Its vascular protective effects have direct influence on arterial wall elasticity and health. Cell membrane permeability, adhesion, leukocyte activity, and other inflammatory factors are positively influenced by Hawthorn.

The fresh plant tincture of the berries has a marked effect on emotional states associated with grief and loss. To varying degrees, gloom, heartache, and depression, are often lifted. It is not uncommon for those who suffer a severe loss to have physical symptoms of heart distress, such as heart palpitation, oppression, pain, and shortness of breath. I have observed Hawthorn to lighten the emotions, as well as related physical sensations.

Lastly, due to Hawthorn's significant flavonoid content, it will be supportive of varicose conditions. Like Rose hips, under its influence tissue permeability will decrease, resulting in im-proved venous return and overall performance. For this purpose take Hawthorn if suffering from venous problems in conjunction with cardiovascular issues. If there is no underling heart problem then try Rose hips, for Hawthorn's cardiovascular effects are unneeded.

INDICATIONS
♦ Arrhythmia
♦ Tachycardia
♦ Angina pectoris
♦ Valvular regurgitation
♦ Hypertension
♦ Atherosclerosis
♦ Varicose conditions

COLLECTION
Leaves, flowers, and berries are all medicinally active. Collect young leaves and flowers (equal proportions) in the spring and the ripe berries in late summer. Use fresh or dry for tea/tincture preparations.

PREPARATIONS
Whole plant preparations, made from fresh or recently dried material, will prove superior to standardized extracts. Heavy processing and the negation of many secondary compounds limit these extract's claim of superior results. Standardization is all the rage, but don't let their popularity dissuade from traditional, whole plant use. I have seen the fresh plant tincture (berries alone, or combination of leaf/flower/berry) or berry infusion give equal and even superior results.

DOSAGE
♦ FPT/DPT (60% alcohol): 30–60 drops 2–3 times daily
♦ Berry/Leaf/Flower infusion: 4–8 oz. 2–3 times daily

CAUTIONS
If combining with conventional heart drugs dosage may need to be adjusted, otherwise Hawthorn is a heart nutritive with little caution.

HOPS

Cannabaceae/Hemp Family

Humulus lupulus var. neomexicanus
Western hops

Humulus lupulus var. lupulus
European hops

DESCRIPTION

Hops is a perennial twining vine. It tends to loosely creep over and blanket support plants, but disappears in colder seasons due to its herbaceous nature. Occasionally it can be found growing in the open without any support. In these cases the plant appears mound–like.

Western hops has opposite, coarsely serrated, palmate leaves that are 3–7 parted and 1⅕"–4" long. The upper sides are very rough; the lower sides are distinctly yellow–gland dotted. The substantial leaf petioles are about as long as the individual leaves. The small male flowers are 5–parted and held in loose panicles. Female flowers are borne in twos and are surrounded by numerous, persistent bracts, that when mature appear cone, or catkin–like. Like the leaves, they are gland dotted (base of cone bracts). Interspersed throughout the foliage they hang downwards and are rarely upright.

European Hops generally is the same in appearance, with some minor differences. The plant is larger and a darker shade of green than its native relative. Leaves are 3–5 parted. Both plants are aromatic. The flowers especially stink, and indeed their potency depends on this volatile oil content.

DISTRIBUTION

Now divided into three main biotypes, North American, Asian, and European Hops, China is agreed upon as the plant's prehistoric birth place.

Western hops' range stretches from western Texas, the Rocky Mountains, south to New Mexico and Arizona. It is a plant of the mountains and is always a pleasure to see growing along stream sides, where slightly apart from the surrounding conifers, it stretches for the sun. I have seen it practically as a ground cover traipsing its way over dry streambed rocks or mountainside scree.

European Hops, due to its cultivation for beer production, is now found in temperate regions world–wide. In the United States, fond of disturbed soils, occasionally it is found as an escapee.

The other two native varieties that are found throughout North America are Humulus lupulus var. lupuloides and var. pubescens. They are regionally common and also make fine medicines.

CHEMISTRY

For Humulus lupulus var. lupulus: terpenes: β–caryophyllene, farnesene, humulene, myrcene; bitter acids: α–acids: humulone, cohumulone, adhumulone; β–acids: lupulone, colupulone, adlupulone; chalcones: xanthohumol, isoxanthohumol, desmethylxanthohumol, prenylnaringenin; flavonol glycosides: kaempferol, quercetin, quercitrin, rutin; catechins: catechin gallate, epicatechin gallate.

MEDICINAL USES

Hops is an age–old sedative. It is indicated for uncomplicated central nervous system excitability. The plant is well used to allay sleeplessness, insomnia, and nervous tension, particularly in menopausal women. Some find its sedative effects similar to Valerian's, particularly if dried, for upon drying lupamaric and lupulinic acids are converted to isovaleric acid. Furthermore Hops combines well with Valerian.

Hops belongs to a family known for its hormonal–like influences. Traditional lore has it that female collectors would start menses early after several days of gathering the stobiles. Although Hops is not an estrogen duplicate by any stretch of the imagination, the plant has been established to hold some sway over estrogen–oriented complaints. After taking Hops menopausal women typically see a reduction in associated issues – hot flashes, irritability, sleeplessness, etc. As with most "estrogenic" herbs there is no concise pattern of influence. Hops decreases symptoms of estrogen deficiency, but also research indicates the plant reduces proliferation of estrogen dependant breast cancer cells lines due to its aromatase inhibition. Certainly there is an estrogen receptor–site interaction taking place as well as a potent enzymatic blocking activity – but exactly what occurs and at what dose – is still open to debate. Even a number of prostrate cancer cells line have shown inhibition when exposed Hops' flavonoids.

Relatedly, for younger men who suffer from wet dreams (nocturnal emission) and who have a nervous disposition, Hops often is an unsurpassed remedy. Associated mental irritability and distress often are eased under the plant's use, as is the genital/bladder irritation that may accompany any issue.

Hops is also an aromatic bitter. Those who suffer from gastritis or general indigestion, especially if triggered by stress will benefit from Hops. Taken before meals it is used to stimulate mouth and gut secretions that are essential in proper food digestion and assimilation. The plant's influence on the central nervous system, especially its lessening effect on sympathetic discharge, combined with its influence over the gastric environment, fits certain physiological dispositions. Related peptic ulcer formation is diminished from the plant's aforementioned qualities as well as its substantial antibacterial volatile oil content, which undoubtedly retards Helicobacter pylori infection.

Effective against an array of gram–positive bacteria (some species of Micrococcus, Staphylococcus, Myobacterium, and Streptomycetes) and fungi (Candida albicans, Trichophyton, Fusarium, and Mucor species), use Hops as an antibacterial/antifungal wash for cuts, scrapes, and as a general disinfectant. The leaves made into a tea or a powder are well applied to these conditions.

Hops can be broken down into three related but distinct parts. They are as follows: strobiles (female flowers or the "hops"), foliage, and resin glands (lupulinum or lupulin). The flowers, certainly the most well known part, contain the most balanced mix of attributes. They are equally sedative, stomachic, and antimicrobial. Although the principal tea item, one drawback to flower use is its sheer bulk. Intimidating to some, two tablespoons seem to take up about 8 oz. of space. Hops foliage, primarily composed of leaf material, is less sedative, but more stomachic and antibacterial. Lastly lupulinum: the resin glands found on the strobile and leaf. Easily dislodged from the dried plant, this yellowish powder is most noticeable at the bottom of the bagged or jarred flowers. The recently dried resin is by far the strongest part of Hops.

INDICATIONS
♦ Insomnia/Nervous tension
♦ Menopausal complaints
♦ Nocturnal emission
♦ Gastritis/Indigestion
♦ Ulcer, peptic
♦ Cuts/Scrapes (external)

COLLECTION
The female strobiles mature mid to late summer, making a trip to the mountains not a hard decision. Be thankful if the stand gathered from is somewhat accessible and not perched on a steep hillside, making collection like painting from a high scaffold. Murphy's law occasionally comes into play when collecting the plant: don't be discouraged if only male plants are found, keep looking for the elusive females, they are present, just being coy.

Using your hands will be the most efficient way to collect the flowers, which should be sticky with resin. The foliage can be collected from either male or female plants. Hops resin glands are sifted from the dried foliage and flowers. Put the dried herb in a plastic bag or jar and shake vigorously. The yellowish sediment at the container's bottom is separated, then prepared as indicated below.

PREPARATIONS

Hops, be it the flower, foliage, or resin gland powder, degrades quickly after drying. Use dried material within 6 months of collection. Prepare the resin gland powder as a dry plant tincture. The fresh plant tincture of the flowers will have the most subtleties and broadest effect, whereas the dry plant tincture of the resin glands will be the strongest sedative.

DOSAGE

- FPT/DPT of flowers/foliage (60% alcohol): 30–60 drops 2–3 times daily
- Fluidextract of flowers/foliage: 10–30 drops 2–3 times daily
- DPT of resin glands (70% alcohol): 20–40 drops 2–3 times daily
- Flower/Foliage infusion: 3–6 oz. 2–3 times daily

CAUTIONS

Use of the plant during pregnancy or while nursing should be avoided due to its effect on the reproductive environment. Although the plant's "estrogenic" qualities are minor, be sensitive to its use in tandem with reproductive issues.

OTHER USES

A Hops pillow, made with the flowers, for the young, old, or sensitive, can be nearly miraculous at producing sleep. Doubtlessly the plant's aromatics are responsible for its effect.

HOREHOUND

Lamiaceae/Mint Family

Marrubium vulgare
White horehound, Marrubio, Mastranzo, Concha

DESCRIPTION

As a short–lived perennial, Horehound is 1′–2½′ tall and generally erect and bushy. Along with the plant's classic mint characteristics it is distinguishable from other related plants by its woolly–white fuzz covered stems. Leaves are toothed, rounded, green above, and lighter beneath. Where they join the stems, the small–white tubular flowers form in dense clustered whorls. The calyxes are toothed and after drying as a group, are bur–like. The seeds are small, egg–shaped, and brown.

DISTRIBUTION

Originally from Europe, Horehound is an opportunistic non–native found throughout nearly the entire country. It frequents places of disturbed soils such as roadsides, trailsides, and drainage areas.

CHEMISTRY

Flavonoids: luteolin, apigenin, vitexin; labdane; diterpenoid: marrubiin; phenylpropanoid esters: (e)–caffeoyl–l–malic acid, acteoside, forsythoside b, arenarioside, ballotetroside.

MEDICINAL USES

Horehound is truly a multi–faceted plant. Because it affects several organ systems, it is a prosaic tool worthy of understanding. As a stimulating expectorant it tends to break up impacted bronchial mucus. Regional secretion is enhanced and mucus is thinned, encouraging easy expectoration. Horehound also has a time–honored reputation in constricted lung conditions. Its decongesting effect is noticeable in humid asthma with associated phlegm. The plant's cyclooxygenase inhibition may play a role in its therapeutic effect here. As a remedy for hoarseness and coughs, the syrup allays throat and bronchial irritation.

The room temperature tea or tincture taken before meals is used to stimulate an array of gastric, hepatic, and small intestinal secretions. The plant enlivens these areas and is useful in dyspepsia with poor protein and fat digestion. Moreover, Horehound is stimulating to appetite, often turning indifference to food into hunger. The tea drunk hot is diaphoretic and is appropriately used when there is a low to moderate fever with dry skin. Drunk cool the tea is mildly diuretic and can be helpful in eliminating fluid retention from non–organic causes.

INDICATIONS
- ♦ Bronchitis
- ♦ Asthma with phlegm
- ♦ Indigestion/Lack of appetite
- ♦ Fluid retention

COLLECTION
In the spring, collect the upper half of the plant. Strip the leaves and flower clusters from the stem. Discard the stems, as they are medicinally ineffective.

PREPARATIONS/DOSAGE
- ♦ Leaf infusion: 4–6 oz. 2–3 times daily
- ♦ FPT/DPT (50% alcohol): 30–60 drops 2–3 times daily
- ♦ Syrup: 1 teaspoon 3–4 times daily

CAUTIONS
Idiosyncratically, Horehound can cause short–term hypoglycemic episodes and in large quantities may slightly elevate blood pressure.

HORSE CHESTNUT
Hippocastanaceae/Buckeye Family

Aesculus hippocastanum
Spanish chestnut

Aesculus glabra
Ohio buckeye, Smooth buckeye, Western buckeye

DESCRIPTION
A moderate sized tree, Aesculus hippocastanum[24] bares large palmate leaves, generally forming in groups of seven. Upright flower racemes are notable, often reaching 8" in height. Flowers are mostly white with reddened bases. The tree's green fruit capsule is prickly and contains 1 to 2 chestnut–brown "nuts".

---

24 Aesculus is completely unrelated to Castanea, or true Chestnut.

Aesculus glabra[25] is a large shrub or small tree, reaching heights of 12'–15'. Its palmate leaves are oppositely arranged with leaflets numbering 5–11. They are variable in number and tend to be lanceolate to obovate with margins eventually becoming serrated. Upper surfaces are glabrous, lower surfaces are pubescent to tomentose, particularly on the leaflet's veins. The perfect, irregular–yellow flowers form in terminal panicles. The tree's spiky (sometimes without spikes), ovoid fruit are $1\frac{1}{5}"$–2" in diameter. The seeds are chestnut–brown.

DISTRIBUTION
Native to the Balkans, Aesculus hippocastanum was once planted extensively as an ornamental throughout Europe and North America. Today it is infrequently planted due to a number of problems – leaf blotch being the most significant.

Aesculus glabra is largely a plant of the mid–western states. From Nebraska and Kansas it ranges south to Texas. In prairie expanses look to streamsides and gully–ravine margins. Wooded hillsides and lower–lying woodlands also host the plant.

CHEMISTRY
For Aesculus hippocastanum: saponins: aescin, desacylescin, prosapogenins; flavonoids: quercetin, kaempherol, and their diglycosyl derivatives; proanthocyanidins; coumarins: aesculin, fraxin; triterpenes.

MEDICINAL USES
Uses for either species of Aesculus profiled here are nearly identical. Even though Aesculus glabra is a lesser–used domestic variety this should not exclude the plant's utilization, particularly among inhabitants within the tree's distribution.

Horse chestnut is firstly a remedy for vascular congestion. The plant has a corrective influence on venous circulation making its traditional application to hemorrhoids and leg varicosities understandable. The activities of aesculin, a cou-

---

25 Aesculus californica is just as useful.

marin derivative, and aescin, a saponin, are at the heart of the plant's application.

Horse chestnut affects venous tissue through two modes. One, it stimulates endothelial contractility via increased ionic calcium permeability. Two, certain tissue–contracting prostaglandins are stimulated within endothelial tissue by aescin, resulting in an orderly movement of blood through the venous circulation.

More orderly fluid or blood movement is paramount to vascular health. In this model Horse chestnut decreases fluid pooling and associated tissue–fluid disarray. As a result capillary membranes are less permeable to extraneous fluids. Also fluid transfer from tissue spaces to capillaries is made more efficient by increased oncotic pressure.

Horse chestnut's reduction of vascular congestion and engorgement, particularly in the pelvic area, will be found of distinct benefit to hemorrhoid suffers. The plant's indication here, rather than pain, will be a feeling of congestion resulting in tightness. Faulty portal circulation is often an underling factor, which the plant favorably influences by strengthening venous tissue. Abdominal fullness, indigestion, and/or intestinal–rectal discomfort related to vascular congestion also indicates Horse chestnut's application.

Use Horse chestnut both internally and topically to diminish problems ranging from major varicosities to minor spider veins. Associated leg heaviness, swelling, and edema respond to the plant as well. All topical preparations will work. Although, because of its surface absorption, the ointment is best suited for this use. Results are quickly seen in virtually all sports–type injuries – falls, sprains, blows, factures, etc. Its influence on swelling from trauma can also be applied to brain and spinal injuries. Even the swelling and tissue edema that occurs post–surgery is diminished by the plant.

Horse chestnut has an interesting effect on the bronchial environment. If asthmatic breathing, spasmodic cough, and a sense of lung constriction are problems, they are often remedied by the plant. Whether Horse chestnut affects the area through its vascular influence, or whether it is from a local effect, is unknown. That said it will be doubly efficient in its effect if other conditions exist such as portal/intestinal congestion, or lower–extremity venous stasis.

INDICATIONS
♦ Venous stasis (external and internal)
♦ Hemorrhoids (external and internal)
♦ Varicosities/Spider veins (external and internal)
♦ Leg heaviness/Edema (external and internal)
♦ Portal circulation, slowed
♦ Injuries/Post–surgery, to reduce swelling (external and internal)
♦ Asthmatic breathing/Cough

COLLECTION
Even though the dried fruit is the traditional portion, the bark of Horse chestnut can also be used.

PREPARATIONS
Both crude and standardized preparations are effective. Standardized products typically are calculated to contain 16–20% aescin.

DOSAGE
♦ DPT (50% alcohol): 5–15 drops 2–3 times daily
♦ Ointment/Oil/Salve: as needed

CAUTIONS
Possible hemolytic issues with heavy use; do not use during pregnancy or while nursing.

OTHER USES
Containing nearly 4% fatty acid, the seeds of Horse chestnut were once utilized for their oil content. The seed oil is used little today.

HORSETAIL
Equisetaceae/Horsetail Family

Equisetum arvense
Common horsetail, Canutillo

Equisetum laevigatum
Smooth scouring rush, Cola de caballo

Equisetum hiemale
Scouring rush, Cola de caballo, Canutillo de lla-no, Caballo

DESCRIPTION
Equisetum arvense, like other Horsetail spe-cies, has underground spreading rhizomes. This perennial has two functionally different stems. Spore–filled cones top fertile stems, which arise in early spring. They are flesh–colored and 6" to 1′ tall. Developing shortly after, infertile stems have numerous whorls of small jointed branch-lets. They appearance as upturned cylindrical feather dusters.

Similar in appearance, both Equisetum laevi-gatum and E. hiemale are scouring rush biotypes. These perennials also arise from spreading rhi-zomes. Their wand–like stems are hollow and jointed. Fertile stems are distinct in appearance in that they also have a small cylinder–like cone terminations. Given its prominent silica formed ridges, E. hiemale's stems are the roughest of the two.

DISTRIBUTION
All Equisetum species profiled here are found throughout most of the United States and much of Canada. They are commonly encountered along streams, moist soils, and drainage areas. Throughout the arid Southwest, they are typi-cally mid to high elevation plants.

CHEMISTRY
Flavonoids: chlorogenic acid, kaempferol, dihy-drokaempferol, hydroxycinnamic acid, equise-tumpyrone, quercetin, protogenkwanin, gos-sypetin, luteolin, apigenin, protoapigenin, gen-kwanin, naringenin; silicic acid, silica, calcium, potassium, phosphorus.

MEDICINAL USES
Mainly a urinary tract medicine, Horsetail is soothing to the area and is of use in diminishing urinary tract irritability and painful urination. Internal preparations are mildly diuretic and will assist in eliminating fluid build up (from non–organic causes) around the ankles, wrists, and mid–sections of the body. Moreover, when taken as a daily tea, kidney stone formation is reduced through the plant's ability of increasing urine volume.

Although its mechanism of action is not clearly defined, as a hemostatic the plant lessens passive hemorrhaging. Use it if there is blood in the urine from physical injury or gastrointestinal bleeding from ulceration and other non–malig-nant inflammatory processes. Internal prepara-tions may even be useful if there is blood–tinged sputum from a severe cough. Topically and in-ternally the plant facilitates wound healing and tissue repair. This is mainly due to Horsetail's flavonoid, silica, and silicic acid content. The plant is also used to strengthen the hair, nails, and skin. Connective tissues throughout the body are augmented. The plant makes a good tea for fortifying bones damaged by injury, or weak-ened from osteoporosis.

INDICATIONS
♦ Painful urination, irritability
♦ Fluid retention
♦ Kidney stones, as a preventative
♦ Passive hemorrhaging
♦ Gastrointestinal ulceration
♦ Weakened hair, nails, skin, bones, and con-nective tissues
♦ Wounds (external and internal)

COLLECTION
Equisetum arvense has the highest quercetin content in its new spring growth – approximate-ly 50% of its total flavonoid content. Other spe-cies are probably similar. As spring changes to

summer, the plant's quercetin content quickly diminishes.

Only collect the infertile stems of E. arvense, as this will ensure the plant's sustainability. Fertile and infertile stems alike can be collected of Scouring rushes. Clip the stems at their bases. Use fresh or dry. After drying, the stems are easily separated into 1"–2" sections for storage.

PREPARATIONS/DOSAGE

- ♦ Fresh juice: 1 oz. 2–3 times daily
- ♦ Herb infusion: 2–4 oz. 2–3 times daily
- ♦ Poultice: as needed

CAUTIONS

It is possible that Horsetail, exposed to common agricultural run–off, produces several toxic compounds. Therefore do not collect and use the plant around contaminated areas. In addition, excessive quantities of the tea or juice may irritate the kidneys.

OTHER USES

The abrasive qualities of Scouring rush are practically legendary, but surely exaggerated. It has been said that the plant has been used to sharpen knives and clean and polish pots and metals – an herbal equivalent to steel wool.

JUNIPER
Cupressaceae/Cypress Family

Juniperus communis
Common juniper

DESCRIPTION

Juniper is usually a shrubby, low–growing bush, although with favorable conditions it is occasionally reported to reach tree proportions. Beyond these exceptional cases, Juniper is usually less than 5′ in height and sometimes double or triple that across. Branches tend to grow laterally and form tangled masses. The evergreen leaves are needle–like and lance shaped. They are whitish above and dark green beneath. The berries take

2 seasons to ripen fully, are bluish–black, fleshy, sweet, and contain 1–3 small, hard seeds.

DISTRIBUTION

Juniper is found throughout temperate North America. In the Southwest it is encountered at elevations of 8,000′ and higher. It is an ubiquitous conifer extensively found throughout Europe.

CHEMISTRY

Prominent volatile content includes: α–pinene, β–pinene, sabinene, myrcene, δ–2–carene, α–phellandrene, β–phellandrene, δ–3–carene, limonene, bornyl acetate, (e)–caryophyllene, α–humulene, α–muurolene, germacrene a, germacrene d, germacrene d–4–ol, γ–cadinene, δ–cadinene, α–cadinol.

MEDICINAL USES

Juniper has centuries of cross–cultural usage behind its application as a urinary tract medicine. A stimulant to the area, it works best to alleviate low–grade, long–standing, subacute, or chronic urinary tract irritability and discomfort. Use it in chronic cystitis and painful urination accompanied by mucus in the urine. Although alcoholic preparations tend to extract Juniper's volatile constituents more completely, the leaf/berry tea is just as useful as a urinary tract antiseptic (both fungal and bacterial strains are inhibited). Small amounts of the tea are useful in imparting cellular stimulation in low–grade, on and off again nephritis, particularly if used in formula.

Due to its aromatics, Juniper tends to be moderately carminative. Several ounces of the tea or 30–40 drops of the tincture can lessen stomach bloating and cramping. Topically Juniper oil or salve can be helpful in resolving long–standing episodes of eczema and psoriasis. Through the plant's interesting mix of antiinflammatory qualities and stimulating aromatics, it often is the right plant for long–standing problems of the urinary tract and skin.

INDICATIONS

- ♦ Urinary tract infections, chronic

- Nephritis, chronic
- Dyspepsia
- Eczema/Psoriasis (external)

COLLECTION

Collect the leaves and/or fruit alone or together. Both parts are equally potent medicines. Dry normally.

PREPARATIONS

For internal use Juniper's essential oil fraction can be prepared as a spirit, or the essential oil can be added to ointment and oil bases.

DOSAGE

- Leaf/Berry infusion: 4–6 oz. 2–3 times daily
- FPT/DPT (75% alcohol): 30–40 drops 2–3 times daily
- Spirit: 20–30 drops 2–3 times daily
- Ointment/Oil/Salve: as needed

CAUTIONS

Due to the plant's potential uterine stimulation, do not use Juniper during pregnancy. Also do not use in acute kidney inflammation.

OTHER USES

Termites that are force fed Juniper sawdust die prematurely.

KAVA

Piperaceae/Pepper Family

Piper methysticum
Kava Kava, Kawa, Gea, Milik, Wati

DESCRIPTION

Kava is a branching, large–leaved, perennial shrub, reaching (when cultivated) heights of 6'–8'. Leaves are heart–shaped, pointed, and smooth; stems are jointed. At maturity roots can be several inches thick, large, and knotted.

DISTRIBUTION

Morphologically diverse, Kava is widely distrib-uted throughout the South Pacific. It is cultivated in Hawaii, Tahiti, Fiji, Papua New Guinea, the Solomon and Polynesian islands, and Vanuatu. Piper wichmannii, generally hypothesized to be Kava's wild ancestor, is found only on the Melanesian islands.

CHEMISTRY

Kava lactones: dihydrokavin, kawain, methysticin, dihydromethysticin, methysticin, kavain, desmethoxyangonin, tetrahydroyangonin, yangonin.

MEDICINAL USES

Doubtlessly clued to its uses by South Pacific Islanders who traditionally employ the plant, Kava was introduced into western medicine by French scientists Gobley (1860) and Cuzent (1861)[26]. Incorporating the plant's early social–medicinal applications, turn–of–the–century (20th) and modern–day practitioners have expanded on Kava's use significantly. The plant's traditional use is best described as a social lubricant, each region having varying customs concerning its use. Almost universally the fresh plant, made into a drink, is used to facilitate communication.

Unlike today, where ceremony is less important, in older times certain rules surrounded Kava's use. Some regions still have strict protocols surrounding its preparation and application, but many do not. Kava was often made by the women folk, to be drunk by the men, as a prequel to discussing matters of some import. Today what unifies Kava use among native South Pacific Islanders is not the how, but the why. In nearly every locale the plant is used as a mildly relaxing drink to ease tensions, aid in communication, and generally make the imbibing parties more comfortable with one another.

In America, and in parts of Europe, a hybrid trend has come to development. Because of its popularity, via the "herbal revival", Kava is almost exclusively used as a relaxant, and in some

---

26   First described by naturalist Johann George Forester while serving aboard the HMS Resolution during Cook's second expedition to the South Pacific (1772–1775).

circles, is doubtlessly abused. Nearly every culture is somewhat obsessed with altered states of awareness, and for various reasons, escapism is not the least of them. Teens in America will sometimes take the powered plant in excess, but the numb mouth, stomach upset, and befuddled dreams are not conducive to extensive reuse. Even in the relatively conservative circles of phytopharmacy, the focus on Kava is in its aforementioned sedative/altering qualities. But Kava has much more to offer.

As a plant for the urinary tract Kava is firstly anesthetic; its pain relieving qualities target the kidneys, bladder, ureters, and urethra. It is effective at reducing the sensitivity of chronic urinary inflammations, especially if there is debility of the area. Pain upon urination is lessened, as is urinary tract/prostrate sensitivity from excessive sexual activity. Kava is found soothing to the localized pain and soreness that often accompanies the act of passing kidney or bladder gravel.

Use Kava as a digestive stimulant when sympathetic nerve impulses, usually from stress factors, cause indigestion, as well as stomach and small intestinal inflammation.

The freshly chewed root, or the gargled tincture is of value in reducing neuralgias of the optic and auditory nerves. This is partly due to the plant's local anesthetic effect.

INDICATIONS
- Restlessness/Anxiety, especially in social situations
- Urinary tract irritability
- Painful urination
- Gastrointestinal debility from stress
- Optic/Auditory nerve irritation

COLLECTION
Lending to its easy procurement, Kava is grown in rich, well–drained soils. The fleshy roots are easily dug and processed accordingly.

PREPARATIONS/DOSAGE
- Root infusion (cold or standard): 4–6 oz. 2–3 times daily
- FPT/DPT (60% alcohol): 30–60 drops 2–3 times daily
- Fluidextract: 10–20 drops 2–3 times daily

CAUTIONS
Under normal use Kava poses little problem. When used in excess by susceptible individuals, both crude preparations and standardized products may cause some liver–skin–vision distress.

Historical accounts of Islanders abusing Kava and consequently developing a number of symptoms are well documented. For instance, Felter in The Eclectic Materia Medica, Pharmacology and Therapeutics (1922) suggests: "Its long–continued use by them has caused more or less obstruction of vision and a dry, cracked, scaly, and ulcerated skin, and lesions closely allied to leprosy."

Modern, western use of Kava has been under scrutiny as of late[27]. Up to 80 "cases" of liver inflammation, of varying degrees, since the 1990s have been "reported". Although there is some reason for concern considering Kava's history of over–use problems, like Comfrey the jury was out before the cases were properly evaluated. Out of nearly 80 cases, only one can be positively confirmed to Kava, all of the other cases had factors such as preexisting liver disease, hepatotoxic pharmaceutical and/or alcohol use.

Dallas L. Clouatre, writing on Kava toxicity in Toxicology Letters 150 (2004): 85–96 states: "Finally, it remains true that kava extracts show good efficacy in the treatment of anxiety. In comparison with prescribed anxiolytics and even many over–the–counter products, moreover, kava extracts continue to demonstrate a far better risk–to–benefit ratio."

Combining Kava, especially the standardized extract, which incidentally contains a different ratio of lactones then what is traditionally used, with pharmaceuticals or alcohol is not suggested. In general consumers are advised to use "crude" preparations, such as the tea, powered

27 Since 2002 legal contention has surrounded Kava on both sides of the Atlantic. The FDA has cautioned against its use. Canada the same; it is banned in France and Germany (ironically the two countries credited with the plant's western medical introduction and expansion).

plant, or the tincture.

Because of Kava's possible dopamine antagonism, the plant should be avoided if suffering from Parkinson's disease. Due to the plant's central nervous system's sedation its use is not recommended in concordance with states of depression or suicidal tendencies. The plant potentiates both alcohol and barbiturates. Kava is not recommended while pregnant or nursing.

In conclusion, with normal use, in healthy individuals, Kava does not pose any health concern. Long term, excessive use (especially of the standardized extract) however, has been shown to affect the skin and vision, most likely through impairing liver function.

KOLA NUT

Sterculiaceae/Cocoa Family

Cola nitida (Cola acuminata, Sterculia acuminata)
Kola, Gooroo nuts, Bichy nuts

DESCRIPTION
Reaching heights of 20'–35', Kola nut is a small to medium sized evergreen tree. Its leaves, alternating along branch stems, are between 4"–6" in length and are generally entire to obovate. The tree has separate male and female flowers. Female flowers are showy and develop into woody fruit. The capsule is composed of 5 tough compartments, each containing 1–3 large seeds.

DISTRIBUTION
Indigenous to tropical western Africa, Kola nut is now cultivated beyond its native range. Extensive commercial growing occurs throughout Africa and South America.

CHEMISTRY
Caffeine, tannin, theobromine.

MEDICINAL USES
As a cardiovascular, respiratory, and muscular stimulant, Kola nut's physiological effects are attributed to caffeine. It is best used in small amounts to slow and strengthen an erratic heartbeat, particularly if associated with weakness and low blood pressure. Heart palpitations will be calmed, as will dyspnea, particularly in asthenic types. Respiration is also increased, as users will note a deepening of inhalation and exhalation. The augmenting effect on these systems will be most noted by individuals who suffer from central nervous system weakness.

Gloominess, depression, and sluggishness of the mind are often lifted by Kola nut. Muscular lethargy, arising out of similar states of cardiovascular and nervous system weakness, will also respond to the plant. The elderly who suffer from hypotension, dizziness, and senility, will perceive a sense of wellness – for these purposes it combines well with white Panax or American Ginseng.

As a cerebral vasoconstrictor, Kola nut, like any other caffeine–containing plant, will be best for the congested and inflamed type of headache. Flushed face, red and irritated eyes, and a throbbing or pounding pain are indicators for its use. Migraines, beyond the initiatory phases of visual disturbance, well on their way to fruition, should respond well to Kola nut.

The plant has a significant tannin content making it valuable for loose stools – but Kola nut's central nervous system stimulation may over–shadow its use as a gastrointestinal tract astringent.

INDICATIONS
♦ Fatigue, muscular/mental
♦ Palpitations/Dyspnea from weakness
♦ Hypotension
♦ Depression/Gloomy state of mind
♦ Senility in asthenic types
♦ Headache, migraine type, congested

COLLECTION
The seeds of Kola nut are collected and dried, then usually powdered. Adulteration with Garnica and other similar seeds does occur. Purchasing the whole seed will ensure that the article is genuine.

PREPARATIONS/DOSAGE

♦ DPT (60% alcohol, 10% glycerin): 30–60 drops 1–3 times daily
♦ Fluidextract: 5–30 drops 1–3 times daily
♦ Seed decoction: 4–6 oz. 1–3 times daily

CAUTIONS

Common with most caffeine sources, issues of hypertension, anxiety, and sleeplessness may occur with excessive use.

OTHER USES

Kola nut is a major soft drink addition. Compared to Coca–Cola's Kola nut/Coca leaf combination of the past, its current ingredient list is tame.

LAVENDER

Lamiaceae/Mint Family

Lavandula angustifolia (Lavandula spica, L. vera, L. officinalis)

DESCRIPTION

A 3'–6' evergreen or semi–evergreen bush, Lavender is a member of the Mint family. Notable for its square stems, opposite leaves, and distinctive aroma, there is little mistaking the plant. Leaves are sessile, linear, and entire. Flowers develop in terminal spikes from branch ends. They are 2–lipped, lavender–colored, strongly aromatic, but bitter tasting. Nutlets are small and brown.

DISTRIBUTION

Lavender's epicenter appears to be northern Spain. Radiating outward it covers vast tracts of dry and barren land throughout the Mediterranean region. It is cultivated extensively throughout its native range as well as in England and America.

CHEMISTRY

Volatile fraction: linalyl acetate, linalool, caryophyllene, terpinen–4–ol, 2–octanone/myrcene, trans–ocimene, α–terpineol, borneol, β–farnesene, 1,8–cineole, camphor, caryophyllene oxide, α–humulene, limonene.

MEDICINAL USES

In the realm of natural medicine Lavender is one of the better known Mint family plants. Due to trendy use its past internal application has been superseded by its association with aromatherapy. Of course the therapeutic use of scents is valid: Lavender's aromatics (found in the essential oil) are absorbed directly through the mucus membranes of the nasal/oral cavity, when upon entering the systemic circulation, their medicinal influence, although weak due to the delivery method, is manifest.

Internal use of Lavender has a whole digestive range not found with the inhaled essential oil. The plant's effect as a carminative is mainly due to its topical contact with gastrointestinal walls. Here like Peppermint, it should be employed for nausea, indigestion with attending gas, and general uneasiness of the area. For children and infants Lavender is of value in curbing colic and vomiting particularly if an agitated state of mind precedes the episode. And if this is not the case, at least through the plant's mild sedative properties, it will help in bringing mental/emotional calmness to the young one. Both young and old can use Lavender for nervousness, anxiety, and emotional weakness, particularly if connected with digestive upset.

Topically the essential oil has distinct anesthetic properties. Applied to the temples and forehead it usually brings some sort of relief for headaches. As a sports rub, it can be used like most other aromatics, i.e., Eucalyptus, Camphor, or Cajeput. It is soothing to the pain of pulls, sprains, and contusions. It can be applied undiluted to burns; relief occurs soon after application. Rotated with Aloe vera or Prickly pear pulp, it makes as excellent therapy.

INDICATIONS

♦ Nausea/Indigestion
♦ Colic/Vomiting
♦ Nervousness/Anxiety, with digestive upset

- Headache (external)
- Pulls/Sprains/Contusions (external)
- Burns (external)

COLLECTION

Flowers yield the highest volatile oil ratios. Both the dried and the fresh flowers/flower stems can be utilized. Dried flower buds are also in commercial demand. They are stripped from the plant's flower spike, dried, and sold in bulk.

PREPARATIONS

Although some liver/biliary effects are more pronounced with the whole plant tea or tincture these preparations are little used today.

DOSAGE

- Essential oil: topical use as needed
- Ointment: as needed
- Spirit: 10–30 drops 2–3 times daily

CAUTIONS

The internal use of the essential oil/spirit is not recommended during pregnancy due to that fraction's possibility of stimulating menses.

OTHER USES

Lavender filled pillows, or eye–packs are known for their relaxing and soothing properties.

LEMONBALM

Lamiaceae/Mint Family

Melissa officinalis
Balm

DESCRIPTION

Lemonbalm is a kindly, small–statured, short–lived, perennial. Usually not more than 2′ in height, the plant is herbaceous in appearance and like other mints, has an opposite leaf pattern and square stems. The 1″–3″ long leaves are generally ovate, wrinkled, and have toothed margins. Flower spikes develop from the upper leaf axils. Each flower is yellow–white. The entire plant is somewhat hairy and if crushed smells distinctly lemon–like. Lemonbalm propagates easily from both seed and clones.

DISTRIBUTION

Originally from the Mediterranean region and southern Europe, Lemonbalm now is extensively planted in gardens and as a pleasant–scented indoor plant. Common and easy to grow, it may be harder to get rid of than to propagate.

CHEMISTRY

Main volatiles: neral (citral b), geranial (citral a), β–caryophyllene, β–cubebene, α–cadinol.

MEDICINAL USES

In many respects Lemonbalm, and the preceding herb, Lavender, share significant attributes. Both belong to the Mint family, both are carminative, and both are mild sedatives.

Lemonbalm is best used as a strong infusion, capsule enclosed essential oil, or spirit. The plant's age–old traditional use is its application to a particular type of dyspepsia ascribed to anxiety and agitation, namely the "nervous stomach". Lemonbalm will benefit individuals who have indigestion or gastritis with nausea or cramps as a result of stress. Most find the plant soothing and sedative.

The plant's relaxant properties are not as strong as some, yet Lemonbalm does make a difference. Its effect on the autonomic nervous system is evidenced by the subtle relaxation that soon occurs after taking the plant. Alone or combined with Wood betony, Lemonbalm makes an excellent tea for the relief of stress–induced headaches. Children usually find the plant's taste agreeable; it is safe for the young and the old alike. A compounded spirit of Lemonbalm can be made by adding equal parts of Nutmeg, Cinnamon, Clove, Lavender, and Lemonbalm essential oils (see Spirit in Preparations). 10–20 drops are taken in a little water. The compound has both calming and carminative properties.

Used undiluted or diluted with a small amount of olive or almond oil. Lemonbalm essential oil will help to resolve HSV (herpes simplex virus) type 1 and 2 outbreaks. To preempt an outbreak apply several times a day upon sensitivity/irritation or use during an outbreak to speed resolution. Lemonbalm tea or the spirit taken internally may have a systemic effect on viral replication, but its potency here has yet to be determined. Regardless its influence will be helpful if stress has been an outbreak trigger. (also see Wormwood for a systemic approach). Chicken pox and shingles' outbreaks also respond to Lemonbalm application.

INDICATIONS
♦ Nervous dyspepsia
♦ Anxiety
♦ Headache, stress–related
♦ Herpes virus group (external and internal)

COLLECTION
Let the plant's taste and smell be a guide to its potency – the stronger, the better. Whether in flower or not, with pruners snip the upper half from the plant. Dry normally. Garble the leaves (and flowers) from the stems. Discard stems due to their lack of oil glands. As long as the dried herb is strong scented it will be an active medication. Lemonbalm, in all forms is commercially available.

PREPARATIONS/DOSAGE
♦ Herb infusion: 4–8 oz. 2–3 times daily
♦ Spirit: 20–40 drops 2–3 times daily
♦ Encapsulated essential oil: 2–4 drops 2–3 times daily
♦ Essential oil: topically as needed

CAUTIONS
None known.

LICORICE
Fabaceae/Pea Family

Glycyrrhiza glabra
Liquorice, Sweet root

DESCRIPTION
Usually 3'–4' in height, Licorice is a deciduous perennial. With both primary stems and secondary branches, the plant is distinctly pea–like with its array of pinnately comprised leaves. A terminal leaflet ends each bunch. They are ovate and petiolate. Flowers are arranged in peduncled axillary spikes; each is pale lavender to violet and about ⅓"–½" long. The mature oblong pod is approximately 1" long and contains 1–6 small kidney shaped seeds. Dense stands occur due to the subterranean stem's ability of sprouting above–ground growth.

DISTRIBUTION
Licorice is indigenous to the Mediterranean region, east to Northern China[28], and overall along the 40th parallel. It is often found growing in abundance where it is occasionally flooded from nearby waterways.

CHEMISTRY
Glycyrrhiza general: licoagrodin, licoagrochalcone b, c, and d, licoagroaurone, licochalcone c, kanzonol y and z, glyinflanin b, glycyrdione a, glabidin, glabranin, glepidotin, pinocembrin, glycyrrhizin, glycyrrhizic acid, glycyrrhetinic acid, dimethoxyhydroxychalone, formononetin, isoliquiritigenin.

MEDICINAL USES
Probably no other herbal medicine and its individual compounds have been researched more than Licorice. Much, but not all, of the plant's influence is due to glycyrrhizin, a triterpenoid saponin, and glycyrrhetinic acid. Over the last 60 years these two compounds[29], used in tandem

28 Glycyrrhiza uralensis or Chinese licorice can be found in western markets, but is more popularly utilized through Traditional Chinese Medicine.
29 Even semisynthetics crafted after them such as car-

or solely, have generated significant interest due to their therapeutic qualities.

As stated elsewhere in this book, it is my intent to expound on whole plants, or their simple concentrations, and how they alter disease or stress states. Framed here, glycyrrhizin and glycyrrhetinic acid work within Licorice as engines, so to speak. Isolated and used in concentrated forms, they essentially become plant–based pharmaceuticals with attending side–effects.

Motivating many of Licorice's effects on seemingly isolated organ systems, is its synergism with the adrenal cortex's corticosteroids, namely aldosterone and cortisol. These particular steroids have numerous influences over the body, hence Licorice's somewhat diverse activity.

Even though most research points in the same direction, specifically how Licorice influences these steroidal departments is still somewhat vague. This is more frustrating for the researcher than the practitioner. One's livelihood is dependant upon the overall picture that Licorice does heal, the other's, why it heals.

How Licorice is proposed to work: the plant inhibits the breakdown of cortisol and aldosterone, allowing endogenous concentrations to effectively linger. Some studies indicate that Licorice directly interacts with cortisol and aldosterone receptor sites, either potentiating these steroids or in some cases, having intrinsic activity of its own. Again the generalities of Licorice we know, the specifics are less clear.

Licorice tea, tincture, or the encapsulated root powder, is an excellent internal moistener and demulcent for irritated mucus membranes. Use it to reduce coughing triggered from irritated bronchial tissue. Most find it useful especially if the cough is dry and troublesome. It combines well with expectorants such as Horehound or Ligusticum.

Dysuria, or painful urination is often curbed as well, be the trouble originating from the kidneys or the bladder. By no means is Licorice significantly antibacterial or a lithotropic agent, but

if there is epithelial irritation, it will be found of benefit.

Wild Licorice (Glycyrrhiza lepidota), see Herbal Medicine of the American Southwest, a plant of the western United States, is better than the variety profiled here, if used when suffering from glomerulonephritis or chronic kidney inflammation. It reduces oxidative stress, inflammation, and subsequent tissue damage from this malady. This activity is largely due to Wild licorice's glabridin content. It is a fact that common Licorice contains this compound as well; the problem in using Licorice in this disturbance though is its other regional effects on the kidneys. The plant's aldosterone synergy proposes a note of caution. Take enough Licorice to reduce inflammation of the area, and that will be enough to affect mineralocorticoids, which could negatively complicate the matter.

Due mainly to its healing influence over gastric and duodenal ulcers, Licorice's effect on the gastrointestinal tract is noteworthy. Through a number of avenues the plant reestablishes normal stomach/duodenal lining. Both mucus secretion and cellular proliferation are stimulated, keeping digestive acids from damaging sensitive gut tissue, and rebuilding what has already been damaged. Licorice increases various prostaglandin concentrations that are responsible for proper gut mucus secretion. The plant's flavonoid content also has a direct topical effect, reducing area inflammation, as well as proving bacteriostatic to Helicobacter pylori, a strain considered a key player in ulcer formation.

As a constitutional medicine the plant fits some individuals superbly. For those who lack proper adrenal cortex functions, not quite Addison's disease, but subclinical tendencies, Licorice will prove valuable. Orthostatic hypotension (dizzy upon quickly standing from a seated position), hypoglycemia, craving for salt (sometimes Licorice for that matter), easily dehydrated and constipated, chronic skin allergies, and greater sensitivity to stressors are just some indications that would suggest Licorice as a valuable tonic.

When using Licorice in this way, do not focus

benoxolone.

on correcting a problem, but on strengthening an area that is weak, or in some cases, sedating an area that is excessive. Everyone has constitutional imbalances – they are the reason why, outside of overt disease, one man must adhere to a strict diet to maintain healthy blood glucose levels, while the other has no problem with hyperglycemia, but is troubled by mild signs of hypothyroidism. Call it genetic predisposition. When a tendency is further influenced by environment, call that illness. If we don't die of infectious disease, accident, or injury, our ripened constitutional imbalances will get us in the end, or at least be a contributing factor. With tonic herbs though we are able to strengthen a dam, instead of plugging leaks.

Topically use Licorice ointment to reduce outbreak and distress from HSV (herpes simplex virus) types –1 and –2 and chicken pox/shingles (varicella–zoster). Internally the plant has little anti–viral activity due to glycyrrhizin's conversion to glycyrrhizic acid in the gut. Injected systemically glycyrrhizin's activity is noteworthy.

INDICATIONS
♦ Cough, with irritated bronchial tissue
♦ Urinary tract irritation
♦ Ulcer, gastric/peptic
♦ Constitutional tonic for adrenal cortex deficiency
♦ Herpes group of viruses (external)

COLLECTION
The plant is extensively cultivated, especially in regions where it naturally flourishes. Both roots and secondary rhizomes are utilized. Glycyrrhiza lepidota, native to North America, is easily collected simply by pulling and following its sub–surface spreading rhizomes. Most species are similar in root morphology.

PREPARATIONS/DOSAGE
♦ DPT (50% alcohol): 10–50 drops 1–3 times daily
♦ Fluidextract: 5–10 drops 1–3 times daily
♦ Root decoction: 2–4 oz. 1–3 times daily
♦ Capsule (00): 1–2, 1–3 times daily
♦ Ointment: as needed

CAUTIONS
Although an occasional cup of tea should not pose a problem, due to the plant's isoflavonoid content unpredictably affecting estrogen and testosterone dynamics, do not use during pregnancy. It is at times used during menopause to alleviate discomforts. Its influence is unpredictable here, some women it helps, some not.

Fluid and sodium retention, hypertension, lowered potassium levels, lethargy, and mental depression are some typical reactions from excessive Licorice use. These effects are due to the plant's synergism with mineralocorticoids. Symptoms quickly disappear once Licorice is discontinued. Do not use Licorice if there is history of cardiovascular or kidney disease, or with any ailment (or pharmaceutical) that may affect sodium or potassium levels.

Incidentally most overdoes of Licorice are due to excessive confectionery consumption. Natural Licorice extract is physiologically active. The quantities needed to develop symptoms of overdoes are large (2–4 oz. daily for a number of days) but certainly possible.

OTHER USES
The plant is used extensively in making Licorice confectioneries; ounce per ounce Licorice extract is many times sweeter than sugar. Each year hundreds of tons of the root are processed for the candy industry, far surpassing world–wide consumption for medical reasons.

LIGUSTICUM
Apiaceae (Umbelliferae)/Carrot Family

Ligusticum porteri
Mountain Lovage, Oshá, Bear root, Colorado cough root, Chuchupate, Raíz de cochino

DESCRIPTION
Ligusticum is a substantial Carrot family peren-

nial. Standing between 1⅔' and 3¼' tall, the plant has a stout stem and is leafy, with large, finely–divided foliage. Leaf blades are between 6" to 12" long; the smaller leaflets are ovate and incised. The white flower clusters form in umbels above the main body of the plant. The mature fruit are oblong, slightly flattened to cylindrical, and ribbed. Ligusticum's roots are distinctive in that they are strongly aromatic with hairy crowns.

Because there are a number of related poisonous plants, some similar in appearance (Poison hemlock) to Ligusticum, positive identification can not stressed more. The following identifier should be applied to Ligusticum, and any other Carrot family plant. It is general but it will at least kept you from making a *really* bad choice. "Vein to the cut, pain in the gut; vein to the tip, everything is hip". Vein refers to leaf vein; pain in the gut, meaning poisonous; cut refers to a trough between outer leaf teeth; tip: leaf tip; hip... good, not poisonous. In my own observations, I have not seen this axiom fail, but I have heard of there being anomalous exceptions to the rule, no surprise when dealing with the natural world. When initially identifying this plant and other Carrot family plants, use several identifiers, as not to make a mistake.

DISTRIBUTION

Truly a western plant, Ligusticum ranges from Wyoming to Colorado, south through Arizona, New Mexico, and into Mexico. Look to the mountains, where Aspen and Conifers are prolific. It is typically not found in the shade of a dense tree canopy, but in the open on slopes and up from stream sides. The plant is a prolific seeder and takes easily to logged and burnt areas. In the Southwest it is found in some of the sky islands, existing in remnant populations.

CHEMISTRY

Phthalide derivatives; furanocoumarins; monoterpenes.

MEDICINAL USES

As a regionally well known medicinal plant, Li-gusticum was a significant article of trade within its class. Used by the Apache, Hopi, Paiute, and Tarahumara, among other tribes, the plant commanded an above–average amount of respect. Due to its strength and stability, Ligusticum traveled well making it a durable trade item. Its appearance outside of its range was somewhat common throughout both prehistoric and historic times.

Ligusticum is firstly a remedy for the respiratory tract. Use the plant to loosen and break up impacted phlegm in beginning–stage bronchitis when the lungs are apt to be hot and dry, or inversely in respiratory afflictions that have left the lungs tired and lax. The timing of Ligusticum is useful, but not imperative. A simple approach is to take the plant from first cough, to the episode's resolution. Chances are this simplistic approach will be more effective than not. If the art form/science of herbalism is to be properly employed then use Ligusticum only when there is a dry cough that is not productive, usually at the start or end of a respiratory infection. If there is accompanying dyspnea or shortness of breath the plant is doubly indicated. Use Ligusticum to energize the area and stimulate expectoration. The plant's array of aromatics are antibacterial as well as antiviral, adding weight to its application of microbial/viral influenced respiratory distresses.

Influenza sufferers will notice a marked improvement after taking the herb even for just a day. Not only is it directly inhibiting to various influenza strains, Ligusticum is helpful in lessening secondary flu symptoms such as, fever, nausea, and aches and pains. It will serve best as a diaphoretic when the skin is dry and the temperate is low to moderate.

Alone, or combined with Yerba mansa (Anemopsis californica), Ligusticum makes a decent gargle for the common sore throat. For strep throat it combines well with Stillingia and White sage. Its anodyne qualities lessen the pain and sensitivity of the area as well. Singers and orators will benefit from Ligusticum's soothing effect on stressed vocal chords. In this case it combines well with Yerba mansa and/or Jack–in–the–pulpit.

In the presence of this element's depletion, Ligusticum has the unique quality of increasing oxygen levels within the blood by nearly 10%. Indicated by its activity, doubtlessly the plant has an influence over alveolar dynamics. Ligusticum will be found of benefit to individuals who suffer from nearly any blood–oxygen deficiency. Emphysema, asthma, and COPD (chronic obstructive pulmonary disease) suffers will especially notice the plant's influence. Another application is to the oxygen depravation of altitude sensitivity and sickness. It is not a cure–all, but the plant makes a difference in that headache and dizziness are lessened when acclimatizing to a higher locale. Climbers or hikers, or anyone involved in athletic activities, at a higher than normal elevation, will benefit from the plant. It will serve as an edge, not a miracle. Little will be noticed if acclimatized and in good cardiovascular shape.

Like other aromatic Carrot family plants, Ligusticum serves as a decent carminative. The tea or tincture is quieting to gas pains. Related fullness and bloating diminishes. Even colicy babies can be given a teaspoon or so of the tea.

Like a mild Angelica in effect, some women will find the plant mildly stimulating to menses. Associated cramping also tends to diminish. It is best used when menses is sluggish or late due to viral infection or climate change.

INDICATIONS

- Bronchitis with dry cough
- Flu with cough and fever
- Pharyngitis
- Vocal cords, stressed
- Emphysema
- Asthma
- COPD
- Altitude sickness

COLLECTION

A distinct spicy–carrot scent should be notable when digging the root; if not, then recheck and make sure the right plant is being harvested, as a mistake with similar looking plants may have dire consequences.

Start about a foot out from the stems arising from the ground, continue around and then down. Mind the tap roots which may travel laterally, as well as vertically. Following a straying tap root can be a chore, but finishing the job properly by collecting the entire root mass reflects favorably upon the wildcrafter. The foliage is of little medicinal value, but can be eaten or cooked with for its carrot–like taste. Gather the plant when it has the least amount of above ground foliage.

Populations throughout the Southwest are disjunct and exist in remnant stands. Many of the "sky island" populations exist fragilely and should not be gathered from. Further north within interior western states Ligusticum is more stable existing in substantial stands.

PREPARATIONS

Wash thoroughly. If drying Ligusticum, split the crown and tap roots length–wise, as to expose larger areas of tissue to the drying effects of air.

DOSAGE

- FPT/DPT (70% alcohol): 30–60 drops 2–3 times daily
- Root infusion (cold or standard): 4–6 oz. 2–3 times daily
- Syrup: 1 teaspoon 3–4 times daily

CAUTIONS

Do not take Ligusticum while pregnant due to the plant's vascular influence of the reproductive environment. Like many medicinal plants some of Ligusticum's constituents will be transferred through breast milk to a nursing baby. For a breast feeding little one with a respiratory infection, having the mother take the plant is an effective way to dose the baby.

Ligusticum's small furanocoumarin content should not pose any type of sun–sensitivity problem. If taking pharmaceuticals that have photosensitizing side effects the addition of Ligusticum may pose an issue, though Umbelliferae such as Heracleum are more problematic.

OTHER USES

The plant seems to be a sort of catnip to bears. They are attracted to the root, which may or may not cause concern to some who are collecting the plant in bear country. Even polar bears, who do not naturally range in the plant's habitat take to the root as if it is in their genetic disposition.[30]

I can not vouch for this but where bears are attracted to the plant, rattlesnakes are repelled by it. If sleeping on the ground, and if concerned with rattlers wanting to bed down with you, try spreading pieces of the dried root around the camp.

LOBELIA

Campanulaceae/Bellflower Family

Lobelia inflata (Rapuntium inflata)
Indian tobacco, Emetic weed, Puke weed

DESCRIPTION

As an annual, Lobelia stands between 8"–2⅔' tall. Herbaceous in nature, the plant's stems are somewhat pubescent, especially on the lower portions. Lobelia's lower elliptic leaves can be sessile or petioled. Upper leaves are sessile, narrow, and smaller than the lower ones. Flowering racemes develop from branch axils. The small, whitish–blue flowers are ¼" long; each calyx is nearly as long as the floral tube. Seed capsules are oval, ¼" in diameter, and contain many small chestnut–brown seeds.

DISTRIBUTION

From the eastern seaboard Lobelia ranges west to Minnesota, Nebraska, and parts of Oklahoma. It is found as far south as Alabama and Georgia. Look to woodlands where there is rich soil and some sun exposure.

CHEMISTRY

Lobeline, lobelidiol, lobinine, isolobinine, isolobinanidine, lobinanidine, lelobanidine, norlelobanidine, norlobelanine, lobelanine, norlobelanidine, lobelanidine, norallosedamine, allosedamine, lobinaline, norlobelol; pyridine alkaloid traces.

MEDICINAL USES

Not many American plants have the distinguished honor of staying in the therapeutic limelight as long as Lobelia. In potency and even mainstream pharmaceutical interest, Lobelia ranks above American ginseng, Echinacea, and Goldenseal. This is due to the plant's interesting and powerful CNS (central nervous system) effects.

Samuel Thomson[31] and Dr. Manasseh Cutler are generally credited with Lobelia's wider introduction, albeit to two opposing systems of medicine. Certainly though the plant had a solid American Indian and folk adherence before gaining in wider status. Following the late 18th and early 19th centuries a rudimentary understanding of Lobelia's chemistry and basic therapeutic activity was ascertained. Lobelia's use as an emetic and bronchial antispasmodic flourished early–on. Its therapeutic nuances were fully explored throughout the mid and latter parts of the 19th century, mainly due to Eclectic and Thomsonian practitioners, and the occasional allopath bucking against the anti–botanical trend.

Purgatives such as Lobelia were in vogue throughout much of western medicine's past. Not only were they used in eliminating ingested toxins but also "cleaning house" in order for oral therapies to have a maximal effect. Unfortunately the use of emetic doses of Lobelia was often taken to the extreme. Poisonings did occur; uncommon, but some proved fatal. Toxic reactions were more apt to occur if the patient did not vomit from the herb, but was left with a large dose of Lobelia within the stomach exerting its CNS effects. The "more is better" approach was

---

30 Ethnobotanist Shawn Sigstedt has conducted some interesting research on bear–Ligusticum interactions. He has clearly documented a number of bear species' attraction to the root.

31 Namesake and founder of the Thomsonian branch of therapeutics: a system of medicine acknowledging the body's vital essence and almost exclusively employing botanical medicines.

as much alive then as it is today, so further un–vomited emetic doses only made a serious situation more grave.

Into the 20th century while whole plant preparations became somewhat dormant, they were replaced by pharmaceutical preparations of lobeline, a chief alkaloid of Lobelia. Beginning in the 1960s researchers turned to Lobelia and its various alkaloids anew, attempting to better understand their nicotine–like structure and effects. As of this writing even pharmaceutical use of Lobeline is considered outdated – although yet again another surge of phyto–pharmaceutical interest is occurring around this Bellflower family plant, mainly in the areas of substance abuse/withdraw and cholinergic/dopaminergic syndromes.

The closest plant/alkaloid set to Lobelia is Tobacco/nicotine. Both plants are strongly acrid if chewed and tend to set off similar physiologic responses: nausea, bronchial expansion, varying sedation/stimulation, etc. Both plants have profound central and peripheral nervous system effects, with Tobacco/nicotine clearly being the better understood of the two. Most likely, if Lobelia was as popular as Tobacco (as a smoking agent), health concerns would be similar. Although the two plants share a core of effects they do have divergent uses and neurochemical influences, as evidenced by specific applications.

Nearly all of Lobelia's activities are dependent on lobeline and related alkaloids. They profoundly affect nAChRs (nicotinic acetylcholine receptors) throughout the central and peripheral nervous systems. The plant's exact influence on neuronal junctures still seems to be an issue of debate, but excitation appears obvious (with some confounding exceptions).

On respiration Lobelia is a profound stimulant, triggering both carotid and aortic bodies, which via the lower brain's respiratory center increases ventilation and bronchial bore. This particular influence has some important ramifications for suffers of oppressive bronchial distresses. When there is a sense of suffocation, shortness of breath, and labored breathing, most

commonly from an asthmatic episode, properly dosed Lobelia will seems nearly miraculous. The ability to breathe more deeply with less constriction is shortly noticed after taking the plant. Its effect on asthmatic inflammation is indirect. Ultimately breathing improves, but not due to a lessening of associated autoimmune reaction. Turmeric for instance, is a better long–term herbal therapy, more closely approaching the core of the matter. But for quick and symptomatic relief, Lobelia has little rival.

When respiration is depressed from alcohol, drug, or pharmaceutical overdose, alcoholic preparations of Lobelia will be quick acting in their stimulation. And in a pinch, the plant's use could prove life–saving. Even when respiration is slowed or impeded from near drowning, electric shock, or smoke/chemical asphyxiation, Lobelia (due to lobeline and related constituents), in the absence of more effective ambulatory therapies, could mean the difference between life and death. It must be stressed that modern medicine has more sophisticated and effective means of dealing with these mentioned traumas, but if I were not breathing due to being struck by lightening, and there was no emergency room nearby, I would want someone to put a couple squirts of Lobelia tincture into my mouth.

Lobelia combines well with Yerba santa for bronchitis with copious phlegm, or with Ligusticum as a stimulating expectorant. Here in combination the dose should be smaller (10–15 drops) than full doses used for more serious issues. Used alone it quickly diminishes a dry hacky cough.

External application over the bronchial/lung region is significant as well. A liniment soaked cloth applied to the area is excellent at reducing pain and sensitivity from pleurisy, bronchitis, and other bronchial inflammations.

For muscular rigidity Lobelia will prove relaxing. Its effect will become evident when used to reduce the intestinal cramps of irritable bowel syndrome, or those of uterine hypertonicity during an especially difficult delivery. Internal use, or even the retained enema are the best applications here. Even ureter/urethra smooth muscle constriction, so evident when passing a kidney stone, is relaxed by Lobelia. A diminishing in the wrap–around flank pain is common with full doses. Soaking in a bath of hot water, while urinating will assist passage as well. Of course it is best not to get to the point of kidney stone development, some of which can be helped by dietary considerations. See Corn silk for a preventative approach.

Excessive CNS discharge resulting in tics and seizure activity is lessened. Even convulsions in children due to fever are reduced. After a full dose, muscular relaxation and a particular calmness of mind is typical. Because of its sedating effect on muscular contraction it was even used to better prepare an area for bone–setting or the alignment of dislocations.

Lobelia is somewhat bipolar in its influence over the heart and related vasculature. Doses generally lower the blood pressure initially, then shortly increase blood pressure. This attribute and others, make Lobelia a better medicine for asthenics, or individuals who have weak circulatory energies.

Where large doses tend to nauseate, small doses (10–15 drops) gently invigorate the gastrointestinal tract. Think of Lobelia's activity as a cholinergic stimulant, activating stomach and intestinal secretions via mucus membrane interaction and nicotinic stimulation[32]. It will be best for individuals who suffer from asecretory indigestion and mild constipation from lack of intestinal and biliary–hepatic secretions, but especially suited for individuals whose digestion is impeded from chronic stress.

As a topical mendicant Lobelia is similar in effects to Tobacco. The continually applied ointment, infusion, or diluted tincture is a tried and true remedy for the rash of Poison ivy/oak exposure. For a variety of painful inflammations, salve, oil, or liniment use will prove relieving. Sport's injuries, contusions, bruises, strains, etc. will all be soothed by external use. Nerve pain from irritation or infection will be found sedated as well. Even the pain and redness/swelling from insect/spider stings and bites will be lessened. The plant does rank among the more reliable topical antiinflammatory/analgesic agents we employ. Lobelia liniment combines well with equal portions of Tobacco liniment.

For some, Lobelia works to curb the physical/mental withdraw symptoms of nicotine/smoking cessation. Although not as handily explained due to shifting models of effect, Lobelia tincture usually has a notable diminishing effect on associated anxiety and craving.

Some interesting work has come out of the University of Kentucky, where it is postulated that lobeline acts as an indirect dopamine antagonist, which has particular interest for abusers of methamphetamines (crystal–meth). Lobeline (or Lobelia) used concurrently with methamphetamines appears to diminish the rewarding effect of this destructive drug.

INDICATIONS

- Asthma (external and internal)
- Breathing, oppressed/labored (external and internal), due to trauma or illness
- Bronchitis, both dry and humid (external and internal)
- Pleurisy/Bronchial inflammation (external)
- Intestinal cramps/Uterine cramps (external and internal)
- Urinary duct cramps with associated kidney stone passage (external and internal)
- Seizures/Convulsions/Muscular rigidity
- Gastrointestinal depression
- Poison ivy/oak rash (external)
- Sport's injuries (external)
- Smoking withdraw
- Methamphetamine abuse

COLLECTION

The whole plant, still verdant, with a mixture

---

32 Somewhat an issue of controversy is Lobelia's, specifically lobeline's, influence over nAChRs. Up until recently Lobelia and its constituents were generally considered medicinally potent due to their specific receptor site interactions. Lately though, with a new series of research, Lobelia's specific effects do not look as certain. Evidence exists showing antagonism as well as agonism, and causative factors completely unrelated to nAChRs.

of flowers and seed capsules makes a fine fresh plant tincture. Collect the entire plant, root and all, and tincture directly. The second method is to gather only seed capsules (August or September). A larger stand of plants in needed for this approach, but a slightly stronger medicine is typically acquired, due to the seed's higher lobeline content. Lobeline content in Lobelia is as follows, ordered highest to lowest: seeds and roots, leaf and flower, and finally stems. Most parts of the plant should be acrid if chewed. Like many other medicinal plants, Lobelia will be most potent if collected and prepared first hand.

PREPARATIONS

With the exception of the seeds, dried Lobelia, commercially purchased, or preparations made from poor source material will be of inferior quality. Although the ingested powder or herb infusion will still be found nauseating, many valuable secondary effects will be lacking. The fresh plant tincture (entire plant) or the dried plant tincture of the seeds are the most potent preparations.

DOSAGE

Due to Lobelia being a "little drug"[33] extra care must be given when using or dispensing this botanical. Dosing ranges can be broken down into two distinct categories.

1. Full dose: Lung centered uses/Spasmolytic uses/Substance issues. Nauseant effects are used as a dosing gauge. A dose that excites nausea will be effective for these more weighty issues. Full doses should *not* induce vomiting. FPT/DPT: 20–30 drops per dose.
2. Tonic dose: Gastrointestinal stimulation/Mild CNS relaxant properties: No or little nausea should be experienced. FPT/DPT: 5–10 drops per dose.

♦ FPT of whole plant (1:4)/DPT of seed (1:10

33 "Little drug" meaning a plant having very potent or distinctly acute uses, with corresponding dangers, essentially analogues to modern–day pharmaceuticals. Lobelia, Aconitum, Datura, and Gelsemium are some examples.

50% alcohol): 20–30 drops 2–3 times daily (Full dose)
♦ FPT of whole plant (1:4)/DPT of seed (1:10 50% alcohol): 5–10 drops 2–3 times daily (Tonic dose)
♦ External preparations: apply as needed

CAUTIONS

Nausea, dizziness, and mild hypertension are common with stronger doses. Proceed with caution when combining Lobelia with pharmaceutically controlled nAChR or dopamine related CNS issues. It may either aggravate or help. Do not use while pregnant or while nursing.

Concerning external applications, remember surface area plus duration equals internal dose. The skin is absorptive. Any poultice used long enough will affect the internal environment[34].

MARSHMALLOW
Malvaceae/Mallow Family

Althaea officinalis
Common marshmallow

DESCRIPTION

Marshmallow is a large, leafy perennial. The whole plant is covered by a fine coating of pubescence hairs, making it soft and velvety to the touch. The plant's branched stems give rise to numerous, large, 3–lobed, ovate leaves; margins are irregularly serrate. The 5–petaled, pink–rose flowers form in clusters and are approximately 1"–2" wide.

DISTRIBUTION

Originally from Eurasia, Marshmallow is now found throughout much of the eastern and central portions of the United States. It is widely cultivated, both as an ornamental and for the root's commercial value. It is found as an escapee along borders of low–lying marshy areas.

34 French herbalist Maurice Mességué almost solely used external applications in treating his clientele.

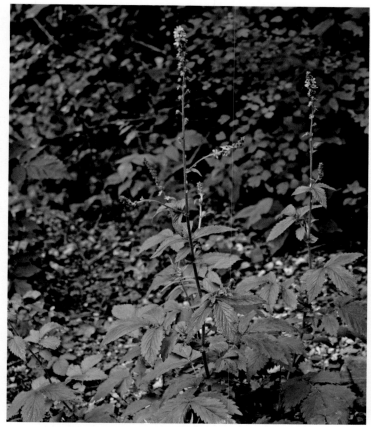
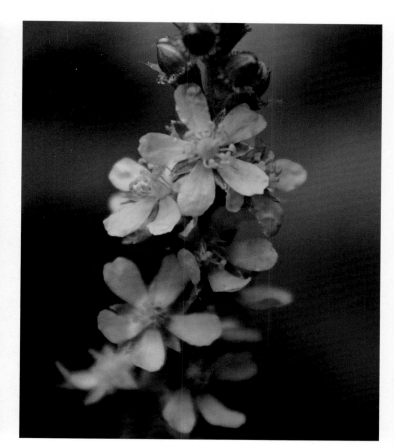

1. and 2. **Agrimony** (*Agrimonia striata*)

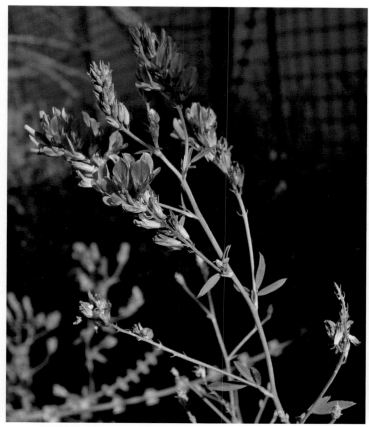

3. **Alfalfa** (*Medicago sativa*)

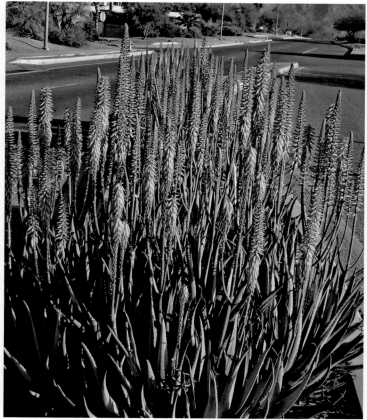

4. *Aloe vera*

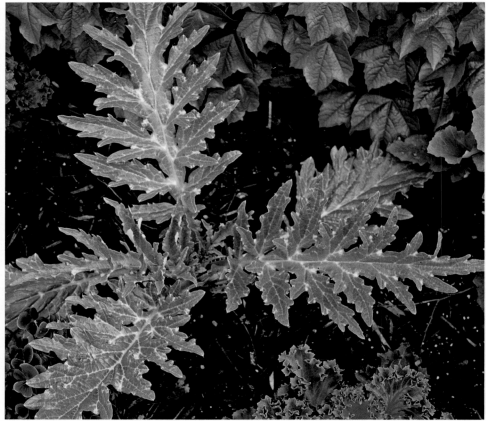

5. **Artichoke** *(Cynara scolymus)*

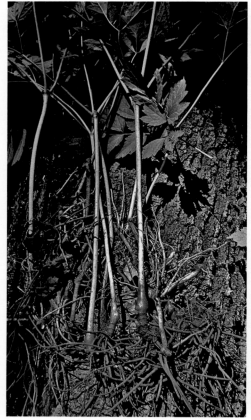

6. **Black Cohosh** *(Actaea racemosa)*

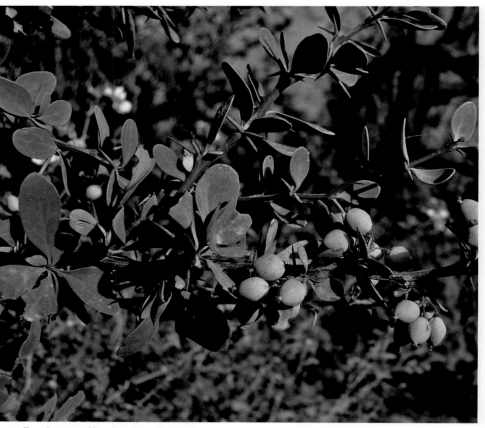

7. **Black Cohosh** *(Actaea racemosa)*

8. **Barberry** *(Berberis vulgaris)*

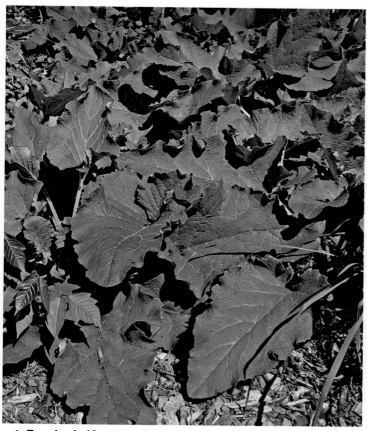

9. **Burdock** (*Arctium lappa*)

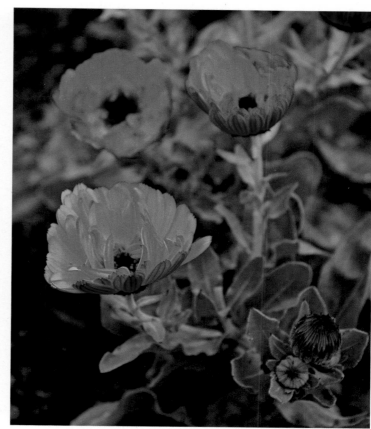

10. **Calendula** (*Calendula officinalis*)

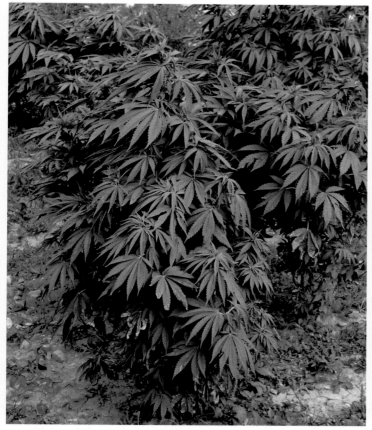

11. **Cannabis** (*Cannabis spp.*) Taken in Afghanistan.

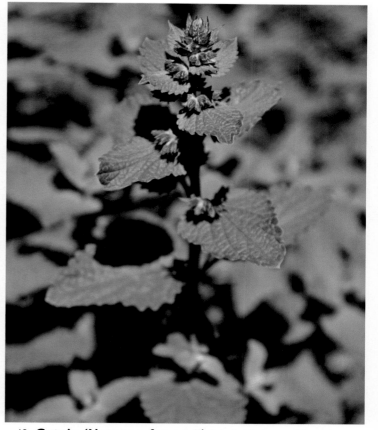

12. **Catnip** (*Nepeta x faassenii*) A hybrid pictured here.

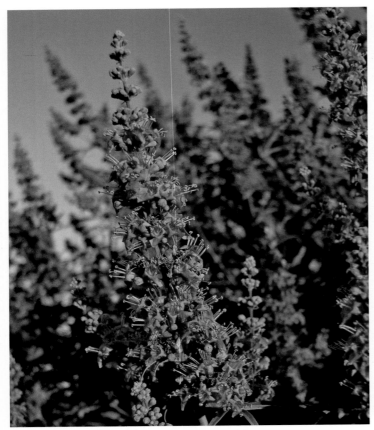

13. **Chaste Tree** *(Vitex agnus–castus)*

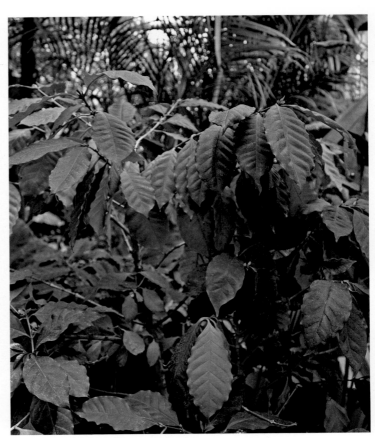

14. **Coffee** *(Coffea arabica)*

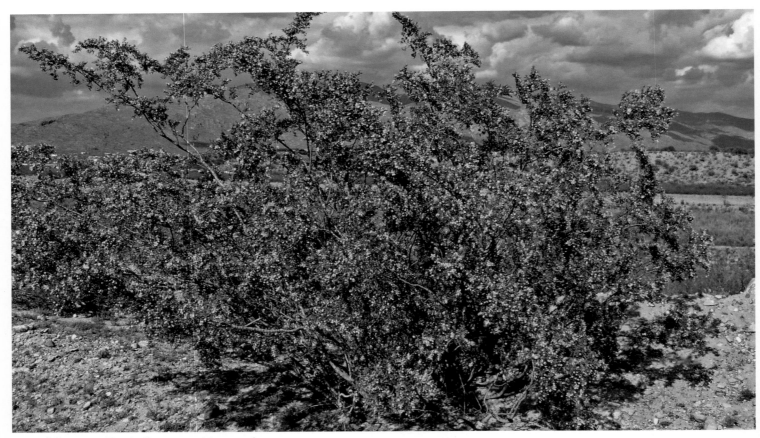

15. **Creosote Bush** *(Larrea tridentata)*

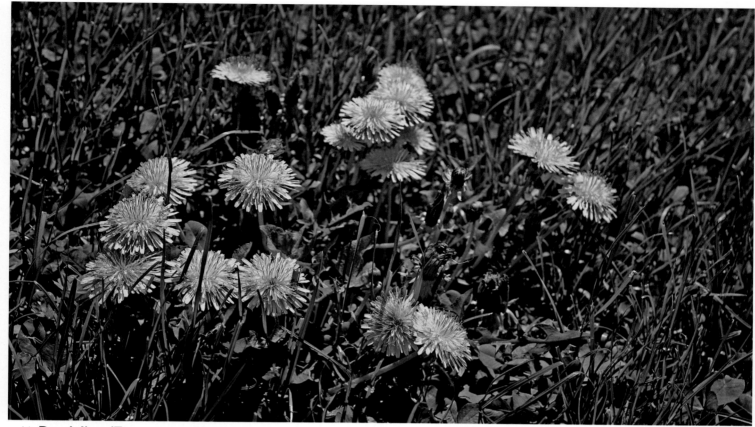

16. **Dandelion** *(Taraxacum officinale)*

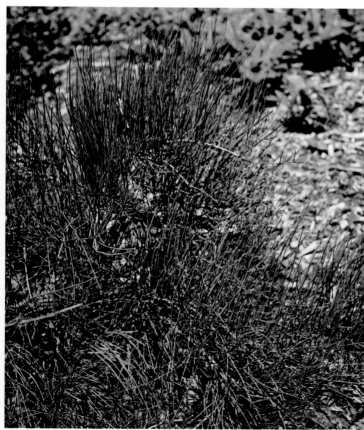

17. **Ephedra** *(Ephedra equisetina)* Another Chinese variety
known as Ma huang.

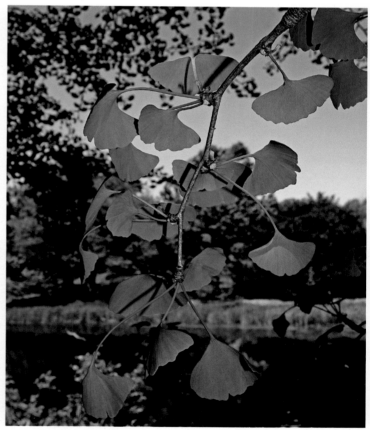

18. *Ginkgo biloba*

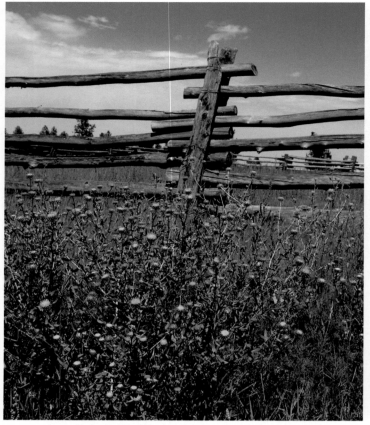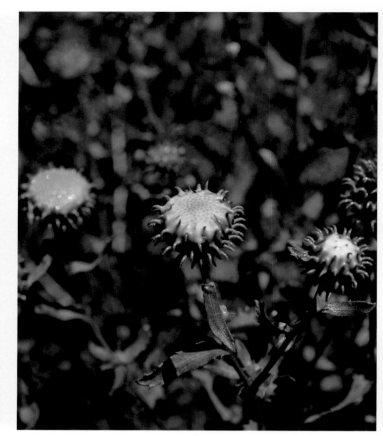

19. and 20. **Grindelia** *(Grindelia nuda var. aphanactis)*

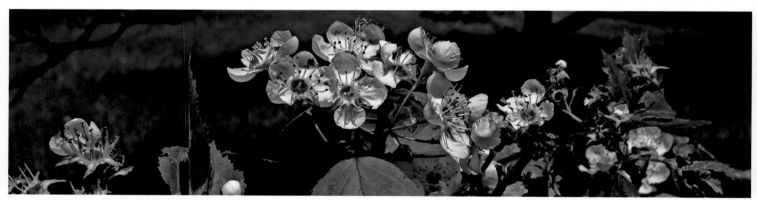

21. **Hawthorn** *(Crataegus dilatata)*

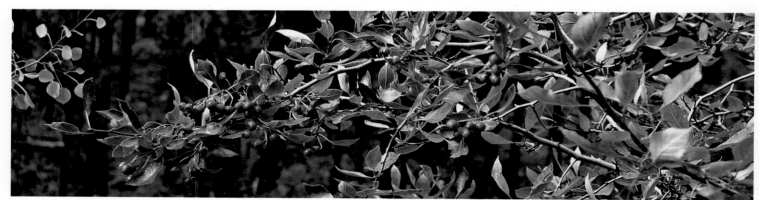

22. **Hawthorn** *(Crataegus rivularis)*

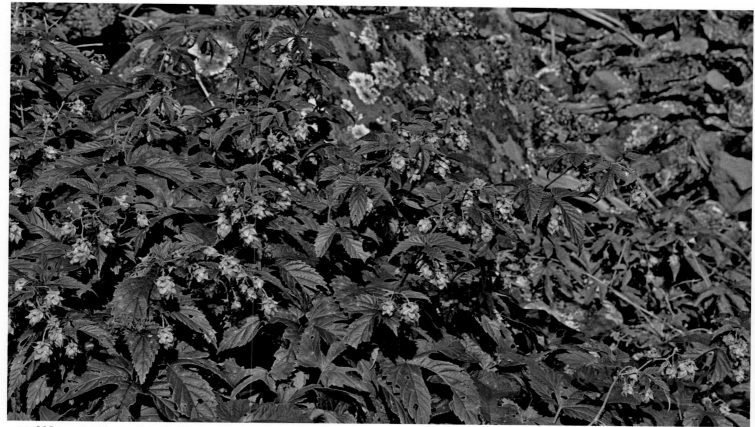

23. **Western Hops** *(Humulus lupulus var. neomexicanus)*

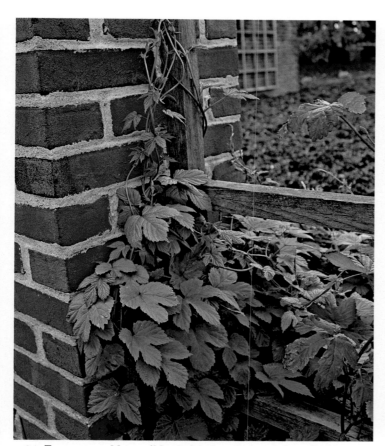

24. **European Hops** *(Humulus lupulus var. lupulus)*

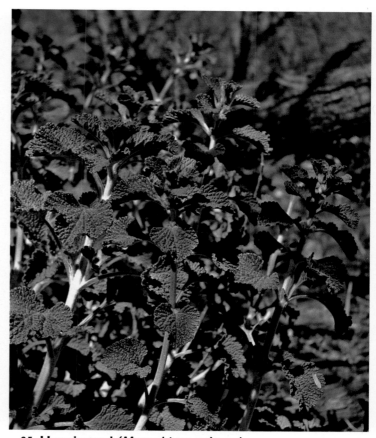

25. **Horehound** *(Marrubium vulgare)*

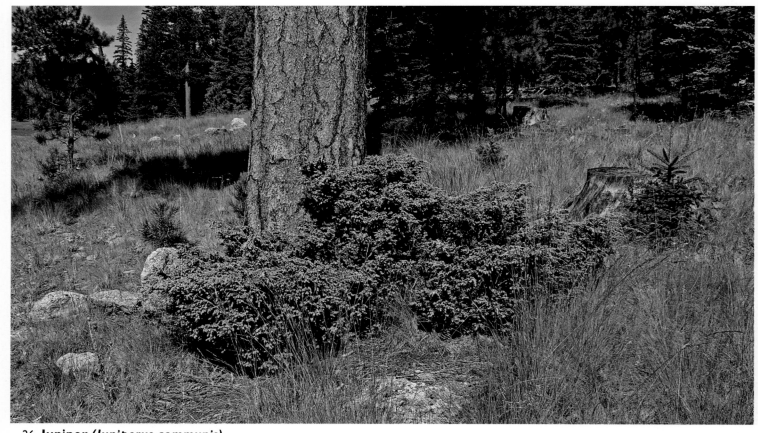

26. **Juniper** (*Juniperus communis*)

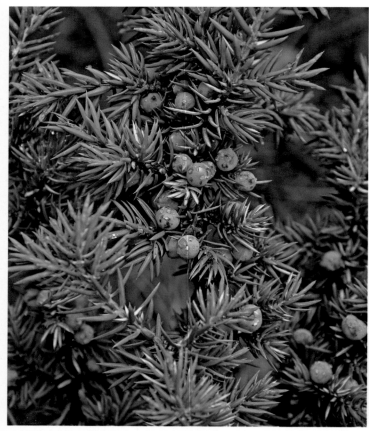

27. **Juniper** (*Juniperus communis*)

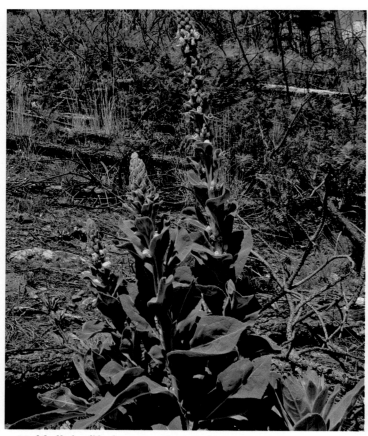

28. **Mullein** (*Verbascum thapsus*)

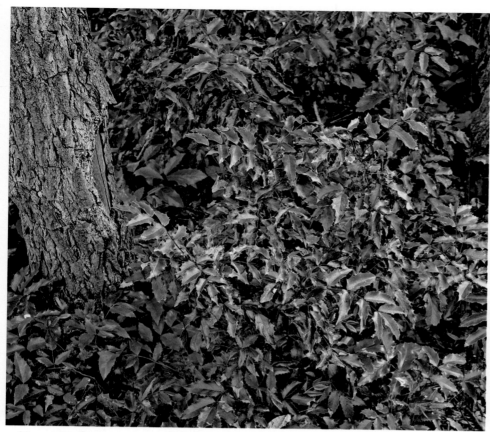
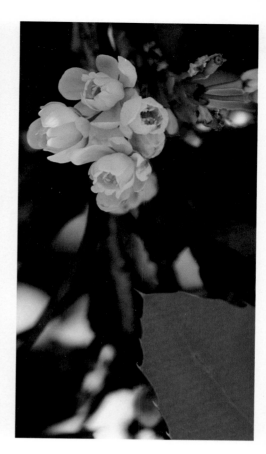

29. and 30. **Oregongrape** (*Mahonia aquifolium*)

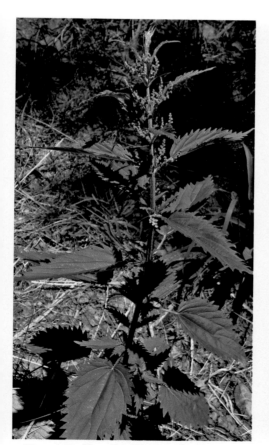
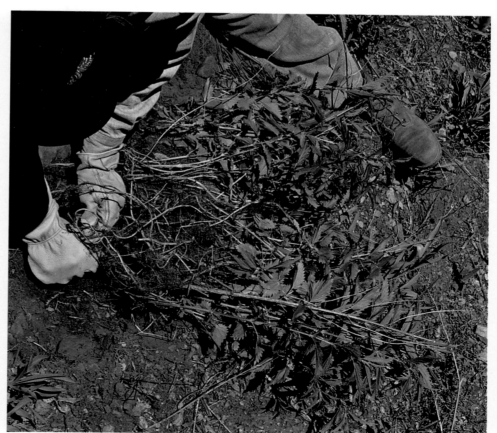

31. and 32. **Nettle** (*Urtica dioica ssp. gracilis*)

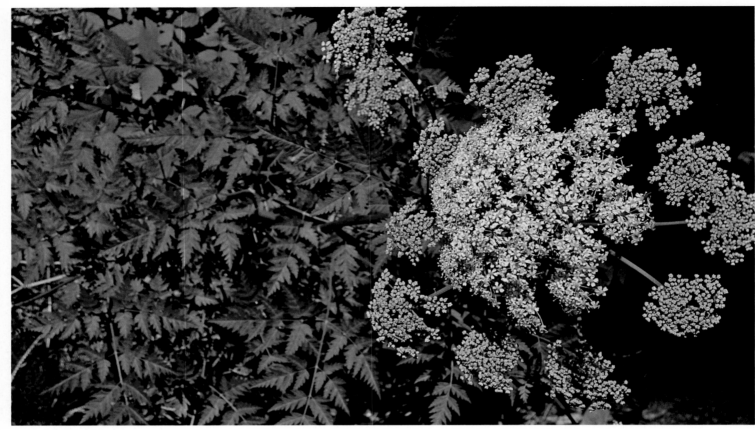

33. *Ligusticum porteri*

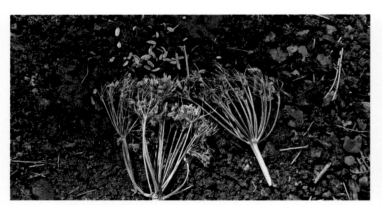

34. and 35. *Ligusticum porteri*
Seeds and seedlings (below).

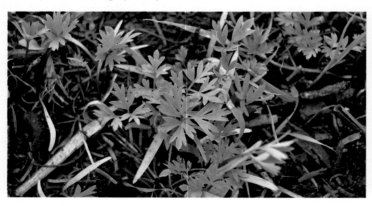

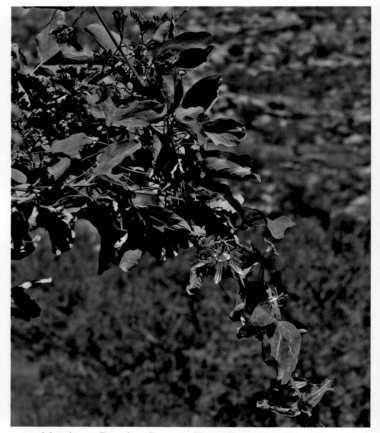

36. **Mexican Passionflower (*Passiflora mexicana*)**
Common to parts of the Southwestern U.S. this variety of Passionflower is interchangeable with more popularly used *Passiflora incarnata*.

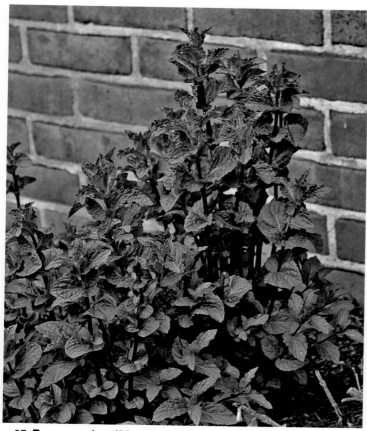

37. **Peppermint** *(Mentha piperita)*

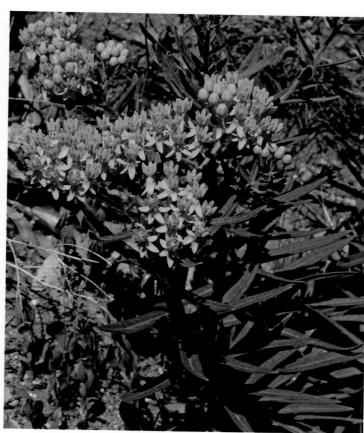

38. **Pleurisy Root** *(Asclepias tuberosa)*

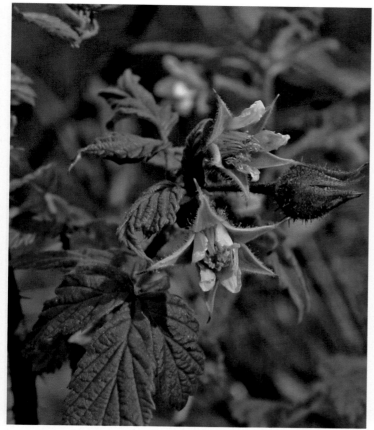

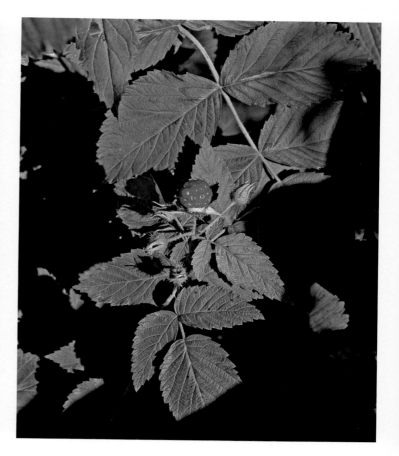

39. and 40. **Red Raspberry** *(Rubus idaeus)*

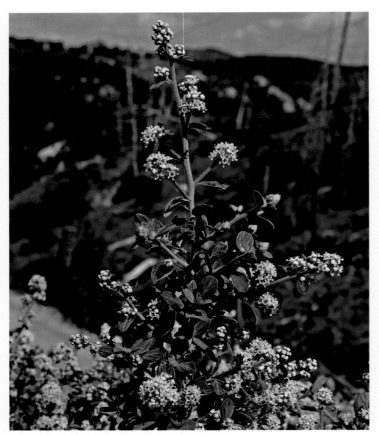

41. **Red Root** *(Ceanothus fendleri)*

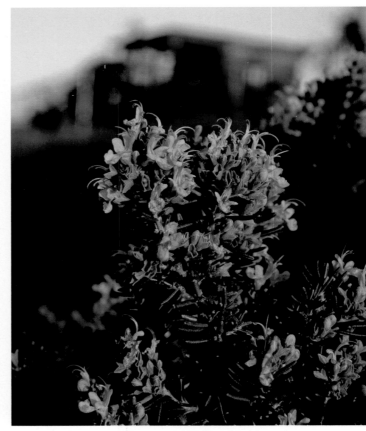

42. **Rosemary** *(Rosmarinus officinalis)*

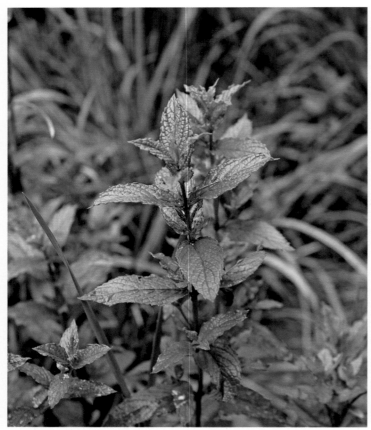

43. **Spearmint** *(Mentha spicata)*

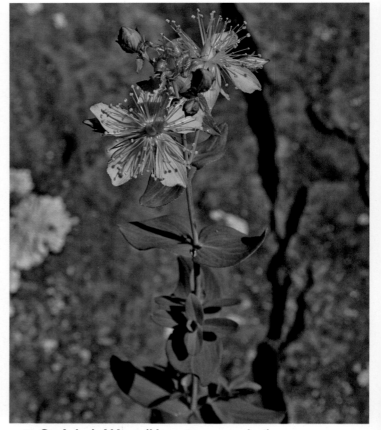

44. **St. John's Wort** *(Hypericum scouleri)*

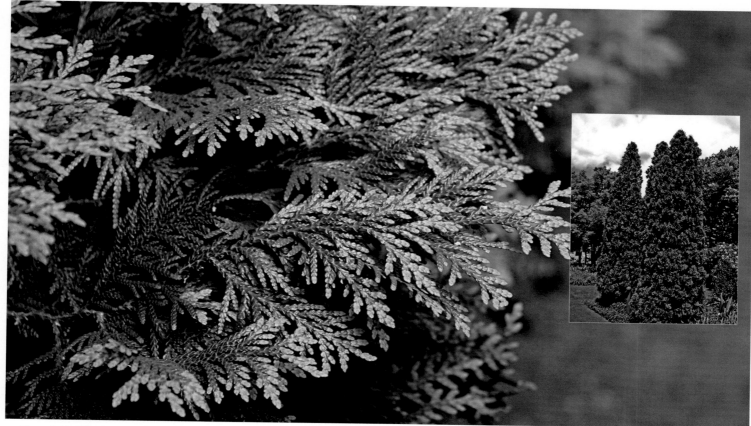

45. and 46. *Thuja occidentalis*

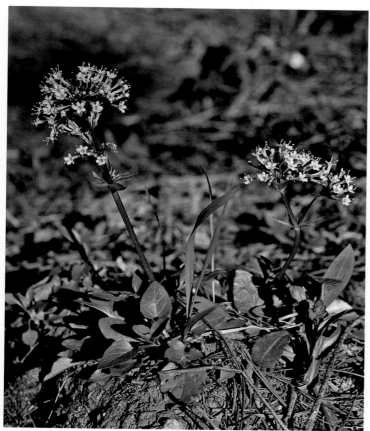

47. **Valerian (*Valeriana arizonica*)** Another medicinal variety common throughout Arizona and New Mexico.

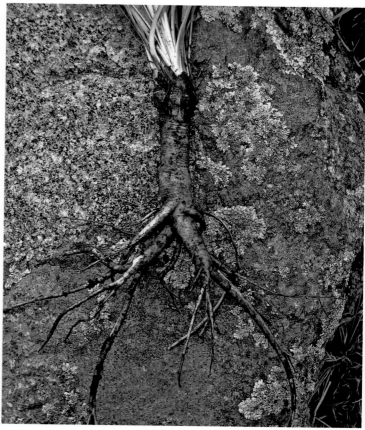

48. **Valerian (*Valeriana edulis*)**

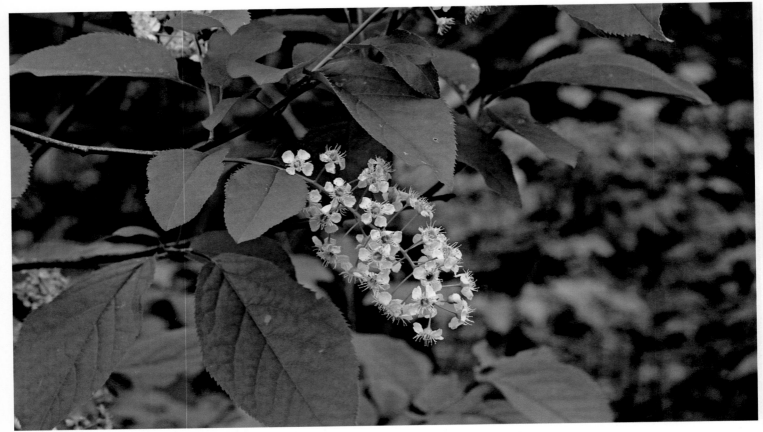

49. **Wild Cherry** *(Prunus virginiana)*

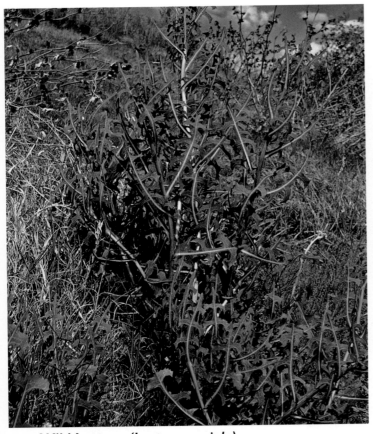

50. **Wild Lettuce** *(Lactuca serriola)*

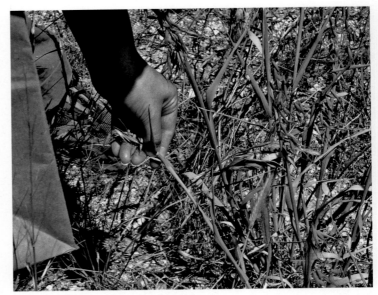

51. **Wild Oats** *(Avena fatua)*

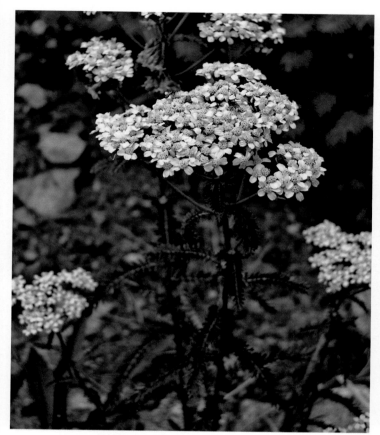

52. **Yarrow** *(Achillea lanulosa)*

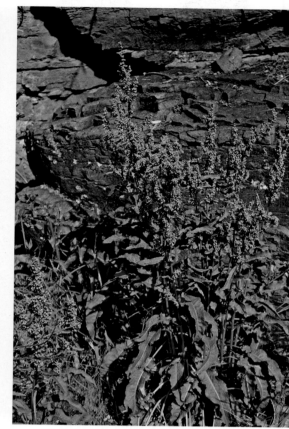

53. **Yellowdock** *(Rumex crispus)*

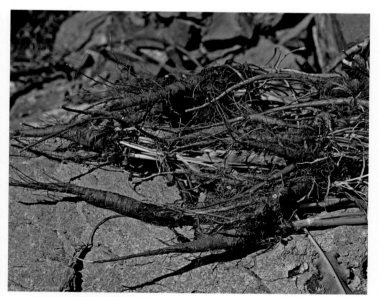

54. **Yellowdock** *(Rumex crispus)*

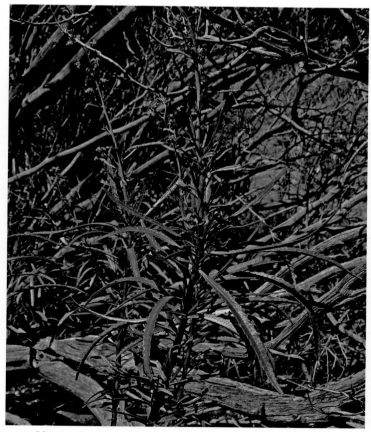

55. **Yerba Santa** *(Eriodictyon angustifolium)*

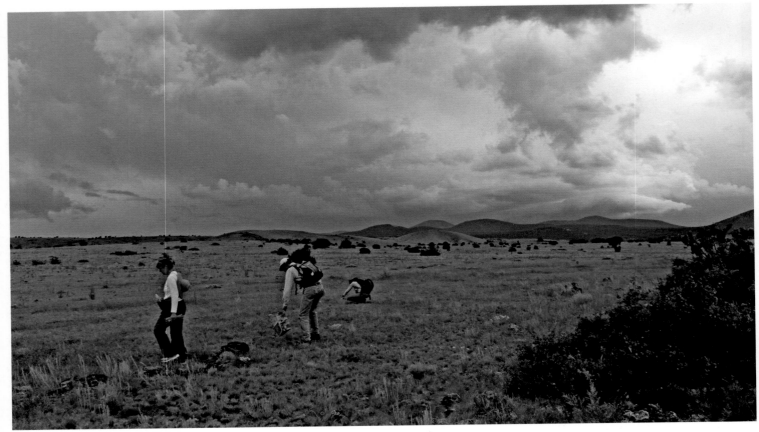

56. Collecting *Artemisia frigida*

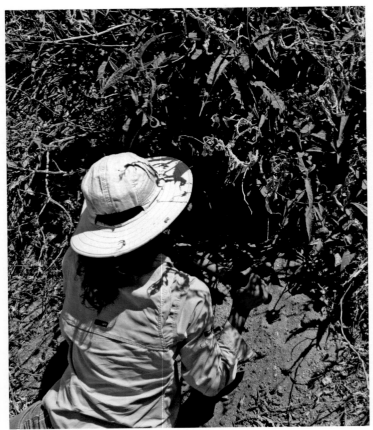

57. Digging for Canyon bursage (*Ambrosia ambrosioides*)

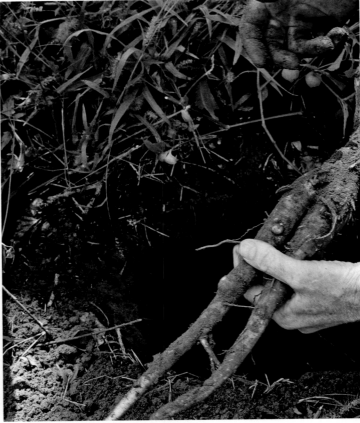

58. Poke root (*Phytolacca americana*)

CHEMISTRY

Polysaccharides: arabinogalactans, galacturonorhamnans; flavonoids; phenolic acids.

MEDICINAL USES

As the most prominent Mallow in therapeutic use today, and in past times as well, Marshmallow's reputation is deserved. The tea holds influence over the urinary tract. Its use is indicated for most irritations of the area. For the pain and inflammation that accompanies cystitis, urethritis, and nephritis, Marshmallow is specific.

The plant does little for an active urinary infection, for its direct bacteriostatic properties are negligible, but in combination with most antimicrobial herbs, such as Heath and Cypress family plants, it will prove effective for both the pain and the infection. Marshmallow also enables antimicrobial therapies to be taken longer without unwanted kidney irritation.

The tea encourages urinary stone breakdown, and is soothing to the tissue irritation that accompanies their presence and passage. Regardless of the stone's composition the tea will be of value. Certainly though acid–based kidney stones are the easier type to break up with internal therapies. Marshmallow combines well with Gravel root. In fact I have seen the combination make operating procedures unnecessary through its ability of breaking up gravel and encouraging its passage.

Surface mucus membranes of the oral region are soothed by the tea. As a gargle, sore throats, be them due to vocal strain or common cold, are soothed. Used solely as a base, the tea made into a syrup is an excellent cough remedy.

In ulcerative/irritable conditions of the stomach and intestines, liberal use of the tea or encapsulated power will be found healing to epithelial tissues. Use Marshmallow if suffering from any type of gastric/peptic ulcer. For intestinal irritation, oral use of Marshmallow will have a marginal effect, due to the gut's digestion and assimilation of the plant's mucilage and starch. Essentially the body will digest Marshmallow before it reaches the large intestine. An enema made from the tea will have the strongest effect on any irritative condition of the area – combine this with the oral use of 2–3 cups of Mugwort/Wormwood tea daily.

Topically the tea is a soothing emollient for the skin. It is healing to rashes, burns, and other similar afflictions. As a douche it is quieting to inflamed vaginal and cervical tissues. If there is bacterial involvement it combines well with Goldenseal, Bayberry, or Oregongrape. The powdered root makes as excellent poultice base for bringing abscesses to a head. The preparation's drawing power is largely dependant upon its ability to stimulate tissue immunity/white blood cells activity[35]. The addition of Echinacea, Astragalus, or Wild indigo to the mixture will dramatically increase the poultice's effectiveness.

INDICATIONS

- ♦ Cystitis/Urethritis/Nephritis
- ♦ Kidney stones/Urinary gravel
- ♦ Sore throat
- ♦ Cough, from irritation
- ♦ Ulcer, gastric/peptic
- ♦ Diarrhea with irritation
- ♦ Skin rashes/Burns (external)
- ♦ Abscesses, topical (external)

COLLECTION

After digging Marshmallow's mucilaginous roots, cut lengthwise and dry in a well ventilated area. If living in a humid environment a dehydrator may be necessary in order to inhibit microbial growth.

The flowers and leaves also make a fine tea for what the root is indicated for. Not quite as strong, but nonetheless if herbaceous material is all that is available, its use will be beneficial.

PREPARATIONS

Marshmallow tea serves as an excellent cough syrup base. Once the Marshmallow–based syrup is made various tinctures or fluidextracts can be

---

35 Marshmallow, like nearly all Mallow family plants, due to its particular polysaccharide/starch arrangement is mildly stimulating to innate immunity.

added to impart other medicinal influences.

To make a base Marshmallow syrup simply follow the instruction under Syrup (Syrup, simple) in the Preparations section. Instead of using water as the base, use the same amount of Marshmallow tea.

DOSAGE

- ◆ Root infusion: 4–8 oz. as needed
- ◆ Capsule (00): 2–3, 3 times daily
- ◆ Douche: 2–3 times daily
- ◆ Moistened powder for poultice

CAUTIONS
None.

OTHER USES
Although little used today, in the past Marshmallow powder was used as the thickening agent in the confectionery industry. The plant was one of the main ingredients in "marshmallows".

It still is occasionally used as a thickening/ binding/filling agent in making tablets and lozenges (certainly here its purpose is two–fold: as a thickening and medicinal agent).

MATÉ

Aquifoliaceae/Holly Family

Ilex paraguayensis
Yerba maté, Paraguay tea

DESCRIPTION
An evergreen small tree to large bush, Maté's waxy–green leaves are 3"–5½" long by 1"–2" wide. Obovate to obovate–oblong, each has a prominent midvein and serrated margins. Flowers are greenish–white and 4–petaled. The mature fruit is a red drupe and a ½" in diameter.

DISTRIBUTION
Maté ranges throughout Brazil, Paraguay, Uruguay, and Argentina, often along streams. Most Maté plantations are within its native range.

CHEMISTRY
Xanthines: caffeine, theobromine, theophylline; phenols: caffeoylquinic acid, dicaffeic acid, coumaroylquinic acid, feruloylquinic acid, quercetin, rutin, kaempferol, caffeoylferuloylquinic acid, tricaffeoylquinic acid; volatiles: furfural, α–pinene, benzaldehyde, myrcene, limonene, linalool, α–terpineol, methyl salicylate, n–decanal, geraniol, geranyl acetone, longicamphenylone, (e)–nerolidol, heptadecane, methyl hexadecanoate, n–heneicosane, n–tricosane.

MEDICINAL USES
As popular as Tea and Coffee is in the United States, Maté is the energizing beverage of choice throughout parts of South America, particularly Brazil, Argentina, and Paraguay. The plant has several interrelated effects which makes its use as a CNS (central nervous system) stimulant multifaceted.

First, Maté contains between 1%–2% caffeine and lesser amounts of related theobromine and theophylline, making it a pronounced caffeine–type stimulant. Although containing less than Guaraná's 5%–6%, Maté's particular array of xanthines are definitely cerebrally energizing. The plant's muted effects on the skeletal–muscular system makes it a useful conversational beverage as well as a study–aid.

The plant's antioxidant quality is substantial. Through an array of phenolic compounds, Maté's free radical quenching activity makes an impact on myocardial and related tissue. Maté just may be the best caffeine–beverage plant for individuals with cardiovascular afflictions. Cellular integrity of the heart is kept more intact making base functions more efficient and less prone to oxygen deficiency. A gentle stabilization occurs with daily use of the tea.

Suffers of hayfever and head–centered allergic response will see effects with Maté. Surely its membrane stabilizing influences are responsible here. Cellular inflammation is reduced and cell wall integrity is preserved, minimizing rhinitis symptoms.

Like Nettle root, Maté is an aromatase inhibitor, making it a specific beverage tea for suffers of estrogen–dependant reproductive cancers, including some forms of breast and prostrate cancer. Even older men afflicted with BPH (benign prostrate hypertrophy) should notice some result. Suffers are recommended to switch from Coffee and Tea (even Green tea) to Maté.

Habitual Coffee drinkers wanting to change to Maté will find its mild choleretic effects relieving to coffee–withdraw constipation. As a biliary stimulant more bile is released from the gall bladder to the small intestine, providing a mild laxative effect.

INDICATIONS

- ♦ As a cerebral stimulant
- ♦ As a cellular antioxidant
- ♦ Supportive tea for estrogen–dependant cancers
- ♦ Benign prostrate hypertrophy

COLLECTION

Gather Maté's leaves and dry for tea. Most commercial material comes from plantation stock. In the wild the tree is collected from for individual, family, and local use.

PREPARATIONS

"Green" Maté, oven–dried without excessive heat, accounts for most of the commercial material. The roasted or toasted form – dried as well as "smoked" – is more commonly found along coastal regions of Brazil. More Coffee–like in taste, it is often sweetened or mixed with other juices, or used as a base in several local soft–drinks.

Toasted Maté maintains its phenolic constituents well. Throughout the heating process some are catalyzed, but overall antioxidant activity remains consistent with "green" Maté.

DOSAGE

- ♦ Herb infusion: 6–8 oz. 2–3 times daily

CAUTIONS

Like any caffeine containing plant excessive amounts may cause anxiety, restlessness, and insomnia. Individuals with moderate to severe hypertension should not use Maté.

OTHER USES

A fairly good source of soluble electrolytes, mixed with fruit juice Maté makes a refreshing replacement drink.

A related holly, Ilex vomitoria, native to the southeastern part of the United States, has a similar caffeine content. Its use as an indigenous stimulant looks promising, and unlike its name – vomitoria – it does not cause vomiting.

MILK THISTLE
Asteraceae/Sunflower Family

Silybum marianum (Carduus marianus)
Marian thistle

DESCRIPTION

Milk thistle is a biannual (or annual depending on climate) and like most other thistles its leaves are basal, clasping, lobed to pinnatifid, and spine–tipped. The plant is aptly named after its most distinctive feature – white leaf veins and blotches of the same color. The stalk–borne, large flower heads are ¾"–2⅓" in diameter. Below the purple inflorescence are spreading phyllaries.

DISTRIBUTION

Milk thistle is native to the Mediterranean region. Throughout the United States it has naturalized extensively and is even considered a weed in many areas. The plant is found in disturbed soils, crop lands, and pastures.

CHEMISTRY

Silymarin containing flavonolignans: silybin, isosilybin, silychristin, silydianin.

MEDICINAL USES

Milk thistle, once known as a bitter tonic and chologogue, now is in the spotlight as one of the more popular medicinal plants used today. This happened with the discovery of silymarin and related constituents and their subsequent application to hepatoxic conditions. Like St. John's wort, Echinacea, and Garlic, the literature on Milk thistle has grown so voluminous, that even the most jaded skeptic must admit the plant is therapeutic. Herbs like Turmeric, Artichoke, and Dandelion share Milk thistle's potency, but chance would have kindly Milk thistle in the forefront.

Milk thistle is the premiere hepatoprotective herb used today. For suffers of hepatitis, particularly hepatitis C, Milk thistle will serve as a valuable botanical therapy. With consistent supplementation, elevated GOT (glutamic–oxaloacetic transaminase) and GPT (glutamic–pyruvic transaminase), both enzymatic markers of liver distress, typically are lowered. Serum bilirubin levels show improvement as well. Chronic conditions are more apt to show betterment than acute flare–ups, making the plant one of a number of choice herbs to use in chronic hepatitis.

Cirrhosis of the liver and fatty liver, whether alcohol related or not, will tend to show improvement under Milk thistle's influence. Here again, enzymatic markers of liver disease are lowered, as is fibrosis activity and insulin resistance. In advanced cases, Milk thistle has been shown to add years before liver failure.

Liver damage from solvents, heavy metals, paints, glues, or nearly any other chemical exposure will be lessened by the plant. Subjective symptoms, such as referred hepatic pain and itchy skin and eyes, tend to also respond. The length and severity of exposure will determine the benefit Milk thistle has on the situation.

Intravenous use of silybin, one of Milk thistle's main flavonolignans, in combination with the usual pharmaceutical regime for Death cap mushroom (Amanita phalloides) poisoning has shown more successful results than just pharmaceuticals alone. The addition of silybin significantly reduces mortality and enhances general recovery from this life–threatening poisoning. Although Milk thistle's bioavailability is nearly cut in half when taken orally (as opposed to

intravenously), take it if there is a situation of mushroom poisoning until regular medical attention is given, and even here joint use of Milk thistle will prove beneficial.

For type II diabetics the seed powder taken several times a day is useful in reducing blood sugar levels. With proper diet and exercise the combination is an effective regiment often able to replace conventional hypoglycemic agents. Likewise elevated LDL–cholesterol and triglyceride levels lower with the seed.

Milk thistle, particularly silymarin, has a substantial chemoprotective/anti–cancer effect, not only for liver centered carcinomas, but body–wide. Numerous cancer cell–lines, are inhibited by the extract, making it a worthy supplement in these situations. As a cellular–protectant against the sickening effects of conventional chemotherapy, Milk thistle and related compounds are beneficial. Particularly in childhood leukemia, it has shown tremendous success in limiting liver toxicities that occur with conventional drugs.

Used both topically and internally Milk thistle moderates the damage from ultraviolet light exposure. Keratinocytes and other skin cells, sensitive to UV rays, are protected from the oxidative stress that normally occurs with exposure. Use Milk thistle both as a skin cancer preventative and to promote healing of already–damaged skin. Both sun and heat burns will heal faster and exhibit less trauma with the plant's application.

As an antioxidant Milk thistle works on a number of fronts. It significantly increases intracellular stores of glutathione. This influence alone makes Milk thistle a broadly acting and powerful free radical scavenger.

The plant's more prosaic uses are similar to Dandelion's. Meaning Milk thistle is a useful bitter tonic and chologogue. Taken before meals it will enhance digestive powers. As a bile stimulant it provides a mild laxative effect, and as importantly, it facilitates lipid breakdown and assimilation.

INDICATIONS

- Hepatitis
- Cirrhosis of the liver
- Fatty liver
- Liver damage, chemical/mushroom
- Hyperglycemia
- LDL–cholesterol/Triglyceride levels, elevated
- Cancer, as a preventative
- Skin damage, UV (external and internal)
- Burns, both sun and heat (external and internal)
- Indigestion
- Poor protein–fat digestion

COLLECTION

After the flower heads have gone to seed, cut and dry whole. With gloved hands work the seeds from the dry involucre.

Good quality organic Milk thistle seed is readily available at natural food stores and through mail–order. Purchasing the seed certainly is an easier route than processing it by hand and realistically the quality will not be much different.

PREPARATIONS

The powdered seed, be it in capsule form or simply mixed into juice or water is the preferred way to take the plant. I recommend purchasing the whole seed, which is stable, and powdering it as needed (a coffee grinder or blender works well here). Tinctures will have some affect, but they, unlike solid preparations, will be diffused systemically. Elimination via the digestive tract/ liver is paramount to Milk thistle's effectiveness, hence the focus on the powdered seed.

Standardized Milk thistle is of course useful, but good quality, whole, Milk thistle seed is still prime. For topical application the fluidextract can be used as a liniment.

DOSAGE

- Capsule (oo): 2–3, 2–3 times daily
- Powdered seed: 1–2 teaspoons 2–3 times daily
- Fluidextract (60% alcohol): 20–40 drops 2–3 times daily
- Liniment/Ointment: as needed

CAUTIONS

Although reports of Milk thistle toxicity are virtually nonexistent, it is possible excessive amounts may cause liver tenderness and nausea. It is also possible Milk thistle may alter pharmaceutical metabolism, so proper dosing may become as issue if used together.

MOTHERWORT
Lamiaceae/Mint Family

Leonurus cardiaca
Lion's tail, Heartwort

DESCRIPTION

This herbaceous biannual or short–lived perennial stands several feet in height. The whole plant is occasionally covered by a very fine pubescence. This is often determined by the locale in which the plant grows – the greater the sun's intensity, the more likely small hairs will be present. Like other Mint family plants, Motherwort's stems are square and its leaves are conspicuously arranged in an opposite pattern.

If there is to be just one prominent characteristic distinguishing this plant from other similar types, it is the large multi–cleft leaves. Upper leaves tend to be smaller and 3–cleft, while the lower ones are 3 to 5 parted, larger, becoming broadly ovate. Flowers form in axillary clusters. The 2–lipped corollas are usually pink, but can be pale–purple to nearly white. They are densely hairy, especially on the back of the upper lip.

DISTRIBUTION

As a native to Eurasia, the plant is extensively naturalized in this country. Temperate regions are the plant's predominate niche, particularly where there is soil disruption. If it is not found self–propagated, it is effortlessly grown, sometimes as a bedding plant.

CHEMISTRY

Diterpenes; volatiles: α–pinene, β–caryophyllene, α–humulene, germacrene–d, caryophyllene oxide, humulene epoxide, n–heptadecane, trimetilpentadecanone–2, dibutyl phthalate, n–octadecane, n–nonadecane, phytol, n–eicosane, n–heneicosane, n–docasane, n–tricosane, n–tetracosane.

MEDICINAL USES

Motherwort is an example of a plant that best fits constitutional types, or physiological personalities, as opposed to outright problems. Unlike related plants, such as Lycopus, which act more strongly to change the body's direction, Motherwort subtly changes certain tendencies. Although the plant affects both men and women, the fairer sex will benefit most from Motherwort usage.

It best fits women who are underweight and emotionally unbalanced largely because of external life stresses. If sleep is problematic, and there is anxiety and restless, particularly in the days preceding the onset of menses, Motherwort will prove relaxing. It is specific for women with long cycles, who have breast tenderness, painful or sluggish onset of menses, and possible heart palpitations during this time of month (or when stressed).

Use the plant if there is a particular central nervous system over–excitability resulting in nerve pain, spasm, and tremor, all manifesting under fatigue and unrest. It diminishes tachycardia also when precipitated by stress or thyroid excesses. Lastly, it curbs the nerve ending irritation of shingles and herpes.

INDICATIONS

♦ Anxiety/Restlessness
♦ Amenorrhea/Dysmenorrhea
♦ Tachycardia
♦ Nerve pain

COLLECTION

Collect Motherwort in its prime, preferably when in flower, typically during the summer months. With pruners clip the upper ¾ of the plant from the stem. Strip the leaves and flowers; discard the stems.

PREPARATIONS

The fresh plant tincture is the preferred preparation, as it will optimally impart the plant's nervous system's effects.

DOSAGE

♦ FPT/DPT (50% alcohol): 30–60 drops 2–3 times daily
♦ Herb infusion: 4–6 oz. 2–3 times daily

CAUTIONS

Pregnancy.

MUGWORT

Asteraceae/Sunflower Family

Artemisia vulgaris
Felon herb

DESCRIPTION

This herbaceous perennial is usually between 3'–6' in height and somewhat shaggy in appearance. Like other Artemisias, Mugwort is identifiable through its pinnatifid, green above, lighter below, leaves. The whole plant is covered by a notable pubescence. Mature stems are purplish–red. Flower panicles form at branch ends and are composed of small, yellow to red petalled flowers.

DISTRIBUTION

Mugwort's range is extensive. Native to temperate regions of the Old World, it is now also found throughout temperate North America. Look to disturbed soils, waste areas, along roadsides, and field margins.

CHEMISTRY

Phenolic acids: caffeoylquinic, caffeic, chlorogenic acids; eudesmane acids; polyacetylenes; prominent volatiles: α–pinene, α–fenchene, camphene, sabinene, β–pinene, p–cymene, α–thujone, β–thujone, chrysanthenone, camphor, borneol, lavandulyl acetate, α–gurjunene, β–caryophyllene, α–humulene, germacrene d, bicyclogermacrene, δ–cadinene, davanone b.

MEDICINAL USES

There are many Artemisias employed today for their medicinal uses. It is truly a wide–acting genus, with different varieties being used by knowledgeable people around the world. Even though each variety (Artemisia absinthium, A. ludoviciana, A. annua, etc.) has secondary attributes that differ from one another, their core usages are basically the same.

Artemisia vulgaris represents a Mugwort archetype that is more gentle than many of the others, i.e. A. absinthium and A. tridentata. It is better tolerated over longer periods of time.

First, Mugwort is a medicine for the gastro-intestinal tract. The tea is a mild gastric stimulant. Like other bitters it will efficiently relieve dyspepsia, with or without bloating. An array of gastric secretions are stimulated by the plant – chiefly hydrochloric acid, pepsinogen, and mucus.

Underlying Mugwort's bitter tonic activity is its seemingly paradoxical cytoprotective effect on gastric and intestinal tissue. The plant has the ability of stabilizing cellular membrane, ultimately protecting gastrointestinal tissues from an array of inflammatory conditions. Most Artemisias have been shown to provide cyclooxygenase inhibition, increased glycoprotein (mucus) synthesis, granulocyte degranulation inhibition, as well as transcription factor NF–kB inhibition. All of these activities protect gastrointestinal tract mucosa from the body's own inflammatory responses. Use Mugwort as a daily tea for ulcerative colitis, gastritis, or other inflammatory conditions affecting the area.

As a liver medicine Mugwort is a choleretic, increasing bile synthesis and release. If prone to gall stone formation Mugwort will thin bile enough to diminish precipitants. It is best used as a preventative. Deeper, these plants have a cooling, antioxidant effect on hepatocyte function. These effects tend to reduce elevated liver enzyme levels – all stress markers evident in viral and general hepatitis. In addition, the plant inhibits glutathione depletion within hepatocytes. Mugwort's hepatoprotective effect can also be of benefit to individuals who consume excess alcohol, rancid oils, and processed foods with their array of artificial ingredients. Several oz. of the cool tea taken before bed is one of the best approaches if prone to, upon waking the next morning, frontal headache, red–irritated eyes, bad breath, and general liver congestion.

The tea drunk hot is a stimulating diaphoretic; drunk cold with no elevated temperature Mugwort is diuretic. The plant also tends to stimulate menses, so is useful in delayed menstruation when the pelvic area feels cold and rigid.

Like most other Artemisia varieties, Mugwort has good inhibition over HSV (herpes simplex virus) strains. Use the tea as an internal approach or the topically applied essential oil for outbreak relief. See also Wormwood.

INDICATIONS

- ♦ Dyspepsia/Gastritis
- ♦ Intestinal inflammation
- ♦ Liver inflammation, with no hepatic/biliary blockage
- ♦ Fever, low–moderate temperature
- ♦ Amenorrhea, with pelvic rigidity
- ♦ HSV–1 and –2 (external and internal)

COLLECTION

Mugwort's foliage is collectable from spring through fall. Gather without the flowers as the pollen can occasionally trigger hay fever reactions in sensitive individuals. Dry well spaced.

Mugwort is easily grown in most temperate regions with only minimal care. Occasionally the potted plant can be purchased through nurseries that cater to garden/herbal buyers. The dried plant is common and commercially available.

PREPARATIONS/DOSAGE

- ♦ Infusion (cold or standard): 4–6 oz. 2–3 times daily

- FPT/DPT (50% alcohol): 30–60 drops 2–3 times daily
- DPT (100% vinegar): 30–60 drops 2–3 times daily

CAUTIONS

Do not use during pregnancy due to Mugwort's dilating effect on uterine vasculature. Due to the plant's chologogue properties do not use if there is a biliary blockage.

OTHER USES

Most aromatic Artemisias can be used to thwart insects and their larvae. Traditionally the herb was spread around or hung near stored food. 10 drops of the essential oil can be mixed with 1 oz. of alcohol; spray as needed. Try it as an insect repellent for people, pets, and plants.

MULLEIN

Scrophulariaceae/Figwort Family

Verbascum thapsus
Common mullein, Woolly mullein, Gordolobo

DESCRIPTION

Like most biennials, Mullein's first year is spent producing basal leaves and a small anchoring tap root. Its large woolly leaves are elliptic to oblanceolate. They radiate outward, with the lower ones being larger and most mature. The upper, younger leaves are particularly covered with a dense coating of fuzzy hair. A tall stalk begins to develop in the spring, and matures with thick spikes of yellow 5–lobed flowers.

DISTRIBUTION

Like many other plants from Europe, Mullein is found in places where the earth is disturbed. This enables foreign seeds an easy foothold to propagate and grow. Roadsides and next to walkways and fields are common areas for the plant. In the West it seeds prolifically after forest fires, in some areas becoming nearly a ground cover during its first year of growth. These stands are typically transitory, disappearing once soil stabilization occurs.

CHEMISTRY

Iridoid glucosides: harpagoside, harpagide, aucubin; flavonoids: hesperidin, verbascoside; saponins; volatile oils.

MEDICINAL USES

Mullein is a mild remedy that influences two main areas: the lungs and the urinary tract. The leaf tea or syrup soothes inflamed mucus membranes of the lungs, particularly those of the bronchi and trachea. Use the plant when there is a persistent dry cough that verges on being spasmodic. Forceful coughs that on occasion bring up blood–tinged phlegm from tissue abrasion, will be equally soothed. The plant is inhibiting to both Klebsiella pneumoniae and Staphylococcus aureus, bacterial strains commonly involved in lung infections. Mullein combines well with expectorants like Lomatium or Ligusticum.

Mullein root has a tonifying effect on the trigone muscle[36]. Its mechanism of action is not clearly understood, but if there is urinary incontinence from bladder weakness, the plant may prove useful. Also if there is irritation from chronic cystitis affecting the urinary situation, Mullein root is often found soothing. In bed–wetting children its effect is less predictable due to psychosomatic issues, but regardless it is worth a try.

Mullein flower oil is an age–old remedy for childhood earaches. 1–2 drops placed in the affected ear is quieting to pain and inflammation. Combined with garlic oil, the duo is both soothing and antibacterial. The flower tincture can be used in the flower oil's place. It evaporates quickly, but still its effect is notable.

INDICATIONS

- Cough, dry and spasmodic

---

36 The trigone muscle functionally composes half of the bladder's ability to store and/or release urine to the urethra. This muscle, which rests at the base of the bladder, is normally contracted. For urine to enter the urethra the trigone must relax.

- Incontinence, from poor bladder tone and chronic cystitis
- Earache, childhood (external)

COLLECTION
Harvest the leaves during the plant's first year of growth, or early into the second, as these will be more vital and healthy then the plant's second year, late–season growth. Gather the slender tap root during the plant's first year. These will be fleshy and medically potent, as opposed to the second year's woody and inert root.

PREPARATIONS/DOSAGE
- Leaf infusion/Root decoction: 4–6 oz. 2–3 times daily
- FPT/DPT (50% alcohol): 30–60 drops 2–3 times daily
- Flower oil/Tincture: 1–2 drops 3–4 times daily

CAUTIONS
None known.

MYRRH
Burseraceae/Torchwood Family

Commiphora myrrha (Commiphora molmol, C. myrrha var. molmol, Balsamodendrum myrrha)
African myrrh, Herabol myrrh, Myrrh gum

Commiphora habessinica (Commiphora abyssinica, C. agallocha, C. lindensis, C. madagascariensis, C. subsessilifolia, Amyris agallocha, Balsamea abyssinica, Balsamodendrum habessinicum)
Arabian myrrh, Abyssinian myrrh, Yemen myrrh, Myrrh gum

DESCRIPTION
Myrrh[37] is an oleo–gum–resin collected from any number of tropical Africa/Asian Commiphora varieties. Officially, C. myrrha and C. habessinica are the species recognized as the main source

plants, but often other lesser–known varieties[38] that produce a similar exudate are gathered from as well. This type of adulteration usually does not pose a problem due to similar constituent make–ups.

Commiphora myrrha is a stout, low–growing small tree. Like many others of the Torchwood family, it is inflated and torturous in appearance. Sparingly branched and leafless much of the year, it is well adapted to arid environs. When in season the tree's thorny branches produce greenish–gray trifoliate leaves. Flowers are small and form from axillary areas. The plant's fruit are two–valved and form a drupe.

Commiphora habessinica can reach 30' in height. Tortuous, pale, and spiny as well, leaves tend to be singularly arranged or grouped in trifoliate bunches. Flowers are small, and produce oval drupes with tipped ends.

Taxonomically the genus is prone to nomenclature upheavals; renaming species seems to be the norm. Equally confounding is that, in reality Myrrh gum is a compilation of exudates from numerous species.

DISTRIBUTION
Arid areas in Djibouti, Ethiopia, Kenya, Oman, Somalia, and Yemen, which receive 8"–12" of annual rainfall are home to Commiphora myrrha. C. habessinica is found from the Arabian peninsula south throughout eastern and central Africa, ending its range in Malawi and Zambia.

CHEMISTRY
Eugenol, cadinene, furanodiene, heerabolene, cuminaldehyde, elemol, various furanosesquiterpenoids; polysaccharides: arabinose, galactose, glucuronic acid, xylose; commiferin, α, β, and γ commiphoric acids, α and β heerabomyrrhols.

MEDICINAL USES
Out of several Torchwood family plants used widely in botanical medicine Myrrh is the most

---

37 Most likely derived from the Hebrew/Arabic word "Mur", which means bitter.

38 Commiphora stocksiana, C. roxburghii, and C. agallocha (including some of the Guggul–types) are also utilized.

well known. Its usage dates far back in history and is intertwined with most of the great religions. It is as much of a physical healer as it is religiously significant. Christians, Jews, and Buddhists use it ritually, usually as an incense. Rural Afghans use Myrrh and a relevant verse from the Koran in amulets to ward off sickness, or help the stricken.

In the realm of physiological medicine, Myrrh is a powerful item, having sway over a number of distinct areas. The diluted tincture as a gargle, or the gum used as a simple tooth powder, is excellent for several chronic oral conditions. Use it for spongy and bleeding gums that are tending to recede – Myrrh's tightening effect is efficacious. Due to the gum's antiseptic qualities it also is effective against a number of harmful oral bacteria responsible for gingivitis and periodontal disease. The classic combination of equal parts of Myrrh and Goldenseal root powder has little rival. As a mouthwash 30 drops of Myrrh tincture alone can be added to several oz. of water (turning the water somewhat opaque); gargle as needed.

Used solely or combined with Echinacea, it makes an excellent application for pharyngitis with swollen tonsils, particularly if the episode is long–standing and has difficultly resolving. As a nasal spray use Myrrh for chronic sinusitis. It will curb any residual infection as well as locally increase the affected tissue's resilience. Specific indications for Myrrh usage are pallid and lax mucus membranes that tend to ulcerate – denoting lack of vitality and circulatory power of affected tissues.

Internally Myrrh affects two main organ systems: the lungs and the urinary tract. It is specific for chronic bronchitis if there is a quality of debility and weakness. If the cough is non-productive, Myrrh will facilitate expectoration; if there is an unhealthy and weakening production of mucus, Myrrh will check secretions. The plant's activity is dependant upon strengthening the bronchial environment by its tissue stimulation. Even in cases of asthma when the patient is frail from age, the gum will improve breath-

ing. Myrrh is not recommended if the situation is acute with active inflammation.

It will be of benefit to long standing bladder and urethra infections that are non–resolving due to area weakness. The plant's affect over the kidneys should not be underestimated. In chronic nephritis, when there is no active inflammation, Myrrh can be used like Juniper – in small amounts to stimulate a healing response in atonic tissues.

Small amounts of the tincture have favorable influence over gastrointestinal complaints. Myrrh remedies the same sort of problems it does throughout the oral–nasal areas. The gum will help to resolve sub–acute and chronic ulcerations affecting alimentary canal mucosa. Hypersecretions related to the complaint tend to lessen. Hyposecretions are corrected as well, provided involved tissues lack some intrinsic vitality. Often Myrrh is combined with bitters, which enhance its tonic activity, particularly on the stomach and small intestine.

On the skin, use the moistened gum, ointment, or oil for poorly healing ulcers and bed sores. Myrrh is distinctly antiseptic, inhibiting a wide array of bacteria and fungi. Using Slippery elm or Marshmallow as a base provides useful emollient properties if making a poultice.

Lesser known is Myrrh's influence over the female reproductive environment. Internally the tincture is of value if there is chronic vaginal discharge with accompanying tissue debility. Due to an intrinsic emmenagogue activity within the gum, used orally, it tends to stimulate menses if there is corresponding uterine/pelvic weakness.

Suffers of endometriosis may see positive results with oral use of Myrrh. Due to its tissue stimulation, improper "seeding" of endothelial tissue tends to diminish.

Much of what Myrrh does is due to its immune stimulation. Both topical and internal parameters are affected via the pant's use.

INDICATIONS
♦   Spongy/Bleeding gums (external)
♦   Periodontitis/Gingivitis (external)

♦ Pharyngitis with swollen tonsils (external and internal)
♦ Sinusitis (external and internal)
♦ Bronchitis with debility
♦ Cystitis/Urethritis, chronic
♦ Nephritis, chronic
♦ Gastrointestinal ulcerations, chronic
♦ Poorly healing ulcers/Bed sores (external and internal)
♦ Amenorrhea, with uterine weakness
♦ Endometriosis
♦ Immunity, suppressed

COLLECTION

Cuts are made into the tree's trunk/stem bark; here a yellowish–white exudate collects. Deposits also occur spontaneously at branch divisions or bark cracks. In time this oleo–gum–resin hardens to a darker yellowish–brown to reddish–brown crystal–like or semi–pliable mass. Called tears, it is then scraped from the tree.

Myrrh is best purchased in mass as Myrrh tears. Worst case scenario is an occasional pebble, shell, or the addition of other Commiphora gums. Adulterants in the powder are more easily disguised, and may not be botanical in origin. Good quality Myrrh should smell aromatic and balsamic and taste aromatic and bitter.

PREPARATIONS

Myrrh is poorly water soluble, making tincture preparations or encapsulated powder preferable. Powder the tears before tincturing.

The essential oil is available in commerce. Although it does not provide Myrrh's full range of effects it is best for external use. The oil and salve can be made from this article.

DOSAGE

♦ DPT of gum (85% alcohol): 15–30 drops 2–3 times daily
♦ Capsule (0): 1–2, 2–3 times daily
♦ External preparations: as needed

CAUTIONS

Myrrh is not recommended during pregnancy, nor while nursing. Large continual doses can lead to gastrointestinal and renal irritation. Otherwise it will cause little problem if dosed properly.

OTHER USES

Myrrh's use as an incense and as an anointing lotion is ancient.

NETTLE

Urticaceae/ Nettle Family

Urtica dioica ssp. dioica (Urtica dioica)
Stinging nettle

Urtica dioica ssp. gracilis (Urtica gracilis)
American stinging nettle

DESCRIPTION

Stinging nettle is a short–lived herbaceous perennial. An opposite leaf arrangement combined with ridged stems makes the plant deceivingly mint–like. The leaves have little scent, but if crushed (without gloves) the sting of the plant's leaf hairs quickly remove it from any Mint family realm. These plants are 2'–3' tall, and usually have multiple long stems arising from their bases. Leaves are lanceolate to ovate, toothed, and dark green. Upon close examination the stinging leaf and stem hairs (trichomes) become apparent. The plant's inflorescence is variable in shape, appearing spike, raceme, or panicle–like. Stinging nettle is dioecious, having both male and female flowers on the same plant.

American stinging nettle tends to be monoecious, having male and female flowers on separate plants. There are less stinging leaf hairs on this species making collection a little less painful. Compared to Stinging nettle this plant is slightly smaller; its leaves are darker green and more consistently lanceolate.

DISTRIBUTION

Stinging nettle is indigenous to Eurasia; it is now found in abundance throughout temperate North

America. Look to disturbed areas, stream banks, and woodlines. American stinging nettle, native to much of North America, is found in similar locales, but enjoys a wider disbursement.

CHEMISTRY

Polysaccharides, sterols: β–sitosterol, kaempferol; flavonoids: apigenin, quercetin, rutin; carotenoids: neoxanthin, violaxanthin, β–cryptoxanthin, lutein, zeaxanthin, lycopene β–carotene; isolectins.

MEDICINAL USES

Due to the plant's readily soluble mineral content, most notably, calcium and potassium, Nettle's most reliable use is as an alkalizing, nutritive tea. It is best used by individuals who are plagued by acidosis – a pH imbalance of the blood, caused by excessive amounts of hydrogen ions. Although there are organic reasons for acidosis, Nettle will be most effective for low pH situations created by dietary indiscretions. If the diet contains large amounts of animal source proteins (Adkins–type diet) then Nettle tea will prove useful due to its buffering effect against acid build–up.

The tea tends to have a mild blood sugar lowering effect. It is surmised that the plant affects both insulin secretion/sensitivity and dietary glucose absorption. There are stronger herbal medicines for such metabolic excesses, such as Prickly pear or Brickellia, but when dietary and exercise approaches are being utilized, and just "a little" more is needed, the tea is often successful.

As an herb used to address constitutional issues, Nettle tea often fits individuals who gravitate to high fat/protein foods, who are sedentary, hypertensive, and hyperglycemic. It is not a tea to reverse an acute situation, but one to buffer the metabolic excesses of a middle–aged mesomorph. These individuals should consider Nettle tea a tonic. For this purpose it combines well with Burdock.

Nettle is one of the vegetable kingdom's most useful teas for nutrient malabsorption. Whether the reason is small intestinal inflammation, functional problems of gastric digestion, or minor parathyroid imbalance affecting calcium levels, the tea will be found nourishing. It is not to be over–looked if in need of a rebuilding tea when recuperating from surgery or illness. The tea combines well with vegetable juices or broths, and especially Yellowdock. The latter has the unique ability of liberating iron stores from the liver, increasing the body's access to this blood–building mineral. Nettle–Yellowdock is a suburb combination, and if used if anemic, the duo will do more good than either plant used alone.

Historically Nettle has been used for chronic bladder irritation with accompanying mucus discharge. Drink the tea when there is irritation and sensitivity of the area, particularly upon urination. Contributing to the plant's effect on the urinary tract, the leaf tea is a well–known sodium leaching diuretic. As a simple approach to sodium–induced water–retention and/or hypertension, 2–3 cups a day should produce a marked improvement.

Nettle root provides a moderate shrinking effect on enlarged prostrate tissue. The tea or tincture will be useful for both aromatase–dependant prostrate enlargement and general prostrate irritation. Urine flow tends to increase and urgency tends to decrease with the plant's use. For this application it combines well with Saw palmetto. Although focus has been on Nettle root with regards to BPH (benign prostrate hypertrophy), most likely the leaf has a corresponding effect given its traditional urinary tract influence.

Recently Nettle has been used as a preventative for the rhinitis of allergy season, mainly in the form of capsules containing the normally dried, or freeze–dried herb. My observation has been Nettle is hit–or–miss in its effectiveness for the watery eyes, nasal discharge, and upper respiratory itchiness of allergic reaction. Most likely any plant with a similar tannin–flavonoid make–up will have similar effects on mucus membranes.

Like bee sting therapy, topically used over painful and arthritic joints, Nettle leaf for some will be a surprisingly effective pain reliever. Until several stings are noticed, the leaves are rubbed against the problem area. The development of small weals or blisters, with accompanying irritation are common and should subside within an hour. Done once or twice a day may seem like a sadomasochistic therapy, but compared to regular Tylenol or Ibuprofen use, the area should shortly feel better and your liver will be healthier. Consider this a seasonal therapy for those who live around the wild, fresh plant. The therapy's mechanisms of action are probably several: placebo (some friendly encouragement from the mind is never unwanted), topical irritation (local vascular dynamics are altered often exercising a relieving influence over deep–seated pain), and lastly, Nettle's compounds (the initial sting may have an analgesic influence, or possibly trigger an innate cellular component that has a beneficial effect). It's anyone's guess, but the application often works for rheumatoid or osteoarthritis.

INDICATIONS
♦ Acidosis, non–organic
♦ Nutrient malabsorption
♦ Cystitis, with mucus discharge
♦ Rhinitis
♦ BPH

COLLECTION
Gloves, a long–sleeved shirt, and pruners are essential when gathering Nettle. Clip the upper stem halves; band together and hang, or spread out on an open flat and allow to dry. Nettle root can be difficult to collect if growing directly in streambeds, not to mention their potency may be slightly less than drier soil roots. Often forming in colonies, one root has many attached above-ground stems.

PREPARATIONS/DOSAGE
♦ Leaf infusion: 4–8 oz. 2–3 times daily
♦ Root decoction: 4–8 oz. 2–3 times daily
♦ FPT/DPT of root (50% alcohol): 30–60 drops 2–3 times daily

♦ Fluidextract of root: 15–30 drops 2–3 times daily

CAUTIONS
The Nettle sting. The weal response usually subsides within an hour. In more sensitive individuals it may take longer. It is rare, but some may be sensitive to the tea, developing a swollen tongue or irritated throat – if this is the case discontinue the plant's use. Due to trichome pieces interacting with the skin, when garbling the dried herb often a mild form of the Nettle sting develops. It is of no concern. The plant is safe during pregnancy and while nursing. Like so many other plants, Nettle will pick up its share of heavy metals from contaminated soils, so care should be taken in where it is collected.

OTHER USES
The fresh young leaves are used as a cooked green. Simmer until cooked and discard (or drink) the water. This process will neutralize (most of) Nettle's stinging ability. Sensitive individuals may want to re–simmer after a change of water.

Up until the mid 1900s Nettle fiber, like Hemp fiber, held a substantial textile positioning due to its abundance and tensile strength. The fiber's dominance peaked in Europe during the early 20th century when Germany outfitted her Army with a majority of Nettle–based clothes, tents, and rucksacks. With Cotton's emerging dominance, Nettle textiles proved too costly to produce, and soon feel into obscurity.

OREGONGRAPE
Berberidaceae/Barberry Family

Mahonia aquifolium (Berberis aquifolium)
Holly grape

Mahonia repens (Berberis repens)
Creeping holly grape

DESCRIPTION

Mahonia aquifolium is a substantial and course evergreen bush. Usually between 3'–6' high, in optimal circumstances it can reach heights of 15'. Thick stands of the plant can develop, often creating near–impenetrable areas.

The plant's shiny leaves are comprised of 5–9 leathery, spinulose leaflets. Yellow, 6–petaled flowers with distinctive sepals develop in several inch–long racemes. The purple–black fruit are grape–like in color and large seeded. They are tart–tasting but edible.

Mahonia repens, M. aquifolium's shorter relative, also has Holly–like, stiff, shiny leaflets, forming in groups of 3–7. Typically no more than 1' in height, the plant is usually walked on, as opposed to being waded through. The yellow flowers form in dense clusters. They are followed by a corresponding clutch of blue–purplish berries. Both species discussed here often hybridize with one another, making concrete identification tedious.

DISTRIBUTION

A plant of the Pacific Northwest, Mahonia aquifolium is commonly found in Douglas–Fir ranges as well as scrub lands. M. repens is found from the Pacific Northwest and the Interior West, south to higher elevation Arizona and New Mexico.

CHEMISTRY

For Mahonia repens, other species are similar: isoquinoline alkaloids: oxyacanthine, berberine, columbamine, corydine, isocorydine, glaucine, jatrorrhizine, magnoflorine, obaberine, obamegine, palmatine, thaliporphine, thalrugosine; lignan: syringaresinol.

MEDICINAL USES

Mahonia aquifolium makes up the bulk of commercial Oregongrape. M. repens (and M. nervosa) adds to the collective store of material; it is both collected as a separate Oregongrape and gathered and processed along with M. aquifolium – technically an adulterant, but one that poses no harm due its equal potency.

Mainly due to Oregongrape's isoquinoline alkaloid content, it is inhibiting to a wide array of pathogens, be them bacterial or fungal. Topically a wash, poultice, or fomentation is applied to infected cuts or wounds. These preparations are also effective for skin and nail fungi. Internally use the root tea or tincture as a systemic support for the same issues. Its use is also indicated in bacterial or mold induced sinus infections and for sore/strep throat.

Thanks to Oregongrape's berberine content, it is directly inhibiting to pathogenic gastrointestinal microbes and their harmful endotoxins. Take the plant if suffering from food poisoning, Giardia infection, amebiasis, and other GI tract parasitic/microbial infections. For these purposes it should be combined with a carminative, which will lessen possible griping associated with these distresses.

As a functional bitter tonic, the tea or tincture is of use in relieving indigestion. Although not as direct in its effect here as Gentian or Swertia, Oregongrape stimulates hydrochloric acid, pepsinogen, bile, and succus entericus secretion facilitating food breakdown in the stomach and small intestine. Some even may experience a laxative effect through the plant's stimulation of these digestive secretions.

Like others in the Holly grape or Barberry group the plant has an interesting effect on the skin and liver. Upon both areas, although through diverging mechanisms, it diminishes inflammatory excesses. Applied externally the ointment or oil slows excessive cellular proliferation and turnover and lipid peroxidation making it valuable in treating psoriasis. Internally the plant's effect on the liver is cooling and protective. It has been shown to normalize liver enzyme elevations, as well as other inflammatory markers associated with hepatitis and liver toxicity from environmental/dietary causes. It is hepatoprotective possibly through its influence of the liver's cytochrome P450 pathway. Traditionally the plant was used for "bad blood" and like Barberry (Berberis vulgaris), it is considered a classic alterative along with plants like Golden smoke, Stillingia, and Echinacea. It is highly indicated in conditions where the skin is dry, red, and heals poorly, or for what were once called, scrofulous conditions.

Moreover, Oregongrape is broadly antiinflammatory and is well used internally in febrile states. It tends to clear pyrogenic compounds within the body. Broadly speaking the tea also has use in inflammatory conditions such as chronic allergies, psoriatic arthritis, lupus, and a range of others.

INDICATIONS

♦ Bacterial/Fungal infections (external and internal)
♦ Sinusitis/Strep throat (internal and gargle)
♦ Food poisoning/Giardiasis/Amebiasis
♦ Indigestion with insufficient protein/fat digestion
♦ Psoriasis (external and internal)
♦ Hepatic inflammation, sluggishness
♦ Fever/Autoimmune inflammation

COLLECTION

The more yellow–pigmented, flexible, and hydrated the roots are, the better. Compared to a number of desert–growing varieties (Mahonia trifoliolata or M. fremontii) both Mahonias profiled here are easy to gather.

PREPARATIONS

Cut the roots into ¼"–½" sections. Tincture fresh or space well for drying. The dried root is commercially available, as are various root preparations. Leaf material can be used in making the oil or salve.

DOSAGE

♦ Root decoction/Cold infusion: 2–4 oz. 2–3 times daily
♦ FPT/DPT (40% alcohol): 30–60 drops 2–3 times daily
♦ Capsule (00): 1–2, 2–3 times daily
♦ Fluidextract: 10–30 drops 2–3 times daily
♦ External preparations: as needed

CAUTIONS

Berberine can cause hemolysis in babies with G6PD (glucose–6–phosphate–dehydrogenase) deficiency. Like other chologogues do not use if there is a biliary blockage.

OTHER USES

The fruit of Oregongrape can be used for jams and jellies, or can be eaten alone. Commonly planted as an ornamental, numerous variants of either species add a shrubby–mass appeal to any yard.

PASSIONFLOWER
Passifloraceae/Passionflower Family

Passiflora mexicana
Mexican passionflower

Passiflora foetida
Corona de cristo

Passiflora incarnata
Maypop, Purple passionflower

DESCRIPTION

All Passionflowers share a majority of unifying characteristics. They are vining plants that trail on the ground or climb into supporting vegetation. Anchoring tendrils are opposite deeply lobed leaves, which alternate along the stem. Flowers form on axillary peduncles of varying length. Depending on species, they are generally a showy affair of different color. Normally there is a base of 5 or 10 tepals. Resting on top of this arrangement is a fringed corona, comprised of numerous filaments. Above this are 5 stamens and 3 styles in whorled patterns. The fruit are many seeded and depending on variety can be sweet and aromatic.

Passiflora mexicana's leaves are deeply 2–lobed, appearing like a pair of pants. The mid–vein area traversing each lobe often has a whitish coloration. The corona is purplish–pink. P. foetida has 3–5 lobed leaves; they are grayish–green and felt–like. Its corona is lilac–colored.

P. incarnate has 3–lobed leaves with pale blue–violet filaments.

DISTRIBUTION

Look for Passiflora mexicana throughout southeastern Arizona between 2,500'–5,000'. The plant is commonly found growing up through Mesquite and Acacia along streams and gullies that run with seasonal water. P. foetida ranges from southern Arizona and southern New Mexico to Texas. It is considered a weed throughout much of the tropical world. P. incarnate grows in warmer temperate regions. It is found throughout the Southeast and as far west as Texas. Other species are planted as ornamentals throughout warmer parts of the West. The bulk of over 300 species exist throughout Tropical America.

CHEMISTRY

For Passiflora incarnata: indole alkaloids: harman, harmine, harmalin, harmol, harmalol; flavonoids: orientin, isoorientin, vitexin, isovitexin; cyanogenic glycosides.

MEDICINAL USES

Passionflower is a multi–faceted sedative. It is well applied to several different stress patterns and if used properly can take the place of complicated herbal regimens. Use Passionflower to take the edge off anxiousness and tension from daily stresses. Taken before bed it can be quite effective in alleviating insomnia.

Passionflower works best in thin, easily stressed, nervous individuals. Other more robust body types may respond well to Passionflower but less predictably. If timed properly Passionflower can diminish mild seizure activity. Take the herb before an episode fully manifests. The plant is also indicated in diminishing tics and muscle spasms from fright, anger, and other vicissitudes of life.

The plant is usually reliable in reducing the cravings and anxiety in substance withdrawal. Make Passionflower a primary herb if quitting Cannabis, opiates, alcohol, or nicotine habits. It is calming to the nerves and soothing to the mind when the body is crying out to be re–intoxicated. It is of particular use in the tremors of alcohol withdrawal.

The plant fits individuals with excessive cardiac force. Look for a strong, bounding pulse, hypertension, and noticeable surface vasodilation – blood movement – around the upper chest and neck. Use Passionflower to lower blood pressure and slow the heart rate. It is one of the best remedies in aborting tachycardia.

The plant is underrated in its application to bronchial complaints when there is an irritative, spastic cough that is difficult to stop. The spasmolytic effect of Passionflower is serviceable in bronchial constriction and shortness of breath when nervousness is exacerbating the episode. The plant is calming to griping and spasmodic diarrhea from food reactions or "irritable bowel syndrome".

INDICATIONS

♦   Anxiety/Tension/Muscle spasm
♦   Insomnia
♦   Mild seizure activity/Tics
♦   Substance withdrawal
♦   Tachycardia with hypertension and forceful pulse
♦   Spasmodic cough/Bronchial constriction
♦   Spasmodic diarrhea

COLLECTION

Passiflora mexicana and P. foetida are summer bloomers and are collected from late summer to early fall when in full flower. Ideally, prune the whole vine with leaf, flower, and immature fruit. Also, collect the cultivated varieties in bloom. Passionflowers that are medicinally potent stink when in flower or when their foliage is crushed. Let their rank smell be an indicator of potency.

PREPARATIONS/DOSAGE

♦   FPT/DPT (50% alcohol): 60–90 drops 2–3 times daily
♦   Fluidextract: 20–40 drops 2–3 times daily
♦   Herb infusion: 4–8 oz. 2–3 times daily

CAUTIONS

Do not use Passionflower during pregnancy due to its weak contractile inhibition of uterine smooth muscle. Although the plant has use in replacing anti–anxiety or sedative pharmaceuticals, full doses of both simultaneously will prove synergistic, likely leaving the recipient overly sedated.

OTHER USES

Passiflora edulis is primarily cultivated in warmer parts of the world for its edible fruit. As a medicine, the plant is inferior. Inversely many other varieties have semi–edible fruit with medicinal/sedative overtones.

PENNYROYAL

Lamiaceae/Mint Family

Mentha pulegium
European pennyroyal, Hilwort

DESCRIPTION

This little perennial mint is usually no more than 2'–3' in height. Variable in growth pattern it can be low–growing to lanky and upright. Pennyroyal has square stems and opposite leaves. They are mildly serrated and ovate; upper leaves are subsessile, lower ones are petioled. The pink to violet flowers develop in dense whorls at upper leaf axil points. Individually they are 2–lipped; the upper lip is notched; the lower lip is 3–parted. The calyx has a hairy throat and is 10–notched. Developing nutlets contain small pale–brown seeds.

DISTRIBUTION

Pennyroyal is native from western and central Europe, the Mediterranean region, finally to Iran and North Africa. Human movement has increased the plant's success – now it is found nearly world–wide. Look to low–lands, creek and stream sides, and generally moist and disturbed soils.

CHEMISTRY

Volatile content: α–pinene, sabinene, β–pinene, myrcene, limonene, cineole, linalool, menthone, trans–isopulegone, neomenthol, α–terpineol, pulegone, piperitone, methyl–acetate, neoisomenthyl acetate, eucarvone, methyl eugenol, β–caryophyllene, β–farnesene, α–humulene, γ–cadinene, spathulenol, cadinol; flavone aglycones: thymonin, thymusin, pebrellin, ladanien, sorbifolin, salvigenin, xanthomicrol, gardenin b, sideritoflavone, apigenin, luteolin.

MEDICINAL USES

Whole plant preparations have predictable effects on a number of systems. Through Pennyroyal's carminative influence, taken with or after meals, it diminishes stomach distension and related gas and bloating. Like others in its class it tends to dilate stomach vasculature, delivering more blood to the area, therefore diminishing stasis and inactivity. Although not as reliable as Peppermint, the plant will be found settling to nausea.

If feverish, the hot tea will stimulate sweating, helping to reduce core temperate via surface heat dissipation. It is best used when the skin is hot and dry.

As a simple stimulatory emmenagogue Pennyroyal will trigger menstruation, suppressed from causes such as stress, sickness, or climate–temperature changes. It is especially valuable when the whole pelvic area feels cold and contracted.

Unfortunately Pennyroyal's prosaic and rational uses tend to be superseded by the dangerous use of the essential oil as an abortifacient. Not even reliable, used this way Pennyroyal is systemically toxic. Take enough Pennyroyal essential oil to possibly abort a baby and poisoning symptoms will be experienced. Fatal poisonings (to the "mother") have occurred from this type of essential oil use.

INDICATIONS
♦ Gas/Bloating/Nausea
♦ Fever, dry skin

♦ Menstruation, suppressed

COLLECTION
When in flower gather the upper half of the plant. Remove the flowers and leaves from the stems; discard the stems. Tincture the flowers and leaves fresh, or dry for tea.

PREPARATIONS/DOSAGE
♦ FPT: 30–60 drops 1–3 times daily
♦ Infusion: 4–6 oz. 1–3 times daily

CAUTIONS
Do not use while pregnant or nursing.

OTHER USES
The essential oil does make an effective insect repellent. Use 10 drops per ounce of alcohol. Apply as a spray.

PEPPERMINT
Lamiaceae/Mint Family

Mentha piperita
Mint

DESCRIPTION
Like all Mint family plants Peppermint has square stems and opposite leaves. Standing between 1′–3′ tall it either reaches upward or is semi–prostrate. Leaves are generally elliptic to ovate with serrated margins and narrowed bases. Flowers form in spikes and are crowded towards branch tips. Each corolla is surrounded by a 5–lobed calyx. Like Spearmint, Peppermint has a dense rhizomal network. Generally the plant is sterile and reproduces by cloning. There is some speculation that Peppermint is a hybrid between Mentha arvensis and M. aquatica or between M. aquatica and M. spicata

DISTRIBUTION
Besides being planted in gardens or plots, Peppermint is often found as escapee throughout the temperate United States. Look for this non–native growing in the sun or shade next to streams, lakes, or other wet areas.

CHEMISTRY
Main volatiles: menthol, menthone, menthyl esters, pulegone, piperitone, menthofurane.

MEDICINAL USES
Peppermint is a superb stomachic–carminative. The tea, tincture, spirit, or essential oil is used with success in reducing gas pains, bloating, and associated gastrointestinal discomfort. To this region it is somewhat anesthetic, reducing area sensitivity. Due to this effect on the stomach walls it is one of our better treatments for nausea and vomiting. Several drops of the essential oil swallowed in a capsule is a quick and effective preparation, especially if any volume of liquid (tea) is found disagreeable. Peppermint will do well to rectify upper gastrointestinal imbalances stemming from deficient stomach wall blood supply and related lack of stomach secretion. Combined with a bitter tonic herb such as Artichoke, Peppermint will even be more effective for secretion deficiencies.

Enteric–coated Peppermint essential oil has become quite popular due to its application to intestinal spasm and bloating. It is particularly marketed to suffers of irritable bowel syndrome. It is certainly effective in the spastic stage of this complaint, but if hepatic underactivity is involved, resulting in constipation, make sure to include the tea or tincture in your regiment.

Peppermint is a chologogue, stimulating bile movement into the small intestine. This is principally why fat/lipid breakdown and assimilation improves under the plant's influence. Similarly, mild constipation from a biliary deficiency is remedied. Combined with Chelidonium, Peppermint is found by some to be almost miraculous in eliminating gallbladder spasms, especially if there is biliary stone involvement.

Like virtually all other Mint family plants, Peppermint affects diaphoresis. The hot tea is a reliable diaphoretic. It is useful in breaking mild to moderate fevers when the skin in hot and dry.

Although Peppermint tea can be used, Spearmint will be better suited for infants and children.

Topically the volatile oils found in Peppermint, particularly menthol, are pain relieving to headaches of any sort. The forehead and temples are the usual areas of application for the essential oil. Rub the oil into the area in circular motions until a tingling sensation is sensed. Used in tandem with internal use of a proper herb for that particular headache will increase the likelihood of the episode's relief.

The essential oil makes a decent muscle rub. Its anesthetic effect will be perceived shortly after application. Use it for sprains, muscle pulls, or other tissue trauma when there is discomfort.

Apply the essential oil topically to HSV (herpes simplex virus) type –1 and –2 outbreaks. Peppermint significantly inhibits the virus's replication and/or attachment. It has a strong countering influence on HSV affecting new host cells. It does little for cells already infected. This means the essential oil will help speed outbreak resolution and also may abort a full episode. It likely will do little for the primary nervous system infection. If tolerable use undiluted. Dilute with a small amount of olive or almond oil if tissue sensitivity develops.

INDICATIONS
- Gas pains/Bloating
- Nausea/Vomiting
- Intestinal spasm/Bloating
- Biliary deficiency
- Fever, skin, hot and dry
- Headache (external)
- Sports injuries (external)
- HSV–1 and –2 (external)

COLLECTION
With pruners snip the upper half from the plant, in flower or not. Younger–growth Peppermint will provide higher amounts and quality of volatile oils, but overall let the plant's taste and smell be a guide to its potency. The stronger, the better. Dry normally. Garble the leaves (and flowers) from the stems. Discard stems due to their lack

of oil glands. As long as the dried herb is strong scented it will be an active medication.

PREPARATIONS/DOSAGE
- Herb infusion: 4–8 oz. 2–3 times daily
- FPT/DPT (60% alcohol): 30–60 drops 2–3 times daily
- Essential oil: 2–3 drops taken in a capsule 2–3 times daily, or applied topically as needed
- Spirit: 20–30 drops 2–3 times daily

CAUTIONS
Essential oil preparations should not be used during pregnancy. Used moderately the tea is fine. In susceptible individuals excessive amounts of any preparation may cause heartburn or intestinal irritation.

When used for fevers Peppermint or any strong diaphoretic may initially cause a small spike in body temperature before promoting diaphoresis. Be aware of this when using with children.

OTHER USES
As a flavoring for chewing gum and confectioneries Peppermint is world–renowned.

PLANTAIN
Plantaginaceae/Plantain Family

Plantago major
Broadleaf plantain, Ribwort

DESCRIPTION
Plantain is a small, low–growing perennial. The leaves originate from the stalkless center of the plant. They are ovoid, dark green, hairless, pleated, and have wavy margins with or without serrations. The flowers are inconspicuous and small. They are clustered in elongated spikes, typically rising upward from the center of the plant. The seedpods contain numerous, small, reddish–brown seeds.

DISTRIBUTION

Plantain is a European native that has naturalized extensively in the United States. Look for it in moist and disturbed soils. Places like lawns, gardens, and roadsides usually host the plant in abundance.

CHEMISTRY

Mucilage composed of polysaccharides; tannins; iridoid glycosides: aucubin, catalpol; silicic acid; protocatechuic acid; flavonoids: apigenin, luteolin.

MEDICINAL USES

The fresh plant chewed or crushed and then placed on insect bites or stings is mildly pain–relieving and antiinflammatory. Like Chickweed, it is also soothing to heat rashes and burns, and will help in wound healing.

Internally Plantain is mild. It is not a major medicine but it is multifaceted. The tea or fresh juice diminishes mucus membrane heat. Use it for intestinal inflammation with corresponding diarrhea. Plantain is a soothing diuretic that lessens urinary tract irritation and burning upon urination. In addition, the plant reduces bronchial irritation particularly when the lungs feel hot and dry.

INDICATIONS

- ♦ Skin inflammations from bites, stings, and rashes (external)
- ♦ Tissue injury (external)
- ♦ Intestinal inflammation with diarrhea
- ♦ Painful urination
- ♦ Bronchial irritation

COLLECTION

Gather the herbage of the plant. Use fresh or dry.

PREPARATIONS/DOSAGE

- ♦ Fresh plant poultice/Oil/Ointment/Salve: as needed
- ♦ Infusion (cold or standard): 4–8 oz. 2–3 times daily

- ♦ Fresh juice: 1 oz. 2–3 times daily or topically as needed

CAUTIONS

None known.

PLEURISY ROOT
Asclepiadaceae/Milkweed Family

Asclepias tuberosa
Butterfly weed, Butterfly milkweed

DESCRIPTION

Pleurisy root is a substantially rooted herbaceous perennial. When mature the plant has a number of vertically rising stems reaching 2′–3′ in height. Leaves are generally linear to lanceolate and pointed. Bases are variable as well, being either truncate, cordate, or obtuse. Margins gently roll to the underside of each leaf. The entire plant is hairy – stems more so than the leaves. Unlike most other Milkweed family plants Pleurisy root exudes no sap when injured.

At the plant's termination flattened clusters of flowers appear. Variable in color, they are usually orange, but can be yellow or red as well. The flower's structure is typical of a Milkweed: 5 petals opposing a 5–parted calyx, forming a unique dumbbell–like shape. Each flower is ⅖″–⅔″ long. Seed pods are puberulent, horn–like, erect, 3″–6″ long, and ½″–⅝″ thick. The oval–flattened seeds have an attached tuft of white hair.

DISTRIBUTION

Except for Oregon, Washington, Nevada, Idaho, Montana, North Dakota, and Wyoming, Pleurisy root is found throughout the lower 48. Though a common plant within most of its range, it is considered vulnerable to endangered in several northeastern states – mainly because the plant exists fragilely on the edge of its disbursement.

CHEMISTRY

Pregnane glycosides (includeing ikemagenin, lineolon); flavonoids.

MEDICINAL USES

Although Pleurisy root does much more than affect the lungs and bronchial environment, its influence on that region is best noted. For the lungs (and also other organs), the plant, through its vagus nerve stimulation, amplifies cholinergic functions.

Pleurisy root is a bronchial membrane moistener. It is one of the best remedies for a dry, persistent cough, especially if dependant upon irritation. Whether a result of an on–going lower respiratory infection or cold/flu involvement, the plant's effect will be beneficial. Even in cases of dry, non–spasmodic asthma, it will be of help. In asthmatic cases if there is bronchial constriction, the addition of Lobelia will counter–act Pleurisy root's minor constrictive effect. In any bronchial affliction when expectoration is difficult Pleurisy root will soften lodged mucus and stimulant necessary secretion.

As its name implies, it is an old standby in nearly any pleuritic condition. The plant is specific for pleural membrane inflammation. Most find the plant soothing to associated chest/lung pain.

As a corrective diaphoretic the plant has little rival. Use it in mild to moderate fevers if the skin is hot and dry. Unlike some diaphoretics its stimulation is reasonable. Rarely will it cause heavy and exhaustive sweating. Inversely if there is colliquative sweating, through Pleurisy root's vagus nerve influence, perspiration will be reduced.

The plant's effect on the vascular system is evident in its influence over the heart, and therefore the pulse. A key indication for the plant's use is a strong, bounding pulse in febrile conditions. Used in conjunction with elevated temperatures Pleurisy root often lowers blood pressure and slows the heart rate. As indicators of vascular excitement of the bronchial vessels look for a flushed face and chest area.

Best of all Pleurisy root rarely can be miss–applied when used in bronchial and febrile conditions. Even if haphazardly dispensed it likely will do good. Although bitter, it is child safe. Results with young ones are seen quickly.

The plant should be considered a constitutional medicine for individuals whose skin is chronically dry, injures/reacts easily, and heals poorly. Typically these people will be adrenalin stress types prone to allergic skin sensitivity, and constipation.

INDICATIONS

- Cough, dry
- Asthma, dry, non–spasmodic
- Pleurisy
- Fever, dry skin, elevated blood pressure, strong pulse
- Poorly healing, dry skin

COLLECTION

The plant's taproot is from 1'–2' deep, forked or unforked, and can be troublesome to dig in calcified/rocky soils. Start digging to the side of the plant and trace the root downward. When the tip has been reached, gently pry the root out. Larger forked roots may necessitate digging around the plant equally. Discard the foliage as it is not useful.

Lesser known than many of the other plants profiled here, Pleurisy root is still commercially available. Although some retail establishments may not stock the plant, it certainly can be ordered. It is easily grown in the garden.

PREPARATIONS/DOSAGE

- FPT/DPT (50% alcohol): 20–40 drops 2–3 times daily
- Cold or standard infusion: 4–6 oz. 2–3 times daily
- Fluidextract: 10–20 drops 2–3 times daily
- Capsule (00): 1–2, 2–3 times daily

CAUTIONS

Excessive doses will be found nauseating and possibly stimulate strong diaphoresis. Do not use while pregnant.

RED CLOVER
Fabaceae/Pea Family

Trifolium pratense
Clover

DESCRIPTION

Red clover is a small, herbaceous, short–lived perennial. With a number of branching stems issuing from its base, it stands between 1'–3¼' high. The plant's alternate leaves are composed of three leaflets (trifoliate) and are palmately arranged. Leaflets are generally elliptic, ¾"–2⅓" long, and have a distinctive red spot on upper surfaces. The pink to reddish–purple flowers form in clusters of 25–80, and are typical for Pea family flowers – banner, wings, and keel. The 1–2 seeded pods are ovate. Seeds are yellowish–brown and sometimes purple–mottled.

DISTRIBUTION

A Eurasian native, Red clover is extensively cultivated throughout the United States. As an escapee it is found in fields, pastures, roadsides, and other disturbed areas where there are moist soils.

CHEMISTRY

Isoflavones: daidzein, glycitein, calycosin, pratensein, pseudobaptigenin, formononetin, genistein, irilone, calycosin, biochanin, prunetin, irilone; flavonoids: quercetin, isoquercitrin, hyperoside; calcium, among other minerals.

MEDICINAL USES

From old Thomsonian and Physiomedicalist involvements to cancer maverick Eli Jones' application of the plant, Red clover's use, at least has been colorful. Much has been ascribed to the plant's influence of carcinoma. Red clover is by no means a cancer cure, but the tea taken daily will retard cancerous growth, or protect as most alteratives will, against reoccurrence.

Secondarily Red clover has an affinity towards the bronchial environment. It is best used to allay a dry, irritable, spasmodic cough. Be it from bronchitis or laryngeal irritability Red clover will be found soothing.

The plant's most practical use is as a nutrient rich tea. Calcium, potassium, and magnesium are found in the infusion in absorbable forms. The tea, alone or with Nettle leaf, will provide good mineral–source nutrition in virtually any state of malabsorption. As a strengthener, the plant is similar to Alfalfa. Weakness and poor appetite are often rectified by Red clover.

Like soy, another Pea family plant, standardized Red clover is being used for its isoflavone content. It is claimed that Red clover reduces an array of menopausal complaints, hot flashes being the most notable. The plant certainly has caught the public's eye as a possible replacement for conventional HRT (hormone replacement therapy).

Supposedly Red clover's phytoestrogens interact with receptive tissue only when there is a lack of native estrogen. Inversely when hormone levels are normal, Red clover interacts little with these sites, having little if no cumulative toxicity.

In reality it is hard to consistently determine how phytoestrogens interact with estrogen receptors. Do they stimulate or block? Fully or partially? Are α or β receptors affected? How does the recipient's hormonal chemistry affect the plant's activity? These variables make Red clovers use unpredictable.

Thankfully the cautions for Red clover (and Soy extracts for that matter) appear minimal. Rationally dosed, even if the outcome is opaque, there is little chance of reproductive tissue proliferation, which unfortunately is a possibility with conventional HRT, disposing the individual to a number of reproductive cancers. There have been several cases of long–term, high–dose Soy extracts (Red clover being similar) causing pre-cancerous concern: a number of women who were part of a six–year study, receiving 1,800 mg./day of Soy extract (soy isoflavones 150 mg./day) were diagnoses with endometrial hyperplasia. Again, common–sense dosage should not cause a problem, even if the therapeutic outcome is questionable.

Red clover extract (Soy and Flax as well) may be a useful prostrate cancer preventative. The use of these isoflavone or lignan containing plants as preventatives is largely based on low incidences of prostrate cancer in Chinese men, who typically have higher levels of these compounds in their plasma and prostatic fluid.

INDICATIONS

♦ As an alterative
♦ Cough, dry, and irritable
♦ Malabsorption

COLLECTION

When in flower the whole herbal portion is gathered. Well spaced it is then allowed to dry. Red clover is commercially available in organic and non–organic forms.

PREPARATIONS

It is important to distinguish between Red clover tea and Red clover standardized extract. Use the tea for non–hormonal applications; the standardized extract, due to its heightened isoflavone content, is used for the other.

DOSAGE

♦ Herb infusion: 4–8 oz. 2–3 times daily

CAUTIONS

Although tea poses no problem, standardized extracts theoretically will influence circulating reproductive hormones, making this preparation's use during pregnancy unwise. Standardized extracts, similar to Soy extracts, may erratically influence normal menstrual cycles.

OTHER USES

Similar to Alfalfa, Red clover is a protein–rich silage plant.

RED RASPBERRY
Rosaceae/Rose Family

Rubus idaeus
American red raspberry, European red raspberry

DESCRIPTION

Red raspberry[39] is a small herbaceous shrub. The plant's erect stems are bristly, but often are smooth when young. Leaves are formed of 3–5 serrated leaflets, one terminating the bunch. They are dark–green above and gray–white, pubescent–tomentose, below. Flowers form in axillary or terminal racemes. Each cluster contains 4–7 flowers. Like most Rose family plants Red raspberry's white flowers are perfect and have 5 petals and 5 sepals. The well known red fruit is hemispherical and ⅖"–½" thick.

DISTRIBUTION

With much of the Southeast and Texas as an exception, Red raspberry is found throughout most of North America. It is common to coniferous forests, along streams, and on rocky slopes and hillsides. The plant is also found throughout similar temperate regions of Eurasia.

CHEMISTRY

Flavonoid glycosides: rutin, isoquercitrin, quercitrin; caffeic acid derivatives; tannins: procyanidins, ellagitannins.

MEDICINAL USES

Red Raspberry is a well known and widely used Rose family astringent. Most medicinal plants in this family (Red raspberry, Agrimony, Geranium, Rose, and Potentilla) are similar in use.

The plant is a mild remedy, and should be treated as such. Basically Red raspberry is a tissue tightener and reduces surface inflammation. Used as sitz bath or douche, the plant reduces the redness and inflammation of vaginitis and cervi-

39 Classifiers split American and European red raspberry into two separate groups (subspecies or varieties), then American red raspberry into two sub–groupings as well. For medicinal and edible purposes they are identical.

citis.

For menorrhagia, if there is red blood when menses should be at its end, the internal tea is useful. Even mid–cycle spotting will be curbed by Red Raspberry. For urinary irregularities such as mild cystitis or urethritis the tea will prove soothing.

Red raspberry is a noted plant particularly if used when it is the woman's first pregnancy. Typically 8 oz. of tea is taken daily as a tonic at the start of the last trimester. Essentially Red raspberry tonifies uterine vasculature, lessening the possibility of miscarriage. Through its effect on area muscle coats, it makes the birthing process more defined and efficient. Also both the internal tea and sitz bath can be used as a postpartum tonic.

Besides Red raspberry's active tissue influence, the tea contains a significant amount of calcium. Although the mineral's volume is not large, because of its soluble form, lesser amounts will remedy deficiencies normally only larger amounts would correct.

INDICATIONS
- As a uterine tonic, pre and post pregnancy
- Vaginitis/Cervicitis (external)
- Menorrhagia
- Cystitis/Urethritis

COLLECTION
When Red raspberry's leaves are in their prime, snip the upper half from the plant, stem and all. Dry well spaced. After drying garble the leaves (and flowers, if collected) from the stems. Discard the stems. Red raspberry leaf is commercially available, although compared to what can be wildcrafted it often is of inferior quality.

PREPARATIONS
The leaf infusion is preferred. Alcoholic and powdered preparations are inferior.

DOSAGE
- Herb infusion: 4–8 oz. 1–3 times daily
- Douche/Sitz bath: 1–2 times daily

CAUTIONS
None known.

OTHER USES
The fruit of Red raspberry is one of the best tasting wild berries we have. Both new and old world varieties are used for syrups, spreads, and confectioneries, or simply for eating. When cultivated for these purposes Red raspberry is of hybrid or cultivar stock.

RED ROOT
Rhamnaceae/Buckthorn Family

Ceanothus americanus
New jersey tea

DESCRIPTION
Red root is a low–growing branched perennial shrub. Its lanceolate to ovate–lanceolate leaves are 2"–4" long and 1"–2⅓" wide. Leaf undersides are pubescent and noticeably 3–nerved. Flower clusters form 1½"–4" long peduncles. Cymes are composed of 5–petaled, hooded, white flowers. Seed capsules are 3–lobed and black, containing dark, red–brown, seeds.

DISTRIBUTION
A successful plant, Red root ranges throughout a substantial area. From eastern seaboard states, west to Texas and Minnesota look for the plant in woodland margins, clearings, and even secondary roadsides.

CHEMISTRY
Triterpenes: ceanothic and ceanothetric acids; flavonoids: kaempferol, delphinidin, cyanidin, quercetin, rhamnetin, chrysoeriol, malvidin, petunidin, luteolin; peptide alkaloids: americine, ceanthamine, ceanthine, adouetine.

MEDICINAL USES
Considering no others of the same group have this plant's unique effect on the lymphatic sys-

tem, Red root is sort of an anomaly within the Buckthorn family. At the core of Red root's therapeutic influence is its effect on lymphatic tissue, immunologic cells, and blood–lymph lipids. The plant is not necessarily a white blood cell stimulant like Echinacea or Stillingia but more of an organizer of these cells and tissues. How Red root does this is most likely through its influence on surrounding cellular charge. Cellular insults that affect the area's charge are myriad: bacteria/viruses and the inflammatory response they trigger, waste materials, and unorganized lipids are just several.

Red root's stabilizing effect is evidenced by the plant's activity on swollen adenoids or in its extreme, tonsillitis. Alone, or more effectively with Echinacea, the reduction in swelling and inflammation is a welcome relief. General pharyngitis, with or without swollen lymph nodes, also responds well to a gargle of the diluted tincture. Where Ocotillo is indicated for trunk/pelvic lymph node enlargement due to poor lipid/lymph relationships, Red root is better for swollen, throat–centered lymphatic tissue if there is a clear immunological issue.

The plant's main application throughout the Revolutionary War period was for splenitis, or "ague cake" as it was once called. Today whether it is related to hepatitis or not, Red root will reduce the congestion and inflammation of the spleen.

For mastitis internal use of Red root in concert with external Poke root oil will prove an effective combination. Poke root, being the stronger of the two herbs, may even cause the area to "sweat"; this being the result of the plant's strong moving effect on lymph. The fresh root of poke applied as a poultice will be the strongest preparation.

Like other alteratives, women may experience benefit through using Red root for fibrocystic breast disease and uterine fibroids[40]. Ex-

40 It is thought that breast/uterine fibroids are hormone metabolite dependant. It is interesting to note that fibroids usually diminish or disappear when a women starts menopause. Relatedly, chronic sympathetic stimulation/stress/ caffeine increases fibroid occurrence.

act mechanisms are unknown but the plant most likely exerts a positive effect through its organizational/clarifying influence over lymph and blood. Hepatic stimulants like Oregongrape or Barberry work well in these situations due to their augmentation of hepatic detoxification pathways.

INDICATIONS
♦ Pharyngitis/Tonsillitis
♦ Splenitis
♦ Mastitis

COLLECTION
Most species of Ceanothus will be good medicines. C. americanus, due to the moister soils in which it is found, is collected without much difficulty. The southwestern Red roots are often more difficult to collect, mainly due to the dry, rocky, and compacted soils they are found in – the drier the environment, the woodier the root. In any case, the root/root bark is gathered; if any part is pink to reddish, use it.

PREPARATIONS
If at all possible tincture the roots fresh. If dried the woodier sections are difficult to powder, plus preparations from dried material tend to be less potent; good for the tannins, but for Red root's lymphatic qualities, lesser so. If making the dry plant tincture be sure to include 10% glycerin in the menstruum. This will inhibit the tannins from forming unwanted complexes.

DOSAGE
♦ FPT/DPT (50% alcohol, 10% glycerin): 30–60 drops 2–3 times daily
♦ Root decoction: 4–6 oz. 2–3 times daily

CAUTIONS
Remote, but there may be possible blood coagulant issues with heavy use.

RHUBARB
Polygonaceae/Buckwheat Family

Rheum officinale
Turkey rhubarb, Chinese rhubarb

Rheum palmatum
Sorrel rhubarb

DESCRIPTION
A large robust perennial, at maturity Rheum officinale can reach heights of 10'. From the meager beginnings of a 6"–10" shoot, the plant arises from the ground to form large, toothed, 3–7 lobed, rounded leaves. Having cordate bases they are somewhat pubescent, can reach several feet across, and attach to the plant's fleshy stalk through inflated petioles. Cream to light green flower clusters form in panicles. They are followed by 3–winged red achenes. Although the plant's deeply palmate leaves are distinctive, R. palmatum is similar in appearance. R. palmatum var. tanguticum, another Rhubarb, differs with its slightly elongated leaf.

DISTRIBUTION
Rheum officinale is native to the high tablelands of Tibet and western China; R. palmatum to northeastern Asia. Both are now extensively cultivated outside of their natives ranges. Still the majority of Rhubarb comes to us from China. The genus comprises approximately twenty five species distributed from central Asia to the Balkan Mountains.

CHEMISTRY
Gallic acid, tannic acid, anthraquinone derivatives: emodin, chrysophanol; calcium oxalate.

MEDICINAL USES
Both species as well as countless varieties (some more therapeutic than others) end up as medicinal Rhubarb. Truly a plant of opposites, Rhubarb is a mixture of laxative anthraquinone and astringent tannin. Its ability to promote intestinal movement as well as astringing gastrointestinal walls is somewhat unique, but certainly therapeutic for a number of problems. Properly dosed, like other emodin–containing plants, Rhubarb stimulates the intestinal mucosa, producing fluid secretion and peristalsis activity. This duo of effects tends to rectify a majority of simple constipative problems. But unlike Cascara sagrada, Rhubarb, through its tannin content, has a follow–up tightening effect[41]. Also unlike harsh purgatives. Rhubarb has little effect over the small intestine.

Rhubarb is best for individuals whose gastrointestinal tracts are weakened through genetic/constitutional factors. This will manifest either as chronic constipation or chronic diarrhea. In such cases there will be a tendency towards indigestion, intestinal tenderness, and associated cramping. Use Rhubarb in long–standing colitis, spastic colon, and in any other intestinal condition if chronic irritation causes intestinal sensitivity.

The tongue is a good indication of when to use the plant. If reddened, pointed, and elongated, and there is attending gastrointestinal distress, Rhubarb will probably do good. For the plant's tonic activity keep doses small; larger doses are distinctly laxative, and may be followed by rebound constipation.

Combined with aromatic herbs such as Ginger or Peppermint, Rhubarb's potential griping effect will be mitigated. In small amounts it is a tonic laxative suitable for the most sensitive of individuals. It is safe for children, the elderly, and even pregnant women.

Rhubarb like Yellowdock holds influence over the hepatic/biliary region. The plant is a known bile stimulant. I have seen Rhubarb tea relieve the hepatic congestion in suffers of hepatitis C. Its effect was short term, but nonetheless, drunk daily, its benefit was evident.

---

41 Rhubarb's rebound astringency can largely be mitigated by the addition of Magnesium. 200–500 mg. of the mineral should be taken at the same time to neutralize the plant's tannin content. Magnesium itself, beyond what is immediately absorbable, is generally laxative. In this case its use is two–fold, both of its activities point towards a more laxative preparation.

INDICATIONS

- ◆ Gastrointestinal tract weakness
- ◆ Chronic constipation or diarrhea with irritation
- ◆ Colitis
- ◆ Spastic colon
- ◆ Hepatic congestion

COLLECTION

Depending on region, Rhubarb is traditionally dug during the fall, spring, or winter. Roots are removed of their outward cortical layer and secondary rootlets and cut either transversely (called "rounds") or lengthwise (called "flats"), then dried. Better commercial grades will be of these two cut varieties – powered Rhubarb often is composed of cortical root shavings or decayed/insect–worm damaged batches. The addition of powdered Turmeric, due to its yellow–orange pigment, does occur. When added to batches of inferior quality it masks poorer colored powdered roots.

PREPARATIONS

To ascertain good quality Rhubarb it is best tasted first. Its flavor should be astringent, bitter, and aromatic. The tongue should be colored yellow, and if chewed a grittiness (due to calcium oxalate crystals) should be sensed.

The tincture, fluidextract, decoction, and syrup are all fine preparations. The addition of magnesium or any other alkali will limit Rhubarb's astringency. Roasting the root or boiling it for longer periods, reduces its laxative effect.

DOSAGE

- ◆ DPT (45% alcohol, 10% glycerin): 20–50 drops 2–3 times daily
- ◆ Fluidextract: 5–15 drops 2–3 times daily
- ◆ Root decoction: 2–4 oz. 2–3 times daily
- ◆ Syrup: 1 teaspoon 2–3 times daily

CAUTIONS

Small amounts of the tea or tincture during pregnancy pose no problem. Although unlikely, larger amounts, due to emodin–anthraquinone content, may trigger corresponding uterine contractions. Rhubarb's effect will be transferred through breast milk to nursing infants. Large doses of the plant will cause excessively loose stools followed by rebound constipation.

OTHER USES

Rheum rhaponticum and R. rhabarbarum, also from central/western Asia, are the culinary varieties commonly found in gardens. From these, stewed Rhubarb or Rhubarb pies are made. Planted as ornamentals, any number of Rhubarb varieties are found throughout Europe and America.

ROSEMARY

Lamiaceae/Mint Family

Rosmarinus officinalis
Rosmarino, Romero

DESCRIPTION

This aromatic mound–forming plant is part herb, part shrub. As a perennial, Rosemary can reach sizes 4′–5′. New growth is distinctly herbaceous and flexible, whereas the plant's central stem/trunk and older branches, are woody and stiff. Rosemary's opposite leaves are an inch or so long, narrow, green above, and lighter beneath. The small 2–lipped flowers are pale blue to lavender and are arranged in groupings among the leaves.

DISTRIBUTION

Of Mediterranean origin, Rosemary is cultivated extensively. As an ornamental it is popular in warmer and drier parts of the United Sates.

CHEMISTRY

Volatile fraction: α–thujene, α–pinene, camphene, β–pinene, β–phellandrene, α–terpinene, p–cymene, limonene, cineole, linalool, isopulegol, camphor, borneol, terpinene 4–ol, α–terpineol, verbenone, bornyl acetate, β–caryophyllene, α–caryophyllene.

MEDICINAL USES

Rosemary's traditional use is fairly straight–forward. Largely due to the plant's volatile oil content, use Rosemary tea, tincture, or essential oil internally as an upper gastrointestinal antispasmodic. Its carminative properties will be found relieving to gas, cramping, and nausea. It is safe to use with infants and children to dispel colic pains. Its anesthetic properties are equally adept at soothing stomach discomfort, particularly from disagreeable food.

If there is an elevated temperate, use the hot tea to facilitate diaphoresis. The same preparation will be somewhat diuretic if taken when there is no abnormal temperate.

Women will find Rosemary dilating to uterine vasculature. If menses is late due to poor vascular tone, undue anxiety, or stress, the plant will be found stimulating. As a mild remedy for premenstrual cramping, its effect will be amplified if combined with Wild yam or Wild peony.

True to Rosemary's reputation as a memory booster, recent research indicates the plant inhibits acetylcholinesterase (AChE), the key enzyme involved in acetylcholine breakdown. This enzymatic approach is one of main conventional treatment strategies for Alzheimer's disease, dementia, and myasthenia gravis. Use Rosemary essential oil or spirit for its cognitive effects. For these purposes it will combine well with Sage and/or Ginkgo.

Externally, Rosemary's array of volatile oils are antibacterial and antiinflammatory. The oil, ointment, or salve made with the whole plant or solely the essential oil, is useful in retarding bacterial growth of infected cuts, scrapes, and other minor topical injuries. The essential oil, used alone, or the spirit used topically, makes a decent rub for sport–type injuries, bruises, sprains, and the like. As a hair follicle stimulator Rosemary achieves its effect by vasodilation of scalp tissues. Some notice new hair growth, some don't; it's not the million–dollar cure for baldness, but worth a try. More favorable results may be seen if used in combination with proper supplementation and an internal peripheral vasodilator, such as Ginkgo.

INDICATIONS

♦ Gas pains/Nausea
♦ Colic
♦ Fever, dry skin
♦ Amenorrhea/Dysmenorrhea
♦ Alzheimer's disease/Dementia
♦ Cuts/Scrapes (external)
♦ Bruises/Sprains (external)

COLLECTION

Gather the new leafing branch ends, in flower or not. Tincture fresh, or dry for other preparations.

PREPARATIONS/DOSAGE

♦ Herb infusion: 3–6 oz. 2–3 times daily
♦ FPT/DPT (60% alcohol): 20–40 drops 2–3 times daily
♦ Spirit: 20–40 drops 2–3 times daily
♦ External preparations: as needed

CAUTIONS

Pregnancy.

OTHER USES

As a notable culinary herb synonymous with Mediterranean cuisine, Rosemary imparts a distinctly balsamic, fresh taste.

SAGE

Lamiaceae/Mint Family

Salvia officinalis
Garden sage

DESCRIPTION

Sage is a small herbaceous perennial, growing to approximately 2'–3' high. Branching with multiple square stems, Sage's leaves are arranged oppositely and are ovate–lanceolate, crenulate, wrinkled, and grayish–green. Blue flowers form in whorled terminal spikes. Seeds are small, black nutlets.

DISTRIBUTION

Sage's native range is throughout southern Europe. Now though the plant is cultivated in gardens on nearly every continent. Numerous horticultural varieties abound.

CHEMISTRY

Volatile fraction: α–thujene, α–pinene, camphene, β–pinene, β–myrcene, α–phellandrene, α–terpinene, p–cymene, 1,8–cineole, α–thujone, β–thujone, camphor, borneol, terpinen–4–ol, bornyl acetate, β–caryophyllene, β–gurjunene, aromadendrene, α–humulene, viridiflorol, δ–cadinene, manool, sclareol, heneicosane, hentriacontane.

MEDICINAL USES

Salvia's medicinal potency is largely dependent on its strong aromatic smell. Like most other Mint family plants, the stronger the smell, the stronger the medicine.

If there is a dry fever and a strong determination of blood a hot cup of Sage tea will be diaphoretic. The room temperature tea or tincture curbs colliquative sweating, particularly when body temperature is normal, the skin is soft and relaxed, and the extremities are cool.

Sage is decidedly carminative. It is useful taken as a spasmolytic for gas pains and flatulence. Its dilatory nature moves blood, hence activity to the stomach walls.

Several different varieties of Sage have been used in English herbal medicine for memory loss, forgetfulness, and to "strengthen the brain". Lately it has been discovered that the essential oil of several varieties of Sage, namely Salvia officinalis and S. lavandulaefolia, inhibit AChE (acetylcholinesterase) in cholinergic neuronal synapses of the brain. This has promise in diminishing the dementia and cognition loss of Alzheimer's disease. Even in non–Alzheimer's study subjects, improved attention and recall has been shown. Apparently, Sage blocks AChE from breaking down acetylcholine into inactive choline and acetate, therefore keeping the compound in the synapse longer. This then improves brain nerve transmission. AChE inhibition through pharmaceuticals is the primary conventional treatment for Alzheimer's disease. The plant's monoterpene content, which is largely responsible for this effect acts strongest as a whole complex. The plant's aromatics are much less potent taken out of context and used in an isolated fashion, even if recombined to mimic the plant's natural essential oil ratios. This is not a new phenomenon. Most plants work best as whole herbal medicines, not standardized extracts.

For ages, Sage has been used to decrease milk production in mothers needing to wean their babies.

Applied externally Sage is strongly antiinflammatory and antioxidant. It is efficacious in relieving pain and redness from burns and other injuries. Its use rivals Lavender in these conditions. The steam can be inhaled from a cup or pot of hot tea for pharyngitis, tonsillitis, and strep throat. This process concentrates the antimicrobial aromatics to the back of the throat where most of the bacterial colonization takes place. This done for five minutes three times a day, along with internal immune stimulating herbs such as Wild indigo, Echinacea, or Myrrh, combined with rest, is a useful plan. Of course the traditional gargle with the hot tea is also useful – it will need to done every couple of hours to assist in recovery.

INDICATIONS

- ◆ Fever, dry, moderate temperature
- ◆ Colliquative sweating
- ◆ GI tract gas and spasm
- ◆ Pharyngitis/Tonsillitis/Strep throat
- ◆ Memory loss
- ◆ Cognition, poor
- ◆ Alzheimer's disease
- ◆ To lessen breast milk
- ◆ Burns (external)

COLLECTION

Due to the plant's characteristic smell, gathering Sage is always a pleasant experience. Collect the leaves and flowering parts only, as these have the greatest concentration of aromatics. Sage in all its forms is easily procured in commerce.

PREPARATIONS/DOSAGE

- ◆ Herb infusion: 4–8 oz. 2–3 times daily
- ◆ FPT/DPT (50% alcohol): 30–60 drops 2–3 times daily
- ◆ Spirit: 20–30 drops 2–3 times daily
- ◆ Essential oil: topically as needed
- ◆ Ointment/Oil/Salve: as needed
- ◆ Steam inhalation: 2–3 times daily

CAUTIONS

Do not use the essential oil during pregnancy or while nursing.

SAW PALMETTO

Arecaceae/Palm Family

Serenoa repens
Saw palmetto berry, Sabal

DESCRIPTION

Generally a low–growing shrub, not more than 5' or 6' high, Saw palmetto forms from a tangled mass of surface stems and underground rhizomes. The plant's evergreen, fan–shaped (15–30 divisions), 3'–wide leaves develop from root crowns. Leaf petioles are notably spiny. Numerous small, cream–white flowers proceed the 1–seeded clustered berries. Technically a drupe, when ripe they are bluish–black.

DISTRIBUTION

Saw palmetto is indigenous to coastal plains of the Southeast. It is commonly found among Pine and Oak Scrub. From southern South Carolina it ranges south to Florida and west to Louisiana and Texas.

CHEMISTRY

Phytoserols: campesterol, cycloartenol, lupe-none, lupeol, β–sitosterol, stigmasterol; other fatty acids: caproic, caprylic, capric, lauric, palmitic, and oleic acids.

MEDICINAL USES

Saw palmetto is the present–day premiere botanical for BPH (benign prostrate hypertrophy/hyperplasia). A number of effects have been clearly demonstrated by the plant, but none can account for its potent influence of the prostrate and of other reproductive tissue. That is works is not questioned, why it works, is.

With Saw palmetto's application to age–related prostrate enlargement, it is typical for the plant's 5–α–reductase inhibition to be cited for its therapeutic influence. Contrary to popular belief, the plant's effect is probably not due to this enzymatic inhibition. Two factors are key in this consideration. One, although present, Saw palmetto's 5–α–reductase inhibition is about 60 times weaker than finasteride's, a popular pharmaceutical used to treat BPH. And two, seen time and time again with other botanicals, the research that is behind the figuring of how this plant works is modeled after pharmaceutical activity and application. That works for drugs (or the few plants that conveniently act like drugs), symptom suppression and the like, but for herbs, often the answer lies outside of the box. Other possibilities abound.

Maybe Saw palmetto's effect on the prostrate/involved ducts is due to its antispasmodic/anti-inflammatory qualities, or its modulation of androgens, prolactin, or estrogen.

With regular Saw palmetto supplementation a majority of BPH symptoms improve. Frequency, flow rate, amount of residual urine, and dysuria all show betterment on par with finasteride's activity. Saw palmetto does not reduce the size of an age–related enlarged prostrate, but also does not have lowered libido and impotence as potential side–effects, again indicating that finasteride and Saw palmetto work through different mechanisms.

Chronic prostatic irritation as well as epididymitis tend to be relieved by the plant, as is the dull ache, discharge, and occasional spasm that accompanies such situations. The plant will especially benefit men who lack normal libido, and who suffer from chronic prostatic, urethral, and testicular irritation.

Incidentally, the Saw palmetto is often recommended as a natural treatment for prostrate cancer. Low doses stimulate androgen responsive cancer cells; higher doses counter malignant cell growth in both androgen dependant and nondependant models. Let Saw palmetto lie as a prostrate cancer therapy until its effect and dose becomes more clear.

For women, Saw palmetto should be considered for its influence of reproductive tissue. Known to increase breast size, libido, and tone overly relaxed uterine tissue, doubtlessly the plant has some hormonal effect. Chronic ovarian irritation and pain, particularly from a reproductive deficiency is often remedied.

INDICATIONS
♦ BPH
♦ Prostatitis, chronic, in the aged
♦ Epididymitis, chronic
♦ Urethral irritation, chronic
♦ Testicular irritation, chronic
♦ Reproductive weakness, both men and women
♦ Uterine laxity
♦ Ovarian irritation, chronic

COLLECTION
Simply gather the ripe fruit from this squatty palm. In order to retard mold growth, dry in a dehydrator, or tincture fresh.

PREPARATIONS
Tea, encapsulated powder, and the fresh and dried plant tinctures are all active preparations. When making the fresh plant tincture be sure to crush the seeds within the fruit before adding alcohol to the plant material (this will expose the lipid fractions to alcohol). Most forms and popular liposterolic extracts are common and commercially available.

DOSAGE
♦ FPT/DPT (75% alcohol): 30–60 drops 2–3 times daily
♦ Fluidextract: 10–30 drops 2–3 times daily
♦ Berry infusion: 4–6 oz. 2–3 times daily
♦ Capsule (00): 2–3, 2–3 times daily

CAUTIONS
Saw palmetto should not be used during pregnancy or while nursing. Until there is a clear picture of the plant's androgen/reproductive effect I recommend against using it in hormonal–based malignancies – for both men and women.

OTHER USES
Considered an important palm throughout coastal scrub regions, it is cultivated for habitat restoration and ornamental purposes.

SENNA
Fabaceae/Pea Family

Senna alexandrina (Senna angustifolia, S. acutifolia, Cassia acutifolia, C. alexandrina, C. angustifolia, C. lanceolata, C. lenitiva, and C. senna)
Tinnevelly senna, Indian senna, Egyptian senna

DESCRIPTION
For some plants it is no easy task keeping up to date with current scientific nomenclature. If revision is the rule then Senna abides like no other.

As a bushy shrub, Senna reaches several feet in height. It is composed of numerous spreading branches, upon which are borne 4–6 sets of ovate–lanceolate leaflets. Flowers are showy and yellow – a banner and keel arrangement. Seed pods are brown, flattened, oblong, and somewhat bowed.

DISTRIBUTION
Senna is indigenous to Africa, the Arabian peninsula, and parts of temperate–tropical Asia. It is extensively cultivated in Egypt, Sudan, southern China, Pakistan, and India.

CHEMISTRY

Hydroxyanthracene glycosides: sennosides; naphthalene glycosides; flavonoids; mucilage (galactose, arabinose, rhamnose, galacturonic acid).

MEDICINAL USES

Senna is a straightforward stimulant laxative. Similar to Aloe, Senna's anthraquinones affect the small and large intestines. By increasing transit time, peristalsis, and decreasing intestinal fluid absorption, Senna is a reliable laxative. Mixing the plant with a carminative herb such as Ginger or Peppermint will limit its potential to cause griping. Taken before bed and dosed properly, Senna will soften the stool and stimulate bowel movement for the next morning. Some of the plant's glycosides are broken down in the colon by bacterial activity. The resulting metabolites, particularly rheinanthrone, are responsible for much of the plant's effect.

Senna is particularly useful if constipation is dependent upon stress and anxiety. It is also important to address dietary and constitutional factors for long–term relief. Fiber and water intake, upper gastrointestinal and hepatic response to food, and psychosomatic factors are all important issues to address when resolving chronic constipation.

Because the pods contain polysaccharide–starches the rate at which Senna delivers its stimulant–anthraquinones is somewhat slowed, making them gentler in effect. The leaves lack these substances, which is the main reason why they tend to be more irritative in nature.

INDICATIONS
♦ Constipation

COLLECTION

The leaves, flowering racemes, seedpods, and immature seeds are all active. The leaves have the largest quantities of anthraquinones. The fully mature seedpods have small amounts and the mature seeds are nearly devoid of these com-

pounds. Collect and dry.

PREPARATIONS

A cold infusion made with the pods is the choice preparation. Although the leaves can also be used, they are considered harsh in activity.

DOSAGE
♦ Cold infusion: 1–2 grams of whole pods to 1 cup of water, taken before bed
♦ Fluidextract (40% alcohol): 5–20 drops before bed

CAUTIONS

Due to the plant's potential sympathetic stimulation of uterine contractions, do not use during pregnancy. Senna will have a laxative effect in nursing infants through mothers drinking the tea. Senna is not recommended in constipation from dehydration, as the plant's effect on intestinal electrolyte absorption will exacerbate the situation. Also muscular tetany has been observed with excessive consumption – electrolyte balance, particularly of potassium, is disorganized by Senna. Excess consumption of the tea or over–the–counter preparations will cause habituation and dependence. Senna is best used for 1–2 weeks at a time, or longer in combination with supporting herbs.

SHEPHERD'S PURSE
Brassicaceae/Mustard Family

Capsella bursa–pastoris
Shepherd's heart, Pickpocket

DESCRIPTION

Shepherd's Purse is a small, herbaceous annual. Its leaves are mainly basal, forming in clustered rosettes. They are varied in shape, entire to pinnately lobed, and usually clasp the stem. The very small, white flowers form in elongated racemes. The plant's most characteristic feature is its wedge shaped seed capsules. They appear as inverted hearts. Each is borne on an individual pedicel.

DISTRIBUTION

Ubiquitous and practically universal, a little soil and water are all that are needed for this little mustard to thrive. It is common to frequently irrigated lawns, garden plots, and grassy areas. Although originally native to Eurasia, it is now a worldly plant, seeking out disturbed soils, only avoiding hot and wet tropics.

CHEMISTRY

Fatty acids; flavonoids; tyramine and fumaric acids, diosmin.

MEDICINAL USES

Shepherd's purse is truly a unique mustard. The plant is a special hemostatic, not acting through any tannin source, like most others, but through another, yet unexplained constituent group. Influencing tissue capillary beds, its astringency is penetrating, yet not gross like Geranium's or Oak's.

For the urinary tract, use the plant in tissue laxity when there is passive hemorrhaging or blood in the urine, particularly if there is accompanying sediment. It curbs chronic irritation of the bladder and urethra, and it is especially indicated if the urine is dark or contains mucus. As a lithotropic agent, Shepherd's purse is well regarded. Use it if there is irritation, hematuria, and general stone formation. If there is a tendency towards elevated uric acid levels or phosphaturia, the plant is doubly indicated. Also if there exists urogenital pain from sexual activity, and for men, seminal vesicle irritation, Shepherd's purse is typically found soothing.

For women the plant is mostly employed to curb menorrhagia. Specifically it should be used if menses is too long, and nearly colorless. The fresh plant tincture will also be of benefit during the first days of menses if bleeding is heavy. During pregnancy if there is threatened miscarriage, and spotting is the main symptom, Shepherd's purse is specific. For mild postpartum hemorrhaging, the plant seldom fails to stop bleeding.

A property of Shepherd's purse that is common to most other pungent mustards, is its menses stimulating potential. Although in opposition to the plant's previously mentioned uses, if taken in large doses it is often stimulating in amenorrhea.

As an astringent, the plant also is useful for gastrointestinal tract bleeding. Mild bleeding from gastric or duodenal ulcers, as well as intestinal injury is lessened. Taken internally with Collinsonia root, the combination allays bleeding and shrinks hemorrhoids.

INDICATIONS

♦ Passive hemorrhage of the urinary tract
♦ Urinary deposits/Sediment in urine
♦ Seminal vesicle irritation
♦ Menorrhagia
♦ Potential miscarriage, with spotting
♦ Hemorrhaging, postpartum
♦ Hemorrhaging, GI tract
♦ Hemorrhoids, bleeding

COLLECTION

Gather the entire plant, small tap root and all.

PREPARATION

The fresh plant tincture is the preparation of choice. Although the recently dried herb, used for tea, is inferior, it is serviceable. The dosage can be easily doubled when used in acute situations.

DOSAGE

♦ FPT: 30–60 drops 2–3 times daily

CAUTIONS

None for normal use.

SLIPPERY ELM
Ulmaceae/Elm Family

Ulmus rubra (Ulmus fulva, Ulmus americana var. rubra, Ulmus pubescens)
Elm bark

DESCRIPTION
At maturity Slippery elm stands 60' high. Its crown is broad and open. The tree's bark on mature sections is thickened, brownish–gray, fissured, and occasionally found in loose plates. The inner bark is lighter in color and distinctly mucilaginous. The serrated leaves are generally ovate to elliptic, 4"–8" long, and 2"–3" wide. Upper surfaces are rough and dark green. Beneath they are lighten green and felty–soft. Flower clusters are unassuming, green, with each calyx bordered by red–brown hairs. Fruit is a single–seeded, winged samara.

DISTRIBUTION
From Florida to Texas the tree is distributed through the Great Plains states; its northwestern extreme being the Dakotas, finally north to Canada. The tree will be found in moist, rich soils of bottom lands and streamsides.

CHEMISTRY
Mucilage: polysaccharides (l–rhamnose, d–galactose, 3–O–methyl–d–galactose, d–galacturonic acid).

MEDICINAL USES
As a demulcent and emollient Slippery elm has little equal in the plant world. The bark, being sought after due to its purity of action, has virtually no secondary effect.

The tea is gargled for mouth and throat irritation. Whether from climate dryness, voice over–use, or the inflammation of pharyngitis, Slippery elm will be found soothing. Even for a dry–irritative cough it will be of help.

Suffers of intestinal inflammation, whether manifesting as constipation, diarrhea, or simply regional discomfort, will benefit from Slippery elm. The tea or encapsulated bark powder is used to ally the intestinal wall inflammation of food poisoning or ingested toxins.

Externally the poulticed bark serves as an excellent emollient. It should be applied to all sorts of inflammations – burns, scrapes, and rashes only are a few issues that will respond well to the plant. As a fine skin softener, it can be used solely for its cosmetic effect, or more seriously to assist abscesses in coming to a head. For this last use its mixture with an immunological stimulant, such as Echinacea or Myrrh, will further the bark's effectiveness. Like Marshmallow the powered bark can simply be used as a poultice base.

INDICATIONS
♦ Sore throat, irritation
♦ Cough
♦ Intestinal inflammation
♦ Skin irritation (external)

COLLECTION
Select a secondary or tertiary branch. Cleanly saw it from the main tree branch. Work the bark from the core wood – if the outer bark is young and unfissured it can be used as well. Do not collect from the main trunk! This will only invite disease and weakness. In fact this type of careless harvesting is responsible for the scarcity of Slippery elm in some regions.

PREPARATIONS
The bark infusion or the encapsulated bark powder are the most popular forms. Besides these, the moistened bark powder can be made into a gruel; 2–3 tablespoons is a typical dosage. Cumbersome, but many find it the most effective preparation.

DOSAGE
♦ Cold infusion (shredded bark): 4–8 oz. as needed
♦ Capsule (oo): 2–3, 2–3 times daily
♦ Gruel: 2–3 tablespoons 2–3 times daily
♦ Poultice (powdered bark): as needed

CAUTIONS
None known.

OTHER USES
Slippery elm is one of the four plants found in "Essiac tea"[42]. In its raw state the inner bark is very fibrous and has been used as the base material for cordage, rope, mats, etc.

SPEARMINT

Lamiaceae/Mint Family

Mentha spicata
Mint

DESCRIPTION
Spearmint is a small herbaceous perennial, reaching heights of 2'–3'. The plant's leaves are lanceolate–ovate, 1"–3½" long, ⅖"–1⅛" wide, glabrous above, and gland–dotted below. Margins are serrated, bases are rounded, and each leaf has a short petiole. Spiked flower clusters form near branch tips. Each flower has a 5–lobed toothed calyx; corollas are white to lavender. Spearmint easily grows through both seeds and clones.

DISTRIBUTION
Although the plant's origin is unknown, Spearmint is found world–wide. Outside of the garden or in a cultivated plot, look to streamsides, ditches, or any wet area, shaded or otherwise. Almost always the plant will be found in proximity to an old farm, homestead, or living area, where it was planted years before.

CHEMISTRY
Main volatile compounds: myrcene, limonene, cis–carveol, carvone, β–bourbonene, β–caryophyllene, β–farnesene, γ–muurolene, n–octacosane, n–tricosane.

MEDICINAL USES
As a "kitchen medicine" Spearmint is ubiquitous, mild, and most importantly, useful. Its close relative, Peppermint, is the stronger of the two and can be used in directly treating a number of gastrointestinal pathologies. Spearmint is more prosaic in application and should be considered a diffuse soother to indigestion, gas pain, and nausea. The tea can be used liberally in these cases.

The hot tea is specifically used in childhood fevers. Not as vigorous as Peppermint, Spearmint will stimulate perspiration, so is indicated in mild to moderate fevers if the skin is hot and dry.

Children usually take to the tea especially if sweetened. The internally used essential oil or spirit may be too strong for little ones, but for adults it is a more active preparation.

INDICATIONS
- Indigestion/Gas/Nausea/Colic
- Fever, skin hot and dry

COLLECTION
With pruners snip the upper half from the plant, whether in flower or not. Dry well spaced. Garble

---

42 Through superb marketing techniques and the greater public's willingness to believe, Essiac tea is one of the most popular lay remedies for cancer. The formula contains Burdock, Slippery elm, Sheep sorrel, and Rhubarb. They are certainly therapeutic in their own spheres of influence, but none, possibly with the exception of Burdock used as a preventative, are considered potent enough to alter malignancies.

The tea hails from dubious origins. Considered a discovery from Ojibwa Indians by a nurse named Caisse (Essiac is Caisse spelled backwards), three out of four plants comprising the recipe are not native to Canada, let alone North America.

Today, Essiac or Essiac–like proprietary formulas are legion, acquiring a hefty share of the herbal market. Generally over–priced, of doubtful potency and quality, they are found in nearly every health food store. From pre–made tea, tea bags, capsules, and tinctures, nearly every maker has an Essiac product.

Miraculous testimonials accompany Essiac's legend. The recipe's therapeutic influence is most likely due to placebo, a phenomenon more powerful than any herb or drug. For the independent minded, do–it–yourself type looking for any stand–alone or complementary cancer therapy, my suggestion is to leave Essiac on the shelf and focus on a better designed combination of alteratives, antioxidants, and immune stimulants. It's better to believe in something that will work outside of the mind.

and discard the plant's stems. Stored in a well–sealed jar, the oils, which give the plant its characteristic smell, remain intact for at least a year.

PREPARATIONS/DOSAGE

- Herb infusion: 4–8 oz. as needed
- Essential oil: 2–3 drops in a capsule 2–3 times daily
- Spirit: 20–30 drops 2–3 times daily

CAUTIONS

Excessive internal amounts of the essential oil may stimulate menses, so should not be used during pregnancy.

SQUAW VINE

Rubiaceae/Madder Family

Mitchella repens
Partidgeberry, Checkerberry, Twinberry

DESCRIPTION

Squaw vine is an evergreen, mat–forming creeper. It is diminutive but perennial. Usually no more than a couple of inches from the ground, it is easily over–looked due to its positioning. The small opposite leaves are ovate and entire or undulate. The dimorphic, funnel–form flowers are white and inconspicuous. They are followed by sets of red, persistent, and edible fruit. Squaw vine is a plant of pairs. Leaves, flower, and fruit all develop in sets.

DISTRIBUTION

A plant of coniferous forests, it ranges from Canada and Minnesota south to Florida and Texas.

MEDICINAL USES

Squaw vine should be used by pregnant women whose full term is threatened by miscarriage. Generally it is of value to women whose last trimester is clouded by distress and irritation. Consider it a uterine strengthener. The plant has a tonifying effect on the reproductive environment, partially through its array of tannins,

but also through other, yet unexplained means. In fact Squaw vine's use in this area spans back before recorded history. The plant's use was adopted from American Indian understanding by Eclectic, Thomsonian, and lay practitioners while the country was still young. It has been used the same way ever since.

Beyond pregnancy, use Squaw vine when there is uterine or cervical irritation, or dysmenorrhea, upon menses. Its calming effect is more subtle than spasmolytics such as Wild yam, but if used consistently its effect will be noticed.

For the urinary tract the plant should be applied if there is pain upon urination. It will be found soothing to the region. Squaw vine is not a noted antibacterial agent for the area, but nonetheless, it is effective for men who suffer from periodic prostatitis.

INDICATIONS

- Miscarriage, threatened
- Uterine/Cervical irritation
- Urinary tract irritation
- Prostatitis

COLLECTION

Gather the whole plant, in flower or not. The creeping rhizome, leaf, stem, and flower are all active. From the edge of a stand work with your hands, or a trowel, removing the plant from the ground. Just as the above portion is found in mats, the roots are that way as well. It is important to collect from the edge of a stand[43], and not its center. This way the remaining portion will be more successful at regeneration.

PREPARATIONS/DOSAGE

- FPT/DPT (50% alcohol): 30–60 drops 2–3 times daily
- Herb infusion: 4–8 oz. 2–3 times daily

CAUTIONS
None known.

43 The author has collected from expansive stands in the Northeast. It often forms interconnected plots stretching for nearly acres on end. Due to it being on the edge of its range it is listed as threatened in Iowa.

ST. JOHN'S WORT

Clusiaceae/St. John's Wort Family

Hypericum perforatum
Klamathweed

Hypericum scouleri (Hypericum formosum)
Scouler's St. John's wort

DESCRIPTION

St. John's wort is an herbaceous perennial. Both varieties profiled here have opposite leaves, with each set offset 90 degrees from one another. Hypericum perforatum is a bushy plant, developing from a central taproot, whereas H. scouleri's stems are few. It is not uncommon for the plant to only have a single stem. Both variety's leaf margins (and select flower parts) are dotted with small black/red glands – the undersides are as well, but lesser so. The quarter–sized, 5–petaled yellow flowers form in terminal cymes. H. perforatum has a greater flower display, making the plant more notable, and easier to collect. The small seed capsules contain numerous tiny seeds.

DISTRIBUTION

Hypericum perforatum, a European native, is found nearly throughout temperate America. Look to disturbed areas, pastures, and field sides. H. scouleri is a plant of the West. From Canada to Arizona and New Mexico look for it along streamsides, springs, and meadows, often in coniferous forests.

CHEMISTRY

Naphthodianthrones: hypericin, pseudohypericin; phloroglucinols: adhyperforin, hyperforin; flavonoids: rutin, hyperoside, isoquercitrin, quercitrin, quercetin.

MEDICINAL USES

Externally St. John's wort is applicable to several situations. Applied to ulcers, wounds, and cuts the herb infused oil is an excellent remedy. The oil combined with fresh Aloe vera leaf pulp makes a superb burn dressing. Sensitivity and inflammation are both reduced, speeding the involved tissue's healing. The plant's qualities are imparted well through this medium. For injuries, if there is some nervous tissue involvement, St. John's wort is specific. Topically applied it assists in nerve repair and quiets neuralgias. Internal tincture use will favorably compound the topical treatment's effectiveness.

The plant is quite healing when used in this two–fold approach for shingles. This unilateral nerve tissue outbreak, caused by VZV (varicella zoster virus)[44], is more quickly resolved with St. John's wort. When topically combined with Chaparral oil, and internally, Skullcap, the combination is thought of by some to be remarkable. Stress reduction is paramount in recovery, as typically Shingles is an occurrence in the aged and stressed. Topically and internally the plant reduces the occurrences of both oral and genital herpes – not a cure but a maintenance. The plant is also indicated in any spinal cord injury or involvement. Within a rational scope, its spurs healing of involved nerve fibers.

More well known are St. John's wort's sedative and mood altering qualities. The plant has been exhaustively researched in its effect on depressive states. Non–standardized preparations of the plant are most useful for mild depression[45]. For moderate depression try the standardized extract. The plant does fit certain nuances more than others: if there is insomnia, an excitable–lost frame of mind that distorts perception, as if no purchase on the rock of life can be held, then try St. John's wort. It has a steading influence on the psyche, particularly when emotions come and go as they please, as if they are the master of us, and not the opposite. Depression that accompanies abrupt changes in life is another of the plant's specifics. I have also seen the plant do

---

44 VZV belongs to the herpes virus group. Responsible for "chicken pox" it can become reactivated later in life causing "shingles" and post–herpatic neuralgia.

45 It is generally agreed upon that St. John's wort is a mild MAO (monoamine oxidase) inhibitor, ultimately keeping serotonin in neuronal synapses longer, therefore providing varying degrees of central nervous system stimulation.

well in lifting the weight of grief or sadness accompanying hypothyroidism.

INDICATIONS
♦ Ulcers/Wounds/Burns (external)
♦ Nerve damage/Neuralgias (external and internal)
♦ Herpes group of viruses (external and internal)
♦ Depression

COLLECTION
When in flower, gather the herb portion of the plant. To insure it has the widest array of potencies collect flowers, flower buds, seed capsules, and new leaf growth. This peak stage is typical of the plant mid to late summer. Another indicator of St. John's wort's potency is its abundance of flower/leaf glands. These small glands contain the pigments hypericin and pseudohypericin and are largely responsible for the plant's effect on depression and possibly other issues.

PREPARATIONS
For internal use, the fresh plant tincture is preferred. Upon drying the plant loses some of its anti–depressant and sedative qualities. For topical use, the traditional approach is to infuse the flowing tops in oil, exposed to sunlight for a week or so. Although this method is certainly tried, a better method, which keeps St. John's wort's factions intact, particularly hypericin, is as follows: take 1 part of wilted flowering tops and infuse them in 7 parts of olive oil. For 8 hours or so maintain the mixture's temperature at 120–130 degrees. This can be done in an oven that registers that low of a temperate, suspended above a wood store, or even placed in the engine compartment of a vehicle over a day trip; get creative. After the flowers have been sufficiently infused, strain the flowers from the oil. There may be a small layer of water at the bottom of the container, if so ladle the oil from the watery portion, then bottle and store. Discarding the watery segment insures the oil's preservation. If there is any remaining water the preparation will spoil due to bacterial growth.

DOSAGE
♦ FPT/DPT (60% alcohol): 30–60 drops 2–3 times daily
♦ Herb infusion: 3–6 oz. 2–3 times daily
♦ Oil/Ointment/Salve: as needed

CAUTIONS
There are a few cautions to be heeded when taking whole plant preparations of St. John's wort. Although remote some of the plant's compounds have shown uterine stimulant activity, making its use unwise during pregnancy. Occasionally animals grazing on the plant develop sun–sensitivity dermatitis. It has been infrequently observed when taking the tincture or tea.

If you find yourself taking the standardized extract, and there is development of a sun–sensitivity rash, switch to the fresh plant tincture. The symptoms should dissipate shortly. Do not mix the standardized extract with pharmaceuticals due to its stimulation of the liver's cytochrome P450 pathway. Drugs will be eliminated quicker than intended, causing dosing problems. This phenomenon has been particularly troubling to patients on chemotherapy and anti–rejection agents. And lastly, do not mix the plant, crude or standardized, with pharmaceutical MAOs.

STONEROOT
Lamiaceae/Mint Family

Collinsonia canadensis
Horsebalm, Richweed

DESCRIPTION
As a tall, stout perennial herb with branching stems, Collinsonia displays large, petioled, ovate to elliptic leaves. They are oppositely arranged, serrated, and can be up 10" long by 7" wide. Leaf sets are perpendicularly offset from one another. Flowers develop in a terminal panicle of racemes. Individually they are small, yellow, and 2–lipped. Mericarps are dark brown and smooth.

Herbage is pleasantly lemon–scented.

DISTRIBUTION

Although spotty in some areas, Stoneroot does have a significant range. From Canada it expands southward through most of the Great Lake and northeastern states (except Maine) to Louisiana and Florida. It is considered endangered in Wisconsin where it exists on the edge of its range.

CHEMISTRY

Flavonoids; flavones; volatiles: β–elemene, δ–cadinene, elemicin, germacrene d, caryophyllene.

MEDICINAL USES

Stoneroot is a peculiar Mint family plant. Medicinally it shares little in common with its relatives. Its main quality is its corrective action towards poor venous circulation. The whole system is affected, but the pelvic region along with the legs, and secondarily, the throat are the two areas that will most surely benefit from the plant's activity. Regardless of the situation, when capillary sluggishness is a main problem, Stoneroot is indicated.

Stoneroot's most well–known application is to hemorrhoids. The plant works best at relieving underlying vascular congestion. If used early on in their formation, Stoneroot will likely prove successful. Take the plant if there is an underling discomfort, specifically a sense of weight and dull pain, with or without perceived heat. Constipation typically accompanies the picture – often with local vascular congestion intestinal function will be slowed.

Leg varicosities with regional fatigue and heaviness is a specific for Stoneroot. If there is accompanying lower trunk, leg, or foot tissue edema, this also will lessen.

Stoneroot appears to provide some stimulation to the parasympathetic nervous system's vagus nerve, which helps to explain its array of effects. Slowed portal vein circulation, resulting in indigestion, loss of appetite, slowed intestinal movement, and constipation will improve. It is well applied to poor gastrointestinal tissue circulation.

Stoneroot should be the first choice for individuals who develop hoarseness, sore throat, and cough dependant upon voice over–use. The plant lessens irritation frequented by singers and speakers. For other constitutional complaints of the throat region, such as chronic laryngitis and coughing from chronically irritated mucus membranes, Stoneroot is indicated. The tincture as a gargle or spray, will be found superior in these cases.

When vascular tone of the heart, especially the left ventricle is lacking, sometimes causing mitral regurgitation, Stoneroot will provide some relief. Its effect is not on the valve itself, but on the surrounding vascular tissue that has become hypertrophied. The chronic cough and shortness of breath or dyspnea that is dependant upon cardiac weakness is often helped. Combined with Hawthorn, or in more serious cases of valvular regurgitation, Selenicereus, appreciable results will often be seen.

The plant was once used for urinary gravel and such, but it is more apt to lessen irritation from these deposits, than actually dissolve stones. Use it in chronic cystitis or urethritis, particularly if these discomforts are a result of improper circulatory activity. It is well applied for men if testicular or epididymis inflammation accompanies hemorrhoids, often tell–tale signs of pelvic congestion. Women too will benefit from the plant through its similar effects. Use it for capillary congestion of the uterus, which may in severe cases result in uterine subinvolution.

INDICATIONS
- Hemorrhoids
- Portal circulation, slowed
- Pharyngitis/Laryngitis
- Cardiac weakness
- Cystitis/Urethritis
- Reproductive area congestion

COLLECTION

The hardness of the plant's roots can be deceiving. Digging the root for the first time I was sure I had come across a section of an old tree branch buried in the ground. They are typically shallow, somewhat circular, knotted, and very dense. Collect the roots and foliage alike.

PREPARATIONS

The root is difficult to cut into pieces. Pruners may need to be used. Use both the foliage and roots for the fresh plant tincture; roots only for the dry plant tincture.

DOSAGE

♦ FPT/DPT (60% alcohol): 30–60 drops 2–3 times daily

CAUTIONS

None known.

TEA

Theaceae/Tea Family

Camellia sinensis
Green tea, Black tea, White tea

DESCRIPTION

An evergreen bush when pruned for cultivation, Tea grows to small tree heights. The plant's dark green, elliptic, and glossy leaves are 2"–5½" long by ¾"–2" wide. Flowers are 1"–1½" in diameter. 7–8 white petals surround the inflorescence's yellow reproductive center. Capsules contain one to several seeds.

DISTRIBUTION

Native to Southeast Asia – India to China – its spread from these lands to other adjacent regions are shrouded by time. Today Tea is cultivated world–wide throughout tropical and subtropical regions.

CHEMISTRY

For Green tea: polyphenols: catechin, gallocatechin, epicatechin, epigallocatechin, gallocatechin gallate, epicatechin gallate, epigallocatechin gallate; flavonols: quercetin, myricetin; purine alkaloids: theophylline, theobromine, theacrine, caffeine; theanine; saponins.

MEDICINAL USES

Second only to water as the most popular beverage consumed world–wide, Tea, simply dried, steamed, and/or fermented (technically oxidized) is an herbal heavyweight. Since the mid–90s, it has received a considerable amount of attention due to its antioxidant properties. Because of its significant polyphenol or tannin content Tea is a decent beverage–source of these compounds, but should not be considered a replacement for other superb antioxidants like Ginger or Turmeric.

Oxidative stress has wide–ranging and fundamental effects on us. It is undeniably linked to the aging process, inflammation, and disease development and progression. As oxidative stress is intrinsic to distress, oxidative process is basic to cellular activity, and essentially life.

The degree to which cellular oxidation takes place, and what tissues are affected, determines if the process is life augmenting or life destructive. Similar to a fever, in most cases the febrile state is necessary for proper infection–fighting. In rare cases though, the fever is severe enough in itself to be life–threatening.

As a moderately–consumed beverage, drink Tea as an antioxidant. Whether or not there is overt disease, its free–radical quenching effects will be of benefit. Specifically drink Tea as a preventative of cardiovascular disease and various forms of cancer.

It is also surmised that the plant is systemically health–promoting by its effect on the intestinal environment. Here the plant's tannins have shown inhibiting influences on several pathogenic microflora strains, all the while keeping beneficial strains such as Bifidobacterium and Lactobacillus intact. Intestinal health improves creating an overall sense of well–being.

The tannins found in Tea are common throughout the vegetable kingdom. From Oak to Alder, from Geranium to Uva–ursi, hydrolyzable tannins exert strong effects on surface tissues;

they tighten and constrict. This is why topically applied Tea (moistened tea bag over a swollen eye for example) will reduce redness and irritation from sunburn and scrapes...and tan hides.

Also tannin–containing plants like Tea are somewhat antimicrobial. Bacterial growth is inhibited due to the polyphenol fraction exerting a membrane–damaging effect on bacterial cell walls. In the case of Tea, gram–negative types are more profoundly affected than gram–positive types.

Out of the three main varieties – green, black, and white – green and black Tea are considered basically equal in antioxidant potential – although their respective compounds differ slightly. Tea does contain a substantial amount of caffeine (40–55 mg. per cup). Unlike Coffee, due to the plant's theanine content, negative effects are rarely seen. This amino acid accounts for 1%–2% of the leaves' dry weight. Mild sedative and blood pressure lowering effects are ascribed to theanine. It also imparts Tea's pleasant taste.

In conclusion, consider Tea useful as an addition to the diet. If thought of as being "nutritional", misunderstandings of its influence will be less. Drink Tea as a beverage with therapeutic overtones, not as a stand–alone therapy. Drinkers of sugared soft drinks will probably notice a significant difference in general health after making a change to unsweetened Tea. Even naturally decaffeinated Tea will provide essentially the same health–enhancing effects as the regular version.

INDICATIONS
♦ As an antioxidant
♦ Scrapes/Sunburn/Irritation (external)

COLLECTION
Immense plantations are devoted to its cultivation throughout the East. China, India, and Sri Lanka are the top producers. Most grades are commercially available.

PREPARATIONS
Green tea is made through wilting and steaming or heating the leaf. Oolong tea is wilted, rolled, crushed, and allowed to oxidize for a short period of time; black tea goes through a similar process, but is allowed to oxidized longer (yielding theaflavin and thearubigins). White tea is the least processed of the group. The young leaves and buds are collected in the early spring. After collection they are steamed and dried immediately.

DOSAGE
♦ Infusion (standard or cold): 4–8 oz. 2–3 times daily

CAUTIONS
Tea's tannin (polyphenol) content, continually applied to sensitive mucus membranes, is capable of causing tissue disruption. Sensitive individuals may find a strong cup of Tea nauseating – this effect is often countered by the addition of milk or cream. Extended use may cause some renal irritation. If this occurs simply reduce quantities or discontinue entirely.

TEA TREE
Myrtaceae/Myrtle Family

Melaleuca alternifolia
Narrow–leaved paperbark

DESCRIPTION
Tea tree is a large, bushy shrub reaching heights of 15'–20'. Its linear leaves are ¾"–1¼" long and tend to be 3–veined. Small oil glands are sometimes visible without a lens. The small flowers are white and form in axillary or terminal spikes. Woody capsules are globose and many–seeded.

DISTRIBUTION
A bush of low–lying, swampy areas, Tea tree occurs in coastal areas of New South Wales and Queensland, Australia.

CHEMISTRY
Volatile fraction: α–tuyene, α–pinene, sabinene,

β–pinene, myrcene, α–phellandrene, α–terpinene, p–cymene, limonene, 1,8–cineole, γ–terpinene, terpinolene, terpinen–4–ol, α–terpineol, aroma-dendrene, δ–cadinene; flavonoids.

MEDICINAL USES

The essential oil distilled from Tea tree[46], better known as Tea tree oil, is the main article of commerce and the base item described for this monograph. Known regionally for some time before recent popularity in America, Tea tree oil deserves a segment because it is a valuable and effective medicinal essential oil.

Applied topically it is superb at curbing numerous bacterial, fungal, and viral strains. Dosing is a main concern: try the pure, undiluted oil on infections where the skin is unbroken, such as nail fungi, ringworm, etc. When there is skin and tissue sensitivity the essential oil can be diluted with olive oil, or prepared as an ointment. Each situation must be evaluated case by case. Some areas/conditions/individuals will be more sensitive than others.

20–30 drops of the spirit, added to several oz. of water, can be gargled and used as a mouthwash for oral Candida albicans infections – often a problem among the immunosuppressed. Bacteria responsible for gingivitis and pyorrhea also are inhibited by a 2–3 times a day gargle.

Vaginal Candida infections are better addressed through the essential oil made into a suppository, as alone the essential oil may be too irritating to these sensitive areas. See Preparation section for full instructions.

Topically applied to antibiotic–resistant staph infections, the essential oil often makes quite a difference. Internal Echinacea and/or Astragalus is indicated when immune system depression is a factor. More common though is Tea tree simply applied to infected cuts and scrapes. Used this way it is equally effective for children.

Undiluted, applied several times a day to the common wart (Verruca vulgaris) is an efficient

---

46   Not to be confused with Cajeput oil (distillate of Melaleuca cajuputi) or Niaouli oil (distillate of M. quinquenervia).

method of removal. Secure an essential oil saturated cotton swab over the wart. Between 7 to 14 days the wart will usually detach itself, leaving a small crater that will heal in time. Calendula ointment can be applied at this point.

Topical application to tissue affected by the herpes group of viruses (HSV, VZV, etc.) is often successful at resolving outbreak. Again, undiluted will be found stronger than the diluted essential oil. Let the sensitivity of the area determine the strength applied. Combined with Mugwort or Wormwood (2–3 cups drunk daily) the therapy will influence outbreak resolution more profoundly due to these plant's systemic effects on the virus.

Recommended by some as an internal therapy, the spirit of Tea tree can be used in a limited way. Like any terpene–containing volatile oil, it will be found carminative and anesthetic to stomach walls. The plant's antimicrobial properties will be primarily limited to the gastrointestinal region, making it useful for bacterial issues related to food poisoning. As a systemic antimicrobial/antiviral agent, so much of the spirit would be needed that toxic side effects may become evident. Here standard immune stimulants will be found more successful and better tolerated.

INDICATIONS
♦   Bacterial/Fungal infections (external)
♦   Warts (external)
♦   HSV/VZV (external)

COLLECTION
Unless the plant is abundant (Australia) the essential oil is common and commercially available. Pure, undiluted qualities are recommended. These then can be diluted or prepared as needed.

PREPARATIONS/DOSAGE
♦   Essential oil, externally applied: as needed
♦   Ointment: as needed
♦   Oil/Salve: as needed
♦   Suppository: 2 daily (one before bed)
♦   Spirit: 10–20 drops 2–3 times daily

CAUTIONS

Tea tree essential oil is well tolerated when used topically. Occasionally tissue irritation occurs with initial application or if used undiluted on sensitive tissues.

Mild to moderate poisonings have been reported for Tea tree when ingested – usually by unknowing children. In the majority of cases toddlers drank a large amount of essential oil (up to 10ml), and upon CNS symptoms, were taken to emergency care, when after treatment they were released within 24 hours.

Topical use is fine for all. Do not use internally if pregnant or nursing. Also Tea tree is not recommended internally for children.

THUJA

Cupressaceae/Cypress Family

Thuja occidentalis
Arbor vitae, Northern white cedar, Eastern white cedar

DESCRIPTION

Growing to heights of 60', Thuja is a substantial tree. As a conifer, its most impressive feature is its scale–like leaves. They form in laterally appressed fans. Both male and female cones develop on the same tree. Female cones are larger than male cones and are $2/5$"–1" in diameter at maturity. Seeds are broadly winged.

Initially thought to be short–lived (80–100 years), Thuja is now being age–reevaluated. Numerous trees in the Niagara area are now asserted to be over 1500 years old. The plant is adept at maximizing available nutrients, partitioning off less vital or diseased parts, while maintaining a very slow growth rate.

DISTRIBUTION

From Canada, the Northeast, and the Great Lakes region, Thuja is distributed south to several of the southern Appalachian States. The tree can be found in a number of varying habitats, but is mostly associated with nutrient–rich, moist soils. Look next to stream sides and around drainage areas. As an ornamental planted throughout the West it is commonly found in proximity to old farms and homesteads.

CHEMISTRY

Volatile fraction: α–pinene, α–thujone, fenchone, borneol, acetic–, formic–, and isovaleric–acids, terpineol, sabinene, camphene, camphor, valerianic acid, occidol; lignans: thujaplicatin, dihydroxythujaplicatin.

MEDICINAL USES

Due to Thuja's aromatic composition the plant's main area of influence is over the genital–urinary and bronchial systems. Secondly, as a topical medicine it will be well applied to numerous microbial involvements. Part stimulant, part astringent with bacterial–fungal inhibiting overtones, the plant is worthy of note.

Suffers of chronic bladder and urethra infections will surely benefit from Thuja tea or tincture. It is best applied to long–standing infections that come and go and seem to be dependant upon general weakness of the area. Corresponding urinary tract pain and irritation will likewise be soothed. If the Heath family group of plants (Uva–ursi, Cranberry, or Manzanita) don't have an impact on the area, most likely Thuja will.

Urinary incontinence, again from tissue weakness (not organic disease), should lessen under the plant's use. For bed wetting children, Thuja combined with Mullein root, is often useful. An emotional component usually needs to be addressed in such cases. In older individuals with poor bladder control Thuja's tonic effect often has perceivable results, particularly when small amounts of urine are uncontrollably voided due to coughing, sneezing, or laughing. If in older men prostate enlargement or irritation of the area is the cause of dribbling of urine, the plant should be reached for first. Thuja's benefit here is due, not any shrinking of prostrate tissue[47] per se, but to its antibacterial/tonic proper-

47 A closely related tree, Thuja standishii contains a

ties.

The tea is the best preparation for addressing intestinal microbial problems, namely traveler's diarrhea (amebiasis) and giardiasis. Thuja's aromatics are inhibiting to Giardia lamblia and the ameba group of organisms, particularly, Entamoeba histolytica. It can be used alone, or more successfully with Castela emoryi or Ailanthus altissima.

Externally Thuja is a valuable treatment for a number of fungal involvements. Various nail and skin funguses are inhibited by the plant. Application of the undiluted essential oil should be used several times a day. The same is well applied to both common (Verruca vulgaris) and genital warts (Condyloma acuminatum). Be the growths upon the genital or anal region continual application is important. Dilute the essential oil with olive oil for more sensitive tissues. Alone or in combination, Thuja makes an excellent vaginal suppository for cervical dysplasia[48]. Over time (6 months) I have observed class 2 and 3 cases resolve completely.

Women will find a douche or sitz bath made with the leaves resolving to vaginal Candida infections. Other areas typical of Candida growth are around the mouth, under arms, and between mid–section rolls of skin. Although more rare, intestinal/systemic infections can result in more severe cases. For such situations combine Thuja with Desert willow or Pau d'arco. Use externally and internally. Babies who suffer from thrush (oral Candida infections) will benefit from external application of the tea or ointment.

Similar to Thuja's fungicidal properties, the plant is also distinctly antibacterial. External preparations are well applied to poorly healing wounds, bedsores, and other slow–to–heal afflic-

tions. As a mouthwash, Thuja is beneficial to the oral environment due to its inhibition of plaque–forming enzymes. Used in this way, twice a day, especially before bed, the plant is one of our best for gingivitis prevention.

Alone or in combination with Marshmallow, Thuja makes an excellent stimulating poultice. Applied to abscesses it certainly will encourage resolution – through coming to a head or resolving internally. This effect is due not so much to the plant's antibacterial overtone, but to its stimulation of innate immunity.

Although not a systemic immune stimulant like Echinacea, Thuja does stimulate innate immunity, and to a lesser degree, acquired immunity (T–cell activity) within surfaces it contacts. Doubtlessly this is one reason why the plant has such a noted effect on the urinary tract. This is one region where Thuja's aromatics are excreted as waste products to be eliminate from the body. To our benefit these compounds affect the surrounding urinary tissues.

Like the urinary tract, the bronchial environment is likewise influenced by Thuja's aromatics. Used as a potent antimicrobial agent, as well as a local immune stimulant, successful application will be seen in a number of respiratory–centered distresses. In chronic bronchitis when expectoration is copious, mucus is green or yellow, and the lungs feel weakened, Thuja will be of great value. Lingering coughs, as a symptom of a chronic or sub–acute bronchial condition, usually will cease or lessen.

Specifically the plant stimulates resident macrophages or dust cells within the alveoli. These specialized cells are at the center of the lung's infection–fighting process. Like the plant's involvement with the urinary tract, Thuja's aromatics, which are excreted and therefore dispersed throughout the lungs, serve to inoculate the area with antimicrobial/immune–stimulating constituents.

Steam applications of Thuja also affect the respiratory tract. In many ways, this method is more direct, and ultimately more effective than internal preparations. With it, topical exposure is

number of diterpenes that have shown aromatase inhibition. It is possible Thuja occidentalis also has application to BPH and breast cancer prevention.

48   The majority of cases are caused by HPV (human papillomavirus) infection, a viral group responsible for common and genital warts and most cases of cervical cancer. Cervical dysplasia is used to describe pre–cancerous tissue alterations usually caused by HPV. Detectable through a "pap smear" (papanicolaou test) results are ranked in classes: class 1 – normal to class 5 – cancerous.

achieved. It is as if an ointment is being applied to pneumal mucus membranes. For chronic sore throats (pharyngitis), laryngitis, and even bacterial oriented strep throat, Thuja–based stream inhalation will be most beneficial. Both the recently dried leaf or the commercially purchased essential oil are fine articles that will produce a medicated steam.

Thuja has been used with success in treating valley fever, or coccidioidomycosis, caused by the soil mold Coccidioides immitis, commonly found in alkaline soils throughout the hot and dry Southwest. It is responsible for flu–like symptoms of fatigue, fever, headache, aches and pains, and cough. Susceptibility is largely dependent upon immune system condition, overall vitality, and racial/genetic disposition.

Lastly the isotonic tea as an eyewash should be applied several times a day for the elimination of styes. Both budding and mature styes will be affected by treatment, but early–stage styes will more reliably resolve. If the eyewash gives negligible results, try applying a small amount of ointment directly to the stye.

Thuja is best used as an emmenagogue when menses is slowed from uterine laxity or illness/stress.

In conclusion Thuja shares many of its therapeutic qualities with other Cypress family plants, in fact consider them all shades of the same color.

INDICATIONS

♦ Urinary tract infections, chronic
♦ Urinary incontinence/Bed wetting
♦ Prostrate irritation
♦ Traveler's diarrhea/Giardiasis
♦ Fungal infections (external)
♦ HPV/Common warts/Genital warts/Cervical dysplasia (external)
♦ Candida infections (external)
♦ Poorly healing wounds/Bedsores (external)
♦ Gingivitis (external)
♦ Abscesses (external)
♦ Bronchitis, chronic
♦ Pharyngitis/Laryngitis/Strep throat (gargle)
♦ Valley fever
♦ Ocular styes (eyewash)
♦ Menses, to stimulate

COLLECTION

Gathering Thuja is fairly straight–forward. Collect new spring–summertime growth by snipping off outward leafing branch tips. Prepare fresh, or dry first by laying out well spaced.

PREPARATIONS

Most methods of Thuja delivery are commonly known – tea, tincture, etc. The steam inhalation technique, lesser so: in a large pot bring 1 gallon of water to a boil, add 4 oz. of Thuja leaf, reduce to a simmer, and inhale the volatile oil infused steam. If using the essential oil[49], add 10–15 drops of oil to the same amount of water.

DOSAGE

♦ FPT/DPT (60% alcohol): 20–40 drops 2–3 times daily
♦ Leaf infusion: 4–6 oz. 2–3 times daily
♦ Inhaled steam from the infusion or essential oil: 5 minutes 2–3 times daily
♦ Spirit: 10–20 drops 2–3 times daily
♦ Essential oil, topically applied: as needed
♦ Oil/Salve/Ointment/Poultice: as needed
♦ Suppository: 2 times daily, once before bed
♦ Eye wash: 2–3 times daily

CAUTIONS

The plant is not recommended during pregnancy or while nursing due to the leaves' substantial Thujone content. Fatalities have occurred with the essential oil's use as an abortifacient.

Children should not use the essential oil or spirt internally. The volatile fraction is too concentrated for their sensitive systems. In small

---

49 New methods have surely taken over but at least up until the mid twentieth century most Thuja distillation took place in backwood stills in upper state New York. After being stripped from their main branches, leaves would be placed in the boiler. The volatile component would rise with steam to a condenser, then collect in a vessel. 30 lbs. of essential oil would be derived from 2000 lbs. of leaf material.

spot areas external use is fine.

OTHER USES
As a forestry product, Thuja wood is used in applications in which there is continual moisture or water exposure.

TURMERIC
Zingiberaceae/Ginger Family

Curcuma longa
Indian saffron, Yellow root

DESCRIPTION
Arising from a fleshy, lateral root, Turmeric's above ground growth is distinctly tropical–monocot in appearance. Standing 2'–3' tall the plant's large leaves are lanceolate, acute–tipped, with tapering bases. Flower spikes are cylindrical, 4"–6" long, and are composed of large floral bracts. Tubular corollas are yellow. Fruit is a capsule.

DISTRIBUTION
Native to Southeast Asia, the majority is cultivated in India. China, Taiwan, Java, and Peru also produce sizable amounts.

CHEMISTRY
Curcuminoids: curcumin, demethoxycurcumin, bisdemethoxycurcumin; essential oil: β–pinene, p–cymene, β–elemene, germacrone, α–curcumene, β–curcumene, ar–turmerone, α–turmerone, β–turmerone, curcumenol, isocurcumenol, curcumol, curdione, neocurdione, furanodienone, furanodiene, curzerene, curcumenone.

MEDICINAL USES
As a mild antiinflammatory, Turmeric is most useful in reducing the pain and inflammation of rheumatoid arthritis. If it fails to give some relief then add equal portions of Creosote bush, the latter being a stronger antiinflammatory. The pain and swelling of sport–type injuries, contu-

sions, blows, etc. are also reduced. Here, internal Turmeric combines well with topical Arnica (if there is pain on movement).

Like other spice herbs Turmeric affects the upper gastrointestinal tract. Indigestion and fullness will be allayed by its use as a stomachic. It increases gastric secretions, therefore its use is indicated in deficiencies of the area.

Turmeric profoundly influences the liver and some of its intrinsic functions. Overtly the plant is a choleretic and chologogue. Even though bile components are increased, total bile volume is augmented as well, producing an overall thinning effect, ultimately lowering biliary cholesterol concentration. Gall stone (cholesterol type) reduction/elimination is a key indication for Turmeric use.

Supplementation has also shown to reduce serum LDL (low density lipoprotein) and triglyceride levels, in some cases rivalling cholesterol–lowering pharmaceuticals. Turmeric's mechanism of action is still unclear. Possibly it is due to some sort of blocking activity in the gut or an enzymatic effect within the liver.

It appears as though Turmeric's cellular influence on the liver is inherently positive and stabilizing. Research has shown glutathione content is increased within hepatic tissue (among other areas), as is glutathione–s–transferase activity. This is an important detoxification pathway that is largely responsible for eliminating systemic carcinogens. Similarly, a number of other metabolite/carcinogen pathways are altered. Turmeric's effect here is to limit the liver's activation of an innocuous toxin, to a more potent, mutagenic one. The plant influences other parameters as well, suggesting its use as a cancer preventative, or adjunctive therapy, should not be underestimated. Arachidonic acid metabolism, a key inflammatory pathway associated with many disease states, including cancer development, is inhibited by Turmeric. The plant's antioxidant properties stabilize cellular membranes within the liver, making that organ more able to withstand stresses.

Turmeric's antimutagenic properties can certainly benefit a vast range of precancerous conditions affecting topical mucosa and the skin. From the lesions of oral submucous fibrosis and oral leukoplakia to poorly healing reddened patches of sun–exposed skin, the plant has a definite corrective influence over mutagenic cells. Even in advanced cases of topical cancer, Turmeric often has a marked effect, reducing lesion size, thickness, and exudation.

Eczema and psoriasis both respond well to the plant's healing ability. As stated earlier, light and oxygen exposure will serve as an activator. A whole range of external preparations – ointment–oil–salve – can be used for these purposes.

Used externally Turmeric is antibacterial, particularly against gram–positive bacterial strains. Increasing its power against pathogenic organisms, including fungi, is its potentiation by light and oxygen. These elements make Turmeric genotoxic to the organism's DNA, subsequently killing the pathogen.

Although Turmeric's antioxidant and anti-inflammatory properties are beneficial body–wide, due to its effect on blood platelets, the herb can be thought of as cardiovascular tonic. Catecholamine and arachidonate induced aggregation or stickiness is inhibited by it, as is this metabolic condition's effect on vascular walls. Although probably not as potent as Ginkgo, Turmeric affords protection against clot formation. It has been shown that in regions where curries are regularly used, incidence of cardiovascular disease is less.

One of Turmeric's traditional uses, as a simple root poultice or slice placed against an insect bit or sting, points to a wider area of activity. A number of studies have shown the root to be significant in reducing the destructive effects of poisonous snake venom. The neurotoxic and hemotoxic effects of cobras and pitvipers (rattlesnakes) are strongly inhibited by Turmeric. Combine it with Echinacea and use liberal amounts internally and externally if conventional antivenom treatments are not available. It can also be used in conjunction with conventional treatments.

INDICATIONS

- ◆ Rheumatoid arthritis
- ◆ Sport injuries
- ◆ Indigestion
- ◆ Hepatic stasis
- ◆ Biliary stones
- ◆ Elevated LDL and triglyceride levels
- ◆ Inflammatory/Oxidative stress, liver centered
- ◆ Cancer preventative, systemic
- ◆ Precancerous lesion (external and internal)
- ◆ Eczema/Psoriasis (external and internal)
- ◆ Bacterial/Fungal infections (external)
- ◆ Platelet aggregation/Clot formation
- ◆ Cardiovascular disease, preventative
- ◆ Insect/Snake bite

COLLECTION

Though the "long" type is more common, at least in western markets, both round and long tubers develop from the same plant and are found in commerce. Turmeric's yellowish–orange to reddish–brown internal color is distinctive.

PREPARATIONS

It is interesting to note that standardized Turmeric products are based on the pigment curcumin. The bioavailability of curcumin is so small that after ingestion most is found intact in the stool. It is the full spectrum of the plant's compounds, including its non–polar essential oil factor, that renders it medicinally active. Whole plant preparations are recommended.

Water based preparations, such as teas, are inferior due to Turmeric's insolubility in that medium. ½–1 teaspoon of power can be mixed into 8oz of water and ingested that way.

DOSAGE

- ◆ FPT/DPT (60% alcohol): 30–60 drops 2–3 times daily
- ◆ Capsule (00): 2–3, 2–3 times daily
- ◆ Oil/Salve/Ointment: as needed

CAUTIONS

Routine use of curries/Turmeric may irritate the stomach lining. It is best not use if there is a history of stomach irritability or gastritis.

OTHER USES
Along with other spice plants such as Cumin, Turmeric is a main component of various curries. It is also used as a natural coloring agent.

UVA–URSI
Ericaceae/Heath Family

Arctostaphylos uva–ursi
Bearberry, Kinnikinnick

DESCRIPTION
Uva–ursi is a mat–like shrub with low–growing to occasionally prostrate stems reaching heights of 1'–1½'. The plant roots at stem nodes, so older colonies can become well established and quite dense. Leaf blades are entire, oval to oblong, with upper glabrous and dark green surfaces. Lower surfaces are lighter green, somewhat puberulent, becoming glabrous with age. The small flowers form in racemes. They are distinctly urn–shaped and white or pinkish. The small berries are ⅓"–⅖" in diameter and bright red.

DISTRIBUTION
Uva–ursi ranges through much of mountainous North America. It is found from Alaska, south to California, throughout the interior western mountains, to the eastern ranges, extending as far south as Georgia and Arkansas. Look to coniferous forests, sandy soils, and rocky slopes.

CHEMISTRY
Phenolic glucosides: arbutin, methylarbutin, hydroquinone; tannins: caffeic acid, gallic acid, catechol, ellagic acid; triterpenoids: uvaol, ursolic acid, lupeol, α–amyrin, β–amyrin, erythrodiol, oleanolic acid; anthocyanidins: delphinidin, cyanidin; quercitrin, quercetin.

MEDICINAL USES

Uva–ursi inhibits lower urinary tract bacterial strains that thrive in alkaline urine. In the presence of alkaline urine, arbutin, a main constituent of Uva–ursi, is broken down into hydroquinone and subsequently is responsible for the plant's antibacterial qualities. Escherichia coli, a typical urinary tract pathogen, thrives in alkaline urine. In the presence of normal acidic urine, or Uva–ursi influenced urine, this bacterium finds attachment to cell walls difficult. Combining the use of Uva–ursi or most other Heath family plants, such as Madrone or Cranberry, with diet changes that include more animal source proteins, along with limiting simple carbohydrates, can promptly resolve alkaline urinary tract infections.

Uva–ursi is also a urinary tract astringent. The plant's tannin complexes responsible for this tone lax urinary tract tissues by imparting a local tightening effect. Use it when there is dragging urinary pain in combination with dribbling of urine and mucus discharge.

As a postpartum sitz bath, Uva–ursi is useful in tonifying and soothing vaginal and cervical tissues. Since Uva–ursi is moderately inhibiting to Candida albicans it is well worth combining topical applications with internal use of Thuja or Garlic.

INDICATIONS
♦ Lower urinary tact infection with alkaline urine
♦ Vaginitis with or w/o Candida involvement
♦ As a postpartum sitz bath

COLLECTION
Gather Uva–ursi leaves from late spring to summer after flowering when the ripe fruit is present. The arbutin content is most concentrated at this time, less so when the plant is in flower.

PREPARATIONS
Several things can be done to facilitate the breakdown of arbutin and methylarbutin into hydroquinone, therefore increasing the plant's effectiveness. Simply drying the leaf starts the conversion. Hydroquinone is also increased by

rehydrating the leaves in a small amount of water for 3–4 hours. After this initial soak, decoct normally.

DOSAGE

♦ Leaf decoction: 4–6 oz. 2–3 times daily
♦ DPT (40% alcohol, 10% glycerin): 60–90 drops 2–3 times daily
♦ Fluidextract: 30–50 drops 2–3 times daily
♦ Sitz bath: as needed

CAUTIONS

Uva–ursi may have a vasoconstricting effect on uterine lining, so it is contraindicated during pregnancy. The plant's tannins can have an irritating effect on gastric mucosa and the kidneys; limit consecutive use to two weeks. With the addition of Marshmallow and/or Corn silk length of usage can be increased.

OTHER USES

Uva–ursi's edible fruit are good for making jams and jellies.

VALERIAN

Valerianaceae/Valerian Family

Valeriana officinalis
Garden valerian

Valeriana acutiloba (V. capitata ssp. acutiloba)
Western valerian

Valeriana edulis
Mexican valerian

DESCRIPTION

A sizable herbaceous perennial, Valeriana officinalis can reach heights of 5′–6′ feet. Most of its size is due to lengthy stem growth. Large pinnate leaves are oppositely arranged and are composed of 3–25 leaflets. They are linear to elliptical and entire to toothed. Flowers form in compounded panicles. Generally pink to white, each floral tube is about ¼″ in length. Like many other Valerians, V. officinalis's roots are primarily sub–surface runners.

Compared to the other varieties profiled here Valeriana acutiloba is a small plant. Its long petioled basal leaves are spatulate, oblanceolate, or obovate, and typically entire. The leaves that develop on the 6″–18″ flower stalk are paired and entire to pinnately divided. The white–pink, ¼″ long flowers form in dense panicles. The plant's creeping rhizomes are anchored just below the ground's surface by fine hair–like rootlets.

Valerian edulis is quite different in appearance. It too is comprised of basal leaves for most of the growing season. Although they are highly variable in form, they generally are oblanceolate, but can be divided as well. Stalk leaves are paired, and are usually divided into 3–7 divisions. The small whitish flowers form in open panicles. Underground, V. edulis is a stout plant, sending down a robust and fleshy, 1′–1½′ tap root.

DISTRIBUTION

Of Eurasian extraction, Valeriana officinalis is a successful weed (considered invasive in Connecticut) through much of the Northeast. From Maryland and Iowa it is found north into Canada. It is also common throughout the Pacific Northwest.

Valeriana acutiloba is a plant of mountainous regions throughout the West. Look to coniferous forests, often among Douglas Fir stands, and almost always on hillsides. It is fond of moist, rich soils, usually with a mountain stream beneath. From the interior western mountain states, such as Wyoming, V. acutiloba is found south to Arizona and New Mexico.

Valeriana edulis, another plant of the West, is also found in some of the same places where V. acutiloba grows. Mountain stream sides are a common area for the plant. It is also often found among rocks, making the plant's tap root snake around unpredictably. Meadows with bordering Pine and Fir, where the soil is moist and rich, is another favorite of V. edulis. The plant also ranges throughout many of the interior mountain states; from Montana south to Arizona.

CHEMISTRY

Monoterpenoids; sesquiterpenoids: valerenic acid and its derivatives: valeranone, valeranal, kessyl esters; valepotriates: valtrate, didrovaltrate, acevaltrate, isovaleroxyhydroxyvaltrate; flavonoids: methyl apigenin, hesperidin, linarin; triterpenes, lignans, alkaloids.

MEDICINAL USES

Valerian presents an interesting mix of effects, some of them even countering its use as a sedative. Like so many other herbs that fall somewhere between nutrition and drug, the plant is special in that it remedies the person with his or her physiological tendencies. It is a plant that fits people better than conditions.

Valerian works best for those with lowered innate vitality. The aged, those weakened from sickness, or those whose health is compromised from constant stress and worry will benefit from its use. In these people the plant works well to bring on sleep and relaxation. It is not unusual for the plant to usher in a sense of clarity and peacefulness of mind.

Depression arising from long–term over–work and worry is often lifted, as is hysteria arising from similar states. I have seen impaired thinking or a cerebral fog of sorts, dissipated by the fresh plant tincture. Valerian helps to lift the depression of hypothyroidism. It is plausible that some fraction of Valerian has a thyroid influencing effect.

If circulation is enfeebled (cold hands and feet, trouble adjusting to the cold), usually seen in the aged or less robust, Valerian as a calming agent, is choice. Heart palpitations, from over–work and worry, especially combined with Passionflower are lessened. Neuralgias with mild spasm or tremor are quieted as are headaches from excessive worry or mental effort.

As a carminative Valerian is useful particularly if indigestion is from emotional upset. The plant's volatile oil content is largely responsible for its action. Gas and bloating are eased, as are headaches that are so commonly caused from imperfect upper gastric digestion.

Not all Valerian species or preparations act the same. The fresh plant tincture tends to be as stimulatory as sedative. Dried, Valerian is more singularly sedative, especially the root infusion.

Valeriana officinalis is the strongest sedative, particularly if dried. V. acutiloba and V. edulis[50], although decent sedatives, are best used if there is obvious CNS (central nervous system) depression and debility. They have fairly well pronounced spinal/cerebral stimulatory properties.

As for how Valerian produces its CNS effects and what group of constituents is responsible, there is still much debate on the issue. It was originally thought that the plant's valepotriate content was largely responsible and this compound group inhibited GABA (gamma–aminobutyric acid) re–uptake. Now other mechanisms are coming to light which are attributed to altogether different compounds.

The plant's adenosine receptor modulation may have much to do with varying effects of different species and preparations. Alcohol preparations contain more lipophilic constituents, such as isovaltrate, and tend to serve as inverse agonists for adenosine A_1 receptors, causing CNS stimulation. Water based preparations, actually stimulate adenosine A_1 receptors, bringing about CNS sedation.

Calcium channel blocking, serotoninergic, melatonergic, and dopaminergic effects have also been reported making Valerian's CNS influence complex. But regardless of intricacies it is important to understand that Valerian is not the straight forward sedative that it is largely touted to be. It is a CNS modulator, capable of either sedation and/or stimulation depending on preparation, species, and even the individual.

INDICATIONS

♦ Insomnia/Restlessness
♦ Hysteria/Depression from weakness

---

50 Compared to V. officinalis this species has a higher percentage of valepotriates and is often used as a base material for the extraction of these compounds.

- ♦ Heart palpitation, from nervous exhaustion
- ♦ Neuralgia/Spasm/Tremor
- ♦ Indigestion/Gas/Bloating

COLLECTION

Valeriana officinalis is easily cultivated as a bedding–herb garden plant. Roots are easily dug due to their runner–type tendency. V. acutiloba has smaller roots that creep under the soil's surface. The small rootlets cling to forest soils remarkably well. Wash with water to remove excess dirt. The herbage of this variety can be utilized, since it too is medicinal.

Since the leaves are nearly impotent, only the roots of V. edulis should be collected and used. The tap root of this Valerian can be difficult to collect depending on its depth and rocks that it has maneuvered around.

PREPARATIONS

Dried, water–based preparations, of any variety, but especially Valeriana officinalis, tend to be more sedative. The encapsulated dried plant and the dried plant tincture, act as sedatives less predictably. The fresh plant tincture of any variety tends to be more stimulatory in nature. For some people Valerian is a superb sedative, regardless of form, but for others it is equivalent to a cup of coffee before bed.

Forget standardized extracts. With Valerian in particular "standardization experts" are guessing at the "active" compound group. It's the whole plant which comprises Valerian.

Of course no description of dried Valerian would be complete without mentioning its distinctive aroma. Usually described as smelling like stinky, unwashed socks, personally I never agreed with the comparison. Thick, earthy, and a bit musky – yes; maybe an obscure description, but closer to an accurate one.

DOSAGE

- ♦ Root infusion: 3–6 oz. 1–3 times daily
- ♦ FPT/DPT (70% alcohol): 45–90 drops 1–3 times daily
- ♦ Fluidextract: 20–40 drops 2–3 times daily
- ♦ Capsule (00): 1–2, 1–3 times daily

CAUTIONS

Do not take during pregnancy or while nursing. Potentiation may be an issue if combined with sedative pharmaceuticals (especially the benzo-diazepine[51] class of drugs). Sensitive individuals may experience next–morning grogginess after evening supplementation.

WHITE WILLOW
Salicaceae/Willow Family

Salix alba
Golden willow

DESCRIPTION

Reaching heights of 60'–90', Salix alba is a moderate sized tree. While the trunk can be up to several feet in diameter, the tree's bark is deeply fissured and grayish–brown. Leaves are covered with a fine coating of white pubescence. Being more prominent on the underside of each leaf, in a breeze the foliage has a pleasing two–toned appeal. Like others in the Willow family, male and female catkins develop on separate trees. Both types are 1⅕"–2" long. Female seeds are attached to a downy fluff, making wind dispersal more successful.

DISTRIBUTION

White willow, originally from Asia and Europe, is now extensively naturalized throughout much of North America. It is planted as an ornamental and is found feral around moister soils.

CHEMISTRY

Phenolic glycosides: salicin, fragilin, salicortin.

MEDICINAL USES

Of all the phenolic glycoside containing plants, White willow is probably the most widely used.

---

51 Valium is derived from Valerian. This myth has been going around for some time. Both the plant and the drug begin with V and both are sedatives, must be related.

It works as an antiinflammatory due to its salicin content and here only after being systemically (in blood and tissue) hydrolyzed to salicylic acid. Think of White willow and other salicin containing plants (Cottonwood, Aspen, Popular) as pro–antiinflammatory. Its therapeutic benefit is reliant upon the body's transformation of salicin into active salicylic acid[52], or esters thereof.

The bark decoction is a sort of timed–released, aspirin–like therapy, useful for an array of inflammatory conditions. Due to the plant's effect on cyclooxygenase and related inflammatory prostaglandins, White willow's application can vary greatly. Rheumatic issues, tissue injury, and both chronic and acute pain syndromes, usually are relieved to some degree. Whenever there is pain and inflammation try White willow. It is a broadly acting analgesic approach.

For adults White willow is decent at lowering a high fever. Like aspirin, its effect is due to prostaglandin inhibition and diminishment of the CNS's (central nervous system) response to interleukin–1. This ultimately reduces the hypothalamus's temperature elevating action. Vasodilation of superficial blood vessels occurs, enabling heat dissipation. Diaphoresis may initiate in conjunction. For relief of moderate fevers, especially if the skin is dry, add equal parts of Peppermint, Spearmint, or Elder. This will increase diaphoretic activity, enabling the body to "sweat it out".

White willow probably has some effect on platelet aggregation. The plant's increase of bleeding time is almost certain, but is really unexplored due to the efficacy and safety of low–dose aspirin therapy.

As a functional bitter tonic, drink several oz. of tea before a meal. Due to its stimulatory effect on gastric activity, more efficient digestion and assimilation occurs, lessening the chance of gas, bloating, and food–centered malaise.

INDICATIONS

- Pain and inflammation, chronic and acute
- Temperate, elevated
- Indigestion

COLLECTION
On older branches gather the inner bark, beyond the outward, protective fissured layer. Due to outer bark thinness, bark on younger branches can be collected entirely.

PREPARATIONS/DOSAGE
- Bark decoction: 2–6 oz. 2–3 times daily

CAUTIONS
Like aspirin's connection to Reye's syndrome[53], do not use with children if there is a viral infection and/or an elevated temperate. Continued use may influence blood viscosity and clotting time. Long term use with anticoagulants, even low–dose aspirin (80 mg. daily) may cause a problem.

WILD CHERRY
Rosaceae/Rose Family

Prunus virginiana
Chokecherry

DESCRIPTION
Reaching a height of approximately 20′, Wild cherry matures into a large bush or a small tree. The plant's smooth, grayish–brown bark is distinctive and comes in handy when trying to discern it from other trees when leafless. Older, lower trunk bark is usually fissured. Wild cherry's elliptic to obovate leaves are 1⅙″–2⅓″ long. They have finely serrated margins, rounded bases, and generally acute tips. From shiny to slightly hairy, the leaves' undersides are variable. Flower clusters form in racemes (2″–4″ long) at branch ends. Each round, white flower has 5 petals, 5 sepals, and is between ¼″–½″ in diameter. The dark red or nearly black fruit hang in drupes. Each cherry

---

52 Relatedly aspirin (acetylsalicylic acid) is hydrolyzed into acetic acid, salicylate, and salicylic acid in the blood (as well as partially remaining intact as acetylsalicylic acid).

53 Even aspirin as a trigger is not absolutely proven, but it's better to be safe than sorry.

contains a large, smooth seed.

DISTRIBUTION

Wild cherry is common throughout most of the United States. It is absent in the extreme Southeast and low desert regions of the West. Prunus virginiana is principally divided into three varieties: var. demissa (Western chokecherry), var. melanocarpa (Black chokecherry), and var. virginiana (Chokecherry). All can be used in the same way.

CHEMISTRY

Cyanogenic glycosides: amygdalin, prunasin, prulaurasin; flavonoids; tannins.

MEDICINAL USES

Use bark preparations if there is a dry–irritative cough. Whether associated with bronchitis, influenza, or other lung afflictions, Wild cherry works best in bronchial conditions with associated rapid pulse, quickened breathing, and fever. It is a sedative for bronchial mucus membrane irritation, dependant on excitable cardiac activity. Rapid breathing, usually with attendant fever, calms nicely with Wild cherry. It often is the perfect fit for children who exhibit these tendencies when sick with wintertime viruses. The plant should be considered a necessity when recovering from pleurisy or pneumonia with attendant colliquative sweating. In this respect Wild cherry acts Sage–like and is able to reduce fever–dependant perspiration.

The plant's hydrocyanic acid content, a compound common to many seeds/barks within the Rose family, is mainly responsible for the plant's sedative activity on the pneumal and cardiovascular systems. Even for straight–forward heart palpitations dependant on debility, psychosomatic responses to stress, or overexertion, Wild cherry is often effective.

Whether related or not to the above cardio–pulmonary framework, the plant is also indicated in gastritis. Here it will be found soothing to inflamed mucosa.

INDICATIONS

◆ Cough, dry and hectic
◆ Bronchitis
◆ Heart palpitations
◆ Gastritis

COLLECTION

Select a good–sized secondary branch. It should have little or no older, fissured bark. After removing it from the trunk, discard the smaller branchlets and leaves. Remove the bark from the selected branch. It usually peels easily once started.

PREPARATIONS

Although drying the bark is essential, heat degrades the value of Wild cherry. For tea the cold infusion method is choice. The syrup, if made without heat, is an excellent preparation. When making the dried plant tincture be sure to include glycerin in the menstruum. This addition will inhibit the plant's tannins from binding with other constituents, making the tincture unusable.

DOSAGE

◆ Cold infusion: 4–6 oz. 2–3 times daily
◆ DPT (40% alcohol, 10% glycerin): 60–90 drops 2–3 times daily
◆ Fluidextract: 20–40 drops 2–3 times daily
◆ Syrup: 1–2 teaspoons 1–3 times daily

CAUTIONS

Theoretically large amounts may cause bronchial and cardiovascular suppression; none known[54] with normal dosage.

OTHER USES

Certainly edible, I remember as a boy having purple fingers and mouth from eating the bitter–sweet fruit.

---

54 Field guide and poisonous plant "experts" love to talk of Wild cherry – seeds and leaves – due to its glycoside content, as a DEADLY poison. Take it with a grain of salt: hydrogen cyanide is to Wild cherry what cocaine is to Coca leaf. It is a miniscule fraction.

WILD INDIGO
Fabaceae/Pea Family

Baptisia tinctoria
Indigo weed, False indigo, Horsefly weed

DESCRIPTION
Reaching 2'–4' in height, Wild indigo is a bushy, herbaceous perennial. The whole plant can be smooth or on occasion sparsely pubescent. Leaves are trifoliate, obovate, and cuneate. Wild indigo's flowering racemes develop from nearly every stem terminal. Flowers are yellow and are of the typical Pea family wing and keel arrangement. Seed pods are cylindrical and upon drying, turn a deep blue–indigo.

DISTRIBUTION
A common plant throughout most of the eastern half of the country, Wild indigo prefers exposed areas. Roadsides and field margins with sandy or loomy soils are common areas for the plant. From southern Canada it is found south to Georgia, then west to Iowa and Minnesota. Maine, Illinois, Iowa, Wisconsin, Minnesota, and Kentucky considers the plant endangered or "at watch". Although past and current collection for commercial reasons has not helped the plant in sensitive areas, where it is abundant, harvesting make little impact.

CHEMISTRY
Flavones: luteolin, apigenin, dihydroxyflavone, trihydroxyflavone; flavonols; isoflavones: genistein, daidzein, biochanin a, formononetin, orobol, calycosin, pseudobaptigenin, afrormosin, tectorigenin; glycoside substituents: 7–O– and 3–O–glucosides, rhamnoglucosides; arabinogalactan–proteins.

MEDICINAL USES
Wild indigo joins Echinacea and Astragalus as one of the mainstay immune stimulants used in western herbal medicine. Although each plant has its own niche and potency level, Wild indigo tends to be stronger in its effect on acquired immunity; with that more caution should precede its use.

Use Wild indigo in situations if there is acquired (and innate) immune suppression/lack of proper immune vitality. The classic indication for the plant's use is tissue infection or sepsis with impaired circulation, giving the involved area a dark, or even slightly bluish discoloration. Another signature for its application is the same discoloration imparted by capillary/immunological enfeeblement, particularly around the face and mouth. Use it in severe pharyngitis or tonsillitis when there is glandular swelling and a tendency for tissue breakdown. The gargled tincture or tea is best used when accompanied by internal dosage.

Overall the plant should be applied when tissues ulcerate and infect easily, as if it is the body's tendency because of a deficiency or weakness. Apply preparations to abscesses with associated edema, tissue necrosis, and suppuration. Wild indigo combines well with other immune stimulants, such as Echinacea, Astragalus, or Commiphora.

It is important to note that many of Wild indigo's classic indications involve either regional or systemic infection. This is all good and well if stranded out in the middle of nowhere stricken with a raging infection–dependant fever. If you have it, use Wild indigo. But stronger, more effective medicines for these things exist today. Depending on the situation's severity conventional approaches may be necessary.

Combined with Goldenseal or Yerba mansa, use it as a nasal wash when treating persistent sinusitis. Discolored mucus of a fetid nature, usually green or yellow, is an indication for the plant's use.

Apart from Wild indigo's general sphere of influence, the plant has a marked effect on the intestines, particularly the large bowel. Stimulating intestinal (and hepatic) secretions, at higher doses the plant is slightly laxative. Use it in septic conditions of the area, manifesting in diarrhea, or in extreme cases, dysentery. If ulceration is present, and evacuations are fetid, dark, and tarry, than again, Wild indigo is indicated.

INDICATIONS

♦ Immune suppression
♦ Sepsis, with impaired circulation
♦ Pharyngitis, with glandular swelling (gargle and internal)
♦ Tonsillitis (gargle and internal)
♦ Abscess, with or without progression external and internal)
♦ Sinusitis (external and internal)
♦ Diarrhea/Dysentery with microbial involvement

COLLECTION

Do not gather Wild indigo on the edge of its range. Proceed with root collection, only if there is a sufficient population. Roots are two–parted, having an outward brownish–black layer and an inner whitish core.

PREPARATIONS

The root's potency stands up well when dried. The tea or dried plant tincture are acceptable preparations. The root can also be tinctured fresh.

DOSAGE

♦ FPT/DPT (60 % alcohol): 10–20 drops 1–3 times daily
♦ Root decoction: 2–4 oz. 1–3 times daily
♦ External preparations: use as needed

A common dosing technique is to internally take the plant until loose stools occur, then back off until stools return to normal.

CAUTIONS

Diarrhea with accompanying intestinal soreness is the most common side effect with Wild indigo. This is simply remedied by reducing the dose. Theoretically it is possible that the plant, since it is a fairly strong acquired immune stimulant, may trigger auto–immune sensitivities. It is not recommended in the presence of any autoimmune disease or issue. Do not take during pregnancy or while nursing.

OTHER USES

Once considered a secondary dye plant and a ward against flies, Wild indigo today sees little activity in these areas.

WILD LETTUCE
Asteraceae/Sunflower Family

Lactuca serriola
Prickly lettuce

DESCRIPTION

This annual, or sometimes biannual, grows to be 2'–6' high. Leaves are alternately spaced, point upward, and clasp the stem. They are deeply lobed and toothed but occasionally are entire and lanceolate. On the underside of each leaf are spines aligned on the midrib. Flower heads are small, yellow, and Dandelion–like. They are borne on branching flower stalks and close by mid–morning. The seeds, like those of many other composites, are small and have an attached swirl of whitish fibers making wind dispersal effective. When cut or injured the entire plant exudes a white milky sap.

DISTRIBUTION

Introduced from Europe, the plant now exists throughout most of the United States. Like other introduced species, Wild lettuce is found along roadsides, buildings, walkways, and other areas where it is allowed through neglect and soil–disruption to flourish. Throughout drier areas in the West, the plant prefers moister soils and semi–shade.

CHEMISTRY

Lactucin, lactucopicrin, lactucic acid, lactucerin.

MEDICINAL USES

Wild lettuce is a sedative best used for mild insomnia and restlessness. Use it when these states derive from mental and emotional stress, lesser so from the pain of physical injury. It curbs agitation particularly if there is a sensation, either imagined or real, of physical heat, such as elevated core temperature from fever, dehydration, or exertion. As a sedative Wild lettuce has some similarities to California poppy. Although the former is not in the Poppy family, by effect, it can be considered a "sub–opiate", hence the antiquated name, Opium lettuce. Moreover, Wild lettuce is used in allying a spasmodic cough dependent on bronchial irritation.

INDICATIONS
♦ Insomnia and restlessness from overwork and stress
♦ Spasmodic cough from bronchial irritation

COLLECTION
Lactucarium is the name applied to the concentrated milky juice of several Lactuca species. It can be collected through a number of time consuming methods. The first approach: clip the tops off of a good–sized stand of Wild lettuce. Wait until the milky juice hardens slightly, and then scrape the milky beads off with a knife or razor blade. Re–snip each plant ¼"–½" below the original cut, and continue on and on.

The second method is similar to the first. Strip the leaves from the plant, then with a razor blade make vertical cuts along the plant's stalk. The exudate can be collected after it hardens or can be sponged up and squeezed out using a small amount of water. Finally, the last method is to collect the whole plant, before flowering, and juice it. Although the resulting juice is not technically lactucarium, the effect of the preparation is practically identical. Whatever method is utilized, dehydrate the milky liquid or juice. This hardened material, typically reddish–brown in color, is lactucarium or close to it.

PREPARATIONS
Although the whole plant tincture and leaf infusion are feeble in effect compared to lactucarium, they still have value. When making the tincture of lactucarium the hardened milky material

should dissolve completely.

DOSAGE
♦ DPT of lactucarium (80% alcohol): 30–60 drops 2–3 times daily
♦ FPT/DPT (60% alcohol): 60–90 drops 2–3 times daily
♦ Leaf infusion: 4–8 oz. 2–3 times daily

CAUTIONS
None known.

WILD OATS
Poaceae/Grass Family

Avena fatua
Oatstraw, Oatgrass

DESCRIPTION
Wild oats is a robust annual, 2'–4' tall with jointed, hollow stems and corkscrewing leaf blades. Inflorescences form in wide panicles. Individual spikelets droop tassel–like. With rearward stretched awns appearing as spindly legs, they resemble green cockroaches. The small oat seeds mature from late spring to early summer and can remain viable in the ground for nearly 10 years. Cultivated oats (Avena sativa) is another commonly found oat. Often it is difficult to tell the two apart, but upon close study, unlike Wild oats, the bracts of this variety are not hairy.

DISTRIBUTION
With exceptions pertaining to the Southeast, Wild oats, a European native, is ubiquitous throughout North America. Look for the plant in disturbed, rich soils, and around drainage ditches and culverts. Occasionally it can be found along streams and canyon sides.

CHEMISTRY
Vitexin, apigenin, d5–avenasterol, avenacosides a and b, nuatigenin.

MEDICINAL USES

Wild oats primarily exerts its effect on distresses arising from nervous system debility. Think of Wild oats as a nervous system stabilizer. It counteracts agitation from over work and prolonged periods of stress. There is some difficultly in describing what Wild oats actually does. It is not an overt sedative, nor is the plant overtly stimulating, but this detracts little from the fact that if you are physically and emotionally "rode hard and put away wet" the plant imparts a sense of stability.

Depressive states arising out of pushing through workloads on the job or at home are lifted. The edginess and frayed–end feeling of kicking nicotine, opiate, or alcohol habits is also lessened. As herbalist Michael Moore succinctly states: "this is crispy critter medicine".

INDICATIONS
♦ Depressive states
♦ Nervous system debility from overwork, stress, or substance withdrawal

COLLECTION
It is important to establish an understanding of Wild oats. Starting in the spring visit a stand several times a month as to not miss the oat in "milk stage". There is a window in which this plant is pickable for 1–2 weeks. The oat seed matures quickly so keep a close eye on it. When the spikelets are green and just starting to yellow, pick several and squeeze them. While squeezing the spikelet, you should feel a "pop" between your thumb and forefinger. This is followed by the milky–preformed seed coming out of the opposite end. At this point, they are prime for tincturing. Strip the spikelets from the rising stalks. Leave at least half of the immature oats on the collective group, so next year they will be equally abundant.

PREPARATIONS/DOSAGE
♦ FPT: 30–90 drops 3–4 times daily

CAUTIONS
None known.

OTHER USES
The whole dried plant, also know as Oatstraw, prepared as a tea is a good source of readily absorbable electrolytes, particularly calcium.

WILD YAM
Dioscoreaceae/Yam Family

Dioscorea villosa
Colic root

DESCRIPTION
A perennial and deciduous vine, Wild yam arises from a substantial root. The cordate leaves are 2"–4" long, tend to be glabrous, and have prominent underside veins. Being dioecious[55] Wild yam has separate male and female flowers. Staminate flowers develop in axillary clusters; pistillate spikes are axillary as well. Both are greenish–white in color. The ½"–1" long, 3–winged capsule, develops 2 seeds in each segment. Often Wild yam does not flower. This is likely due to sunlight blockage by overstory trees.

DISTRIBUTION
Wild yam is a woodland vine, found from mid–plain states, east to the coast, north to the Great Lakes region, New Hampshire, Canada, and finally south to Florida and Texas. From full sun to shade in both low and high elevation areas, it does well in a variety of conditions. Some significant stands exist along roadsides, where soil disruption allows better germination.

CHEMISTRY
Sapogenins: diosgenin, protodioscin, methyl protodioscin, parrisaponin, dioscin, progenin II, epiafzelechin; phenolics: catechin, epicatechin, procyanidins.

MEDICINAL USES
Geared towards gastrointestinal, biliary, and re-

---

55 The plant is highly variable. On occasion Wild yam has been reported to be monoecious or even perfect.

productive tissue, Wild yam excels as a smooth muscle relaxant. Its use here dates back beyond 19th century vitalist use, doubtlessly to various Indian tribes who lived in proximity to the plant.

Intestinal spasms, often related to stress or intestinal infection[56] are reduced through the plant's use. The addition of an intestinal antimicrobial, such as Tree of heaven or Castela emoryi is necessary to affect the cause of the problem. Use Wild yam solely if the regional spasm is a result of food sensitivity, indigestion, or heightened cholinergic function.

I have observed good results with applying the plant to the spastic stage of IBS (irritable bowel syndrome). In these cases food sensitivities/allergies, as well as psychosomatic response to food, are important factors involved in the disturbance. In most cases stress is at least partly responsible. A calm state of mind when eating is important, as this sets proper parasympathetic influence for gastrointestinal function. The plant's use towards stomach cramps and nausea outside of IBS will be found soothing. Combining Wild yam with stomachic Mint family plants will often prove more efficacious.

For the gallbladder, Wild yam typically excels at reducing or eliminating spasms of the area. Once called bilious colic, associated pain and discomfort, from stones or dietary irritation, can radiate outward and affect the entire region. With intense gallbladder attacks even upper back and shoulder pain is noticed. Fatty and rich foods are common triggers.

Stones are more serious, and are especially painful when being passed along the biliary duct to the small intestine. Wild yam acts to quiet the smooth muscle cramping of the gallbladder and duct leading to the small intestine. By relaxing the sphincter/duct tissue that surrounds the mass, Wild yam also helps in the passage of gall stones.[57]

The best gall stone treatment is in their prevention. As a daily tea use Dandelion or any bile thinning herb. Possible weight loss and dietary changes usually are warranted. Gall stones can also be gradually reincorporated into the surrounding bile. The key is to thin bile by hydration and increasing its production; here Dandelion tea will also be effective.

Although secondary, compared to the plant's effect on the liver/gallbladder systems, use Wild yam to relax smooth muscle of the urinary tract. Kidney or bladder colic, which typically comes when passing urinary gravel, is lessened. The tubular tissue of the ureter is relaxed as well, and like the plant's influence of the biliary duct leading to the small intestine, it will assist in the passage of urinary tract stones.

Menstrual cramps are sedated by Wild yam, as is ovarian sensitivity during ovulation. And more specifically if pregnancy is being threatened by premature uterine spasms the plant is likely to reduce the contraction–like activity.

Wild yam contains a number of steroidal saponins, namely diosgenin. This particular saponin was once used as a base material for the synthesis of progesterone and other pharmaceutical–grade steroids.[58] This conversion – steroidal saponin to pharmaceutical steroid – occurs in the lab via various chemical processes.

Confusion arises with the entrance of "Wild yam cream"[59], sold through health food stores, on–line, etc. Most of these creams are promoted as a natural form of progesterone, to be used dur-

---

56 Food and/or water borne bacteria are the likely causes of such distress. Bacteria such as Escherichia coli, Bacillus cereus, or Salmonella sp. are some of the more common varieties encountered.

57 Is it wise to attempt gall stone passage with Wild yam and other botanicals? In most cases, with proper guidance and materials, the outcome will be successful. In other cases the stone/s may be too large to pass and may cause a biliary blockage, and that is a problem. If the situation arises when herbs must be used to expel gall stones: in 8 oz. of Wild yam tea add, 20 drops of Lobelia tincture (made with the fresh plant or seeds), and 20 drops of Chelidonium. Drink hot, every 3 hours until the stone's passage. If after several days the pain has not receded, or signs of a biliary blockage are apparent (light colored stools, dark urine, whites of the eyes are yellowish) see a doctor.

58 From around 1950 to the early 1970s, Dioscorea mexicana or Barbasco was the main diosgenin source plant, suppling international markets with needed steroids.

59 A number of Dioscorea species will be found in "Wild yam cream".

ing menopause or for a number of menstrual issues. That the diosgenin in Wild yam (whatever species), when applied topically (or taken internally) is somehow converted to progesterone (or DHEA) is completely untrue and misleading.

Fortunately most "Wild yam creams" contain added USP progesterone. But some do not, they only contain Wild yam extract and various secondary ingredients. USP progesterone, applied topically does have some coherent application. Wild yam without added progesterone does not.

Because of this misconception I have even seen Wild yam promoted as a natural form of birth control (pharmaceutical estrogen and progesterone are used this way, why not an herbal equivalent?). The most dedicated zealot, informed through a cheap booklet, something to the effect of: "Wild Yam: Nature's Birth Control", was a single mother nine months later. The plant's internal uses are independent from any pseudo–progesterone effect[60], and should be considered apart from "Wild yam cream".

"Though Dioscorea has been used for nearly a century, its true place in therapeutics is still undetermined, probably because so many impossible claims have been made for it." Felter said this nearly 100 years ago, and sadly, for a different set of reasons, it still holds true today.

INDICATIONS
♦ Intestinal spasms
♦ Spastic stage of IBS
♦ Nausea
♦ Stomach cramps
♦ Gallbladder and duct spasm
♦ Kidney, bladder, or ureter colic
♦ Cramps, menstrual/ovarian
♦ Miscarriage, threatened

COLLECTION
Wild yam is a root medicine. When abundant, gather the gnarled and pitted tuber. Unfortunately in some areas wild populations have declined

60 If there is any hormonal affect from Wild yam, or various creams made from Dioscorea spp., it probably is slightly estrogenic, and not progesterone–like.

due to over collection mainly for a false use. It is one thing for a plant to diminish because it is being properly used. It is entirely another when a plant becomes rare because its use is based on a fabrication.

PREPARATIONS/DOSAGE
♦ FPT/DPT (65% alcohol): 60–90 drops 2–3 times daily
♦ Fluidextract: 30–60 drops 2–3 times daily
♦ Cold infusion: 3–6 oz. 2–3 times daily

CAUTIONS
Apart from spasmolytic applications do not use during pregnancy.

WITCH HAZEL
Hamamelidaceae/Witch Hazel Family

Hamamelis virginiana
Witch hazel

DESCRIPTION
Typically a small tree or large bush, Witch hazel has oval to obovate, serrated–wavy leaves. They are densely pubescent when young and 6" long by 4" wide. Flower clusters form from leaf axils and do not fully expand until October or November – a late bloomer. Seed capsules are 2–celled and woody, each segment containing a single shiny black seed, fully ripening the next season.

DISTRIBUTION
An abundant and common tree of the eastern part of the United States, Witch hazel ranges from Canada to Florida and Texas. It is found in a variety of environments: stream banks, hillsides, both rich and dry soiled woods.

CHEMISTRY
Polyphenols: epicatechin, catechin, epigallocatechin, prodelphinidins; polysaccharides.

MEDICINAL USES

Out of all of the astringent tannin plants, Witch hazel is by far the most well known. Not only does the plant contain between 2% and 10% tannin in various parts, but also a fair balance of both condensed and hydrolyzable tannins types, making its astringent application somewhat broad.

As a mouthwash and gargle, Witch hazel will be found soothing to a whole range of oral problems. Use the tea for sore throats or pharyngitis – whether acute or chronic it will be of benefit. Bleeding and sore gums will tone nicely with the tea made into a mouth rinse. For sinusitis, when nasal membranes are obviously inflamed, a nasal wash, made isotonic with salt, is helpful. After just one application, discharge, stuffiness, and vascular congestion are lessened.

Its activity towards hemorrhoids is of importance. If there is a sense of vascular congestion, weight, and discomfort, Witch hazel will be found healing. Apply the salve after each bowel movement. An old handkerchief, or a piece of flannel can be soaked into a strong tea of Tobacco or Datura and applied as a warm compress as well. These two plants will be more pain relieving, and in combination with the internal use of Stoneroot or Ocotillo, the regiment will have little equal.

As for varicosities caused from pelvic and leg venous stasis, Witch hazel ointment applied 2–3 times daily will eliminate some of the discomfort and prominence. Varicosities from both pregnancy and constitutional tendency will be helped. Addressing the problem internally will lead to longer–lasting relief.

Women will benefit if suffering from vaginitis and attending discharge by using a warm douche of isotonic Witch hazel tea. It will be found soothing to irritated tissues. By adding Thuja (or Cypress) the combination will be effective in limiting any bacterial, viral, or fungal involvement.

Witch hazel's most prosaic use is its application to cuts, scraps, and burns. Use a wash, fomentation, or an ointment for these problems. For burns alternate between Witch hazel and Aloe leaf pulp.

Internally Witch hazel tea can be used short–term as a gastrointestinal astringent. Although it is not as strong as Oak bark, it is a successful treatment for uncomplicated diarrhea and intestinal irritation.

INDICATIONS
- Sore throat (gargle)
- Bleeding/sore gums (mouthwash)
- Sinusitis (nasal wash)
- Hemorrhoids (external)
- Varicosities (external)
- Vaginitis (external)
- Cuts, scraps, burns (external)
- Diarrhea

COLLECTION
Unfissured bark, young twigs, and leaves can all be used. Witch hazel is commercially available.

PREPARATIONS
Crude preparation will be the most reliable. Proprietary products of Witch hazel distillate, contain no astringent tannins. Just how therapeutic these preparations are is questionable.

DOSAGE
- FPT/DPT (50% alcohol, 10% glycerin): 30–60 drops 2–3 times daily, or used externally
- Fluidextract: 10–30 drops, 2–3 times daily
- Douche: 2–3 times daily
- Nasal wash: as needed
- Other external preparations: as needed

CAUTIONS
Remote but possible, gastrointestinal irritation and constipation can develop with excessive internal use. There are no cautions for external use.

WORMWOOD
Asteraceae/Sunflower Family

Artemisia absinthium
Madderwort, Mugwort, Wermuth, Absinthium

DESCRIPTION
A shaggy, straight–stemmed, herbaceous perennial, Wormwood grows to 2'–4' tall. The entire plant, particularly the leaves, is canescent. Grayish–green above, lighter below, they are 1–3 times pinnately divided. Floral grouped leaves are entire and linear. Wormwood's small yellow flowers are grouped in rounded heads. Collectively they form in branched panicles. Achenes are small and propagate easily.

DISTRIBUTION
Indigenous to Europe, now Wormwood is commonly found in disturbed soils throughout much of temperate North America. Although it is absent from most of the Southwest and Southeast, it is cultivated with ease.

CHEMISTRY
Prominent volatile oils: sabinene, myrcene, para–cymene, 1,8–cineole, (z)–β–ocimene, linalool, trans–thujone, (z)–myroxide, terpinen–4–ol, trans–sabinyl acetate, neryl isovalerate.

MEDICINAL USES
Like Mugwort although stronger, Wormwood's uses are broad and prosaic. Better at addressing imbalances and mild complaints, the plant can be employed most successfully as a bitter tonic/stomachic. The tea or tincture taken before meals is an excellent way of preparing the stomach and small intestine for pending food. Containing both bitter and aromatic principals, the plant used this way addresses both a lack of digestive secretion and an underlying vascular deficiency of the gut. It will be found particularly helpful for those who are troubled by dyspepsia, gas, and bloating.

As a mild biliary remedy, Wormwood is stimulating to liver and gallbladder function. It is especially indicated when there is bile stasis due to poor hepatic/biliary response to food. If after a rich meal there are corresponding feelings of indigestion, possibly with frontal headache development, try the tea or tincture before or even after meals.

Like most other Artemisias, Wormwood is one of our better remedies for gastritis and heartburn. The room temperate tea taken as needed is an excellent therapy for tissue inflammation and discomfort of the gastric region. Used consistently, due to the plant's antioxidant compounds, tissue healing starts to occur; short term it will be found cooling and soothing; long–term it is repairing.

Possibly Wormwood's most significant use is in its application to ulcerative colitis/crohn's disease. Used alone or combined with Canadian fleabane there is a significant chance the individual will be able to discontinue steroidal/non–steroidal mainstream therapies.

New research suggests crohn's disease may have a herpes virus–type component, as tissue samples from infected regions often test positive for one or more varieties (simplex I/II–EBV–and others). Of a corresponding note I have dispensed Artemisia ludoviciana, prepared as a tea, for the relief of genital herpes symptoms. It is a useful inhibitor of that virus' DNA replication. It is reasonable to assume that most strongly–aromatic Artemisias have similar effects. The essential oil of Wormwood can be applied topically to prevent–resolve outbreaks.

Although its name suggests otherwise, the plant is only a fair worm remedy. Pinworms respond to both tea and enema use. For an average weighted adult, everyday for 2 weeks[61], drink one quart of tea along with the retained enema before bed.

Artemisia cina, A. maritima, A annua, and A. ludoviciana will be stronger vermifuges due to their santoninum/artemisin array of compounds. With one of these Artemisias as a tea base, add a

---

61 Start several days before the full moon due to egg laying/hatching activity corresponding with this peak lunar time.

full dose of Ailanthus, Quassia, or Castela tincture to the infusion. This should also be added to the enema solution as well – proceed with the same dosage schedule as with Wormwood. This will treat a greater array of intestinal parasites, although both tapeworm and hookworm will be beyond even this potent combination's reach.

Wormwood is a decent diaphoretic when used at the onset of a cold or flu. The plant's aromatics tend to provide surface vasodilation. Diaphoresis usually ensues, helping the body to cool and dissipate heat.

Some women find Wormwood stimulating to menses. Not strong in this department but occasionally useful, the warm tea or tincture in warm water taken when the period is stop and start will be found stimulating.

Wormwood is best known for the volatile oil it produces. Combined with Anise and Fennel, among other oils, it was a key volatile ingredient in Absinthe, a liquor associated with bohemian culture in a time of strict Victorian adherence.

INDICATIONS
- Indigestion/Dyspepsia
- Biliary stasis
- Gastritis/Heartburn
- Ulcerative colitis/Crohn's disease
- Herpes virus group, as an inhibitor (external and internal)
- As a mild vermifuge
- Fever, dry skin
- Suppressed menstruation

COLLECTION
For tea or dry plant tincture gather the upper ⅓ of the plant, flowering or not. Dry and garble. Discard the stems. Use fresh for the fresh plant tincture.

PREPARATIONS
The dried herb in commerce will be marginal. It is best to grow and/or collect your own. The essential oil should only be used topically.

DOSAGE

- Herb infusion: 2–6 oz. 1–2 times daily
- FPT/DPT (50% alcohol): 20–40 drops 1–2 times daily
- Enema: once daily, before bed

CAUTIONS
Due to the high thujone content of the essential oil it is not recommend to take the refined substance internally. Although several drops will not pose a problem, reports of delirium, convulsions, involuntary evacuation, followed by unconsciousness, has been reported with ingesting ½ oz. of the essential oil. Thujone poisonings have resulted in death in the past.

Do not even use crude Wormwood preparations if pregnant or nursing. Used with children, dosed properly, for parasite issues is fine.

OTHER USES
See Mugwort's "Other Uses" for a brief outline on how to use most Artemisia varieties as an insecticide.

YARROW
Asteraceae/Sunflower Family

Achillea millefolium
Milfoil, Western yarrow, Plumajillo

DESCRIPTION
As a perennial Yarrow displays wispy and feather–like finely dissected leaves. Most leaves are basal, but some smaller stalk leaves do develop along its length. The flower clusters form in dense panicles. Individually each inflorescence is composed of both ray and disk flowers, usually white, but sometimes tending to pink. The entire plant is aromatic, particularly the leaves and flowers.

DISTRIBUTION
Common and wide spread throughout the Northern hemisphere, look to disturbed soils, forests, and meadows.

CHEMISTRY

Partial list for Achillea millefolium: flavonoids: casticin, santin, apigenin, luteolin, rutin, quercetin; hydrocarbons: n–hexadecane, p–cymene; monoterpene hydrocarbons: camphor, tricyclene, α–thujene, α–pinene, β–pinene, camphene, myrcene, γ–terpinene, terpinolene; monoterpenols: 1,8–cineole, linalool, β–terpineol, borneol, terpinen–4–ol, α–terpineol; monterpenyl esters: bornyl acetate, sabinyl acetate, α–terpinyl acetate; sesquiterpene hydrocarbons: α–copaene, β–caryophyllene, γ–cadinene; sesquiterpene lactones: guaianolides, eudesmanolides, longipinenes, germacrane derivatives; proazulene.

MEDICINAL USES

Neanderthal Man had knowledge of Yarrow demonstrated by pollen samples found in the Shanidar IV flower grave site of present–day Iraq. Six genera are represented by pollen finds in this 62,000 year–old site. Three: Achillea, Ephedra, and Althaea are covered in this work. The remaining three are equally medicinal and still are popularly utilized. There seems to be no doubt that Yarrow is ancient in use and that Neanderthal Man possessed the ability to use this important vulnerary in some capacity.

Because of the plant's tonifying activity it is well used in most conditions when there is tissue laxity and low regional vitality causing unchecked, yet minor, hemorrhaging.

With or without mucus in urine, Yarrow is specific for hematuria with accompanying urinary pain and irritation. Also if menorrhagia is due to atony, be it too lengthy periods or spotting during mid cycle, the plant usually stops blood flow. A number of Yarrow's flavonoids do have at least some influence over estrogen receptor sites. This could explain the plant's influence of the reproductive environment. Although not as strong as other plants with spasmolytic qualities, i.e. Black cohosh or Wild peony, Yarrow used when there is dysmenorrhea, will prove pain relieving. For chronic vaginitis, both as a douche and internally, Yarrow is a simple, yet effective remedy. The plant's antiinflammatory properties are distinct. Applied to chronic inflammation, be it topically for poorly healing wounds, or as a tea for chronic gastrointestinal inflammation, the plant will prove useful.

Ideally, it is a better tea for atonic phases of ulcerative colitis, not for acute flare–ups. But in reality, active and subacute or chronic inflammation often exists side–by–side, affecting related yet different tissue groups. Taking into account Yarrow's astringent and antispasmodic effects, small to moderate amounts of tea will be of benefit even in acute episodes. It will address the spasm, hemorrhage, and ulceration of this painful condition. Yarrow also has a protective and healing effect on gastric mucosa. If suffering from chronic gastritis and/or ulcer formation, consider the tea specific.

As an aromatic bitter tonic Yarrow is serviceable. Taken before meals the tea or diluted tincture will quiet atonic indigestion and dispel gas pains. The plant is also a moderate choleretic. Its stimulating effect on bile release assists in small intestinal fat digestion and assimilation.

Yarrow is a reliable diaphoretic. Thanks to the plant's volatile oil content the hot tea will help break stubborn dry fevers. Like other stimulating diaphoretics care should be taken if the temperate is dangerously high – Yarrow may cause a slight increase in temperate before diaphoresis commences. In these cases the professional use of Aconite, Veratrum, or Gelsemium may be more appropriate.

The plant is also a root medicine. Use fresh Yarrow roots to relieve toothache pain. A shredded piece of root should be applied to the area, and kept along the offending tooth as long as possible. The fresh plant tincture of Yarrow root can also be applied to the area, but be careful not to apply the tincture directly if there is exposed nerve tissue. In these cases a tincture–saturated cotton swab often is effective.

INDICATIONS

- ◆ Hemorrhaging, passive
- ◆ Hematuria
- ◆ Menorrhagia

- ♦ Dysmenorrhea
- ♦ Vaginitis (external)
- ♦ Wounds, poorly healing (external)
- ♦ Inflammation, gastrointestinal/Ulcerative colitis
- ♦ Indigestion with gas pains
- ♦ Fever, dry skin
- ♦ Toothache (external)

COLLECTION
Nearly the whole plant can be utilized – roots, leaves, and flowers. Discard the stems after the necessary parts are stripped away. They lack substantial astringency or aromatic content.

PREPARATIONS
Fresh plant preparations will be most effective. After drying much of Yarrow's potency and subtleties are lost.

DOSAGE
- ♦ FPT/DPT (50% alcohol): 30–60 drops 2–3 times daily
- ♦ Herbal infusion: 3–6 oz. 2–3 times daily
- ♦ External preparations: as needed
- ♦ Douche: 1–2 times daily

CAUTIONS
An occasionally cup of tea, or equivalent tincture, poses no problem during pregnancy or while nursing. However Yarrow used consistently as a daily herb may cause a problem due to its influence of reproductive tissue.

Proceed with caution when using the tea as a diaphoretic in children with high fevers – there may be a predictable temperate spike before sweating commences. In acute gastrointestinal inflammations too much Yarrow may aggravate the situation. Lessen the dose or discontinue if this is the case.

YELLOWDOCK
Polygonaceae/Buckwheat Family

Rumex crispus
Curly dock, Lengua de vaca, Yerba colorado

DESCRIPTION
When in flower, this robust perennial stands 2'–5' tall. Yellowdock's long, lance–shaped leaves have wavy margins. They are mostly basal and form in large rosettes. As the stalk is produced, some leaves are arranged alternately along its length. The small green flowers form in dense clustered spike–like racemes. Unlike many other Docks that exhibit hook–like appendages on seed margins, Yellowdock's are completely smooth. After flowering, the seeds and stalks become reddish–brown.

DISTRIBUTION
Yellowdock is found throughout most of North America. The plant is abundant at a great array of elevations, exceptions including extremely high elevations where low temperatures are a limiting factor. Look for this European non–native along streamsides, fields, ponds, and moist disturbed soils.

CHEMISTRY
Condensed and hydrolyzable tannins; anthraquinone pigments: nepodin, chrysophanol, physcion, emodin; quercetin.

MEDICINAL USES
Yellowdock is an old–school alterative. Its primary use is as a intestinal wall tonic. The plant has the ability, through its beneficial effect on small intestinal fat absorption, to lessen many skin and lymph irregularities. Use Yellowdock if there is a tendency towards eruptive and scaly skin conditions that appear to be linked to intestinal discomfort and stasis. In addition, lymph enlargements are typically reduced due to Yellowdock's lipid–lymph organizational ability. Moreover, the plant improves absorption of fat–soluble vitamins. Through this tonic activity it is

nutritional to individuals who are dealing with functional anemia or sub–anemic tendencies.

Externally a fresh poultice of the whole plant or other topical preparations are used on many of the same conditions Yellowdock treats internally. Poorly healing ulcers and migrating itchy rashes dependent upon "bad blood", stress, poison ivy exposure, or chemical sensitivity are Yellowdock specifics.

INDICATIONS

♦ Skin rashes (external and internal)
♦ Skin eruptions/Acne with poor fat digestion (external and internal)
♦ Fat malabsorption/Nutritional malabsorption

COLLECTION

A general rule when digging Yellowdock: if the roots are difficult to dig and they are pigmented deep yellow–orange, then they will be strong medicine. Stronger plants will be found in drier, clay–laden, dense soils. Yellowdock found partially submerged on streamsides will be inferior.

PREPARATIONS

After cleaning the roots well, either split the taproots in ¼"–½" strips or chop crossways into ¼" pieces, then dry.

DOSAGE

♦ FPT/DPT (50% alcohol): 30–60 drops 2–3 times daily
♦ Fluidextract: 10–20 drops 2–3 times daily
♦ Root decoction: 4–6 oz. 2–3 times daily

The dosing of Yellowdock is important. Like Rhubarb, in small amounts, the plant is tonic to intestinal walls, in larger amounts it is more irritative and tends to be laxative.

CAUTIONS

Large doses should not be used during pregnancy or while nursing due to Yellowdock's anthraquinone–laxative effect.

OTHER USES

The young leaves can be added to salads or cooked as a green.

YERBA SANTA

Hydrophyllaceae/Waterleaf Family

Eriodictyon californicum
Mountain balm

Eriodictyon angustifolium
Narrow–leaved yerba santa

DESCRIPTION

This erect, 3'–9' tall shrub has shedding bark and lanceolate to oblong leaves. They are leathery and 2–toned, with rolled–under margins. Upper leaf surfaces are hairless, or nearly so; lower surfaces are densely hairy between leaf veins. The leaves' dual appearance is striking; above they are yellowish–green, below, fuzzy–white. E. californicum's leaves are several inches longer and somewhat wider than E. angustifolium's. The latter's are the more diminutive of the two.

Yerba santa's flower clusters form at branch ends and are open in appearance. Both varieties have funnel shaped corollas. E. californicum's inflorescence is white to purple and sparsely hairy. It is twice as large as E. angustifolium's white, densely hairy flower.

DISTRIBUTION

The epicenter of Eriodictyon californicum's biomass is northern California. With extensive populations of the plant found in various coastal and inland mountain ranges there is no lack of collectable supply. Throughout southern California it is more sporadically found at mid–elevations. Its northern limit stretches to Oregon. Look to disturbed roadside soil, trailsides, and exposed hillsides where other Chaparral–Scrub shrubs are found.

From southeastern California to Utah, Nevada, and Arizona, Eriodictyon angustifolium is found in mid–desert regions. As the most easterly–growing of the genus, the plant seeds well in disturbed soils, especially those that are burnt by fast–moving chaparral fires. I have seen large stands of the plant stop only where the land had not been burnt years before. Sun–exposed hillsides and trail and road sides are other areas to look.

CHEMISTRY

For Eriodictyon californicum: flavonoids: eriodictyol, luteolin, chrysoeriol, apigenin, hispidulin, luteolin, nepetin, jaceosidin, homoeriodictyol, kaempferol, quercetin.

MEDICINAL USES

Yerba santa has a rich history of use in American herbal medicine. Like Creosote bush, regardless of creed or color, everyone in the Southwest privy to plant usage, utilized it for essentially the same thing – an expectorant with decongestant properties. In the past Yerba santa's high esteem was maintained not only because it worked but because of its stability. For herbaceous material, the plant stored and shipped well. It held up through the ravages of time, travel, and elemental exposure leading to a reliable herbal medicine.

Use Yerba santa when suffering from bronchitis or when in need of an expectorant, not only to loosen phlegm, but also to dry the bronchial environment. Unlike other expectorants that tend to increase pulmonary secretions, Yerba santa has a distinct decongesting quality, yet without stimulating cardiovascular functions such as Ephedra. Compounding the plant's useful lung effects, is its antibacterial property. Yerba santa's leaf resins are distinctly bacteriostatic, particularly against gram–positive microbes: Micrococcus sp., Mycobacterium tuberculosis, Sarcina sp., and Streptococcus pyogenes.

Asthmatic congestion, when breathing is accompanied by mucus, responds well to Yerba Santa. Also use the plant in cases of rhinitis or sinusitis caused by allergies and/or infection.

For urinary tract infections the plant is distinctly antimicrobial. Use it in cases of bladder and urethra infection when there is mucus in the urine. For infections that Uva–ursi does not affect try Yerba Santa as its non–polar compounds tend to eliminate microbes that the latter plant does not. A combination of the two can be used as well.

INDICATIONS

◆ Bronchitis, copious phlegm
◆ Asthma, humid
◆ Sinusitis/Rhinitis, copious mucus
◆ Cystitis/Urethritis, with mucus in urine

COLLECTION

Gather the leafing tips in the spring or early summer when new growth is apparent. They should be resinous and somewhat sticky. The leaves can be dried loosely or in wrapped bundles.

PREPARATIONS/DOSAGE

◆ FPT/DPT (70% alcohol): 30–60 drops 2–3 times daily
◆ Fluidextract: 10–30 drops 2–3 times daily
◆ Herb infusion: 2–4 oz. 2–3 times daily

CAUTIONS

None known with judicious use.

OTHER USES

Due to Yerba santa's interesting taste, extracts of the plant were often added to mask bitter medicines. Some may recognize its taste as cough syrup–like.

YUCCA

Agavaceae/Agave Family

Yucca schidigera (Yucca californica, Y. mohavensis)
Mohave yucca

DESCRIPTION

Developing from thickened subterranean rhizomes, Yucca is a colony plant. Each having one to several above–ground leafing stems, the plant is robust and thick. Leaves are linear, pointed, and 2'–3' long. Old leaf margins have separating fibers. The stalk borne flowers form in dense panicle racemes. Individuals are perfect, white to cream, and often tinged with purple. The 3"–4" long fruit are fleshy and black–seed filled.

DISTRIBUTION
Southern California, southern Nevada, and western Arizona, Yucca schidigera has a limited range, but is locally abundant, growing in expansive stands throughout the Mohave desert.

CHEMISTRY
Sapogenins: diosgenin, gitogenin, neogitogenin, hecogenin, manogenin, sarsasapogenin, smilagenin, stigmasterol, tigogenin, neotigogenin; steroidal compounds: β–sitosterol, stigmasterol, campesterol.

MEDICINAL USES
Many other Yucca species will be similar in saponin content and medicinal effect. Do not be fixated on Yucca schidigera. Y. baccata or Y. elata are also fine choices.

Yucca produces several therapeutic effects mainly through its influence of intestinal tract membranes and related flora. The plant's saponins form complexes with abnormal colonic flora by–products rendering these toxins, to some degree, inert. Since these saponins are indigestible, the formed complexes are removed with other waste matter from the colon. Therefore, bacterial end–products are unable to exert an inflammatory effect because they literally are stuck to Yucca's saponins, making absorption into systemic circulation impossible.

It is interesting to note that constipation is often a factor in many arthritic/inflammatory conditions. When abnormal microorganisms have more time to interact negatively with intestinal waste matter there is a tendency for our internal environment to become pro–inflammatory. This is certainly one reason why laxative and liver stimulant therapies have a place in treating pain syndromes. Also old Mexican and White cowboys alike are known to use the plant to lessen the full body pains of years of hard work and cowboyin'.

Yucca is useful in lowering bile salt and cholesterol re–uptake by the lower duodenum. As above, the binding effect of these saponins can lower blood triglyceride and cholesterol levels.

High protein/high fat/low carbohydrate diet followers will benefit from Yucca's effective binding of ammonia[62] in the colon. This allows it to pass out with the feces and not be reabsorbed through the portal circulation. Thus, liver stress in response to a high protein diet, will diminish.

INDICATIONS
♦ Rheumatoid arthritis
♦ Chronic pain, dependent upon constipation
♦ LDL/Triglycerides levels, elevated

COLLECTION
Collect the roots and lower trunk in the fall. Yucca's saponin content varies in response to season and species. The highest yields are in the fall when the plant draws back in and again starts the cycle of accumulation for next years spring growth.

PREPARATIONS
Chop the gathered material into ¼"–½" pieces. Lay out on a flat to dry if in an arid place or if in a more humid environment use a dehydrator. Either way the root will dry quickly given its porous nature.

DOSAGE
♦ Root decoction: 4–6 oz. 2–3 times daily
♦ DPT (50% alcohol): 30–60 drops 2–3 times daily
♦ Fluidextract: 10–30 drops 2–3 times daily
♦ Capsule (00): 2–3, 2–3 times daily

It is best to approach Yucca as a short–term plant

62 Ammonia, an end result of protein breakdown, is converted from urea in the colon by colonic flora. If the liver is not able to reconvert ammonia back to urea, because of large protein qualities from diet or impaired renal or liver function, resulting ammonia toxicities can ensue.

used concurrently for 3–4 weeks. If longer term use is needed try a rotation of Yucca for 3–4 weeks followed by 1 week of Creosote bush or Turmeric.

CAUTIONS

Used in excessive quantities Yucca can cause intestinal distress. Do not use during pregnancy due to the plant's potential altering effect on reproductive hormones.

OTHER USES

1–2 oz. of the powdered root can be added to water making a usable soap/shampoo. The fruit from the fleshy varieties are sweet and edible. Collect and eat when small brown marks of sugar fermentation are just starting to appear on the outer light green surface of the fruit skin. According to Peter Bigfoot, a mountain man herbalist who lives in the Superstition Mountains of Arizona, the seeds will cause diarrhea.

**APPENDIX A
THERAPEUTIC INDEX**

CARDIO/VASCULAR

Angina pectoris
Hawthorn

Arrhythmia
Hawthorn

Cardiovascular disease, general
Garlic, Ginger, Ginkgo, Hawthorn, Turmeric

Hemorrhoids
Butcher's broom, Ginkgo, Horse chestnut, Stoneroot, Witch hazel

Hemorrhoids, bleeding
Shepherd's purse, Witch hazel

Hypertension, essential
American ginseng, Ginseng, Hawthorn

Hypotension
Ginseng, Guaraná, Kola nut

Oxidative stress
American ginseng, Burdock, Eleuthero, Ginger, Ginkgo, Ginseng, Gota kola, Maté, Turmeric

Palpitation
Passionflower, Valerian, Wild cherry

Portal circulation, slowed
Horse chestnut, Stoneroot

Raynaud's syndrome
Bilberry, Ginkgo

Tachycardia
Hawthorn, Motherwort, Passionflower

Stroke/Ischemia
American ginseng, Ginkgo, Ginseng

Varicosities
Butcher's broom, Calendula, Ginkgo, Hawthorn, Horse chestnut, Witch hazel

Varicosities, with edema and ulceration
Butcher's broom, Calendula, Ginkgo, Horse chestnut

Valvular regurgitation
Hawthorn, Stoneroot

Vascular disorders, general
Bilberry, Ginkgo, Hawthorn

Vascular disorders, peripheral
Bilberry, Ginkgo

GASTROINTESTINAL

Amebiasis
Barberry, Oregongrape

Anorexia
Cannabis, Hops, Horehound, Thuja

Colic
Catnip, Chamomile, Fennel, Lavender, Peppermint, Rosemary, Spearmint

Constipation
Aloe, Black walnut, Cascara sagrada, Coffee, Rhubarb, Senna

Cramps/Spasm, general
Cannabis, Catnip, Fennel, Ginger, Pennyroyal, Peppermint, Rosemary, Sage, Spearmint, Wild yam

Cramps/Spasm, intestinal
Bayberry, Black walnut, Cannabis, Chamomile, Ginger, Lobelia, Peppermint, Rhubarb, Sage, Spearmint, Wild yam

Diarrhea
Bayberry, Bilberry, Goldenseal, Guaraná, Horehound, Marshmallow, Rhubarb, White willow, Wild indigo, Witch hazel

Diarrhea with intestinal cramps
Black walnut, Cinnamon, Passionflower

Dyspepsia
Artichoke, Bayberry, Chamomile, Dandelion, Goldenseal, Hops, Kava, Milk thistle, Mugwort, Oregongrape

Dyspepsia, poor secretion
Cayenne pepper, Coffee, Lobelia, Mugwort

Dyspepsia with bloating
Catnip, Chamomile, Cinnamon, Clove, Eucalyptus, Fennel, Ginger, Juniper, Lavender, Lemonbalm, Mugwort, Pennyroyal, Spearmint, Turmeric, Valerian, Wormwood, Yarrow

Fissure, anal
Goldenseal

Flora imbalance, intestinal
Burdock, Dandelion,

Food poisoning
Barberry, Cinnamon, Clove, Eucalyptus, Oregongrape

Gastritis
Artichoke, Bayberry, Chamomile, Goldenseal, Hops, Mugwort, Rhubarb, Wild cher-

ry, Wormwood

Giardiasis

Barberry, Oregongrape, Thuja

Hemorrhaging, passive

Cinnamon, Goldenseal, Horsetail, Shepherd's purse, Yarrow

Inflammation, intestinal

Black walnut, Mugwort, Plantain, Rhubarb, Yarrow

Infection, Candida albicans

Black walnut

Infection, general

Astragalus, Cinnamon

Malabsorption

Alfalfa, Barberry, Black walnut, Dandelion, Milk thistle, Oregongrape, Nettle, Red clover, Yellowdock

Nausea, chemotherapy/radiation

Cannabis, Ginger

Nausea, general

Bayberry, Catnip, Cinnamon, Clove, Ginger, Lavender, Pennyroyal, Peppermint, Rosemary, Spearmint, Wild yam

Nausea, motion sickness/seasickness

Ginger

Ulceration, lower

Aloe, Bayberry, Chamomile, Calendula, Comfrey, Goldenseal, Horsetail, Myrrh, Rhubarb, Wormwood, Yarrow

Ulceration, upper

Aloe, Bayberry, Chamomile, Calendula, Comfrey, Goldenseal, Hops, Horsetail, Licorice, Marshmallow, Myrrh, Yarrow

Ulcer, rectal

Goldenseal

Vomiting

Catnip, Clove, Lavender, Peppermint, Spearmint

Worms

Wormwood

LIVER/GALLBLADDER

Cirrhosis/fatty liver

Milk thistle

Congestion, liver and gallbladder

Barberry, Cascara sagrada, Dandelion, Oregongrape, Peppermint, Rhubarb, Turmeric, Wormwood

Gallstones, non–acute

Artichoke, Turmeric

Hepatitis, viral

Astragalus, Milk thistle

Inflammation, liver

Artichoke, Barberry, Milk thistle, Mugwort, Oregongrape

Oxidative stress

Eleuthero, Ginseng, Milk thistle, Turmeric

Poisoning

Milk thistle

Spasm, gall bladder/duct

Lobelia, Wild yam

LYMPH/IMMUNE

Enlargements, lymph node

Echinacea, Wild indigo

Immune suppression, general

Astragalus, Echinacea, Myrrh, Wild indigo

Infection, bacterial, general

Astragalus, Barberry, Oregongrape, Echinacea, Garlic, Myrrh, Wild indigo

Infection, viral, general

Astragalus, Echinacea, Garlic, Wild indigo

MEN

BPH (Benign prostrate hypertrophy)

Maté, Nettle, Saw palmetto

Epididymitis

Saw palmetto

Herpes virus group

See Skin section

Libido, decreased

American ginseng, Clove, Ginseng

Libido, excessive

Hops

Prostatitis

Saw palmetto, Squaw vine, Thuja

Seminal vesicle irritation

Shepherd's purse

Spermatorrhea

Hops
Testicular irritation
Saw palmetto
Warts, genital
See HPV in Skin section

METABOLIC

Acidosis, non–organic
Nettle
Adrenal cortex deficiency, sub–clinical
Licorice,
Hyperglycemia–NIDDM
Aloe, American ginseng, Burdock, Cinnamon, Ginseng, Milk thistle
Hypothyroidal, sub–clinical
Oregongrape,
Gout
Burdock, Dandelion
LDL levels, elevated
American ginseng, Artichoke, Garlic, Ginseng, Milk thistle, Turmeric, Yucca

MOUTH/THROAT

Gingivitis/Periodontitis
Myrrh, Thuja
Gums, spongy and bleeding
Bayberry, Myrrh, Witch hazel
Laryngitis
Echinacea, Stoneroot, Thuja, Wild indigo
Pharyngitis
Arnica, Barberry, Bayberry, Cayenne pepper, Echinacea, Goldenseal, Ligusticum, Marshmallow, Myrrh, Oregongrape, Red root, Sage, Stoneroot, Thuja, Wild indigo, Witch hazel
Sores, mouth
Bayberry
Strep throat
Barberry, Echinacea, Sage, Myrrh, Oregongrape, Sage, Thuja, Wild indigo
Tonsillitis
Cayenne pepper, Echinacea, Red root, Wild indigo
Ulceration
Calendula, Chamomile, Wild indigo

NERVOUS SYSTEM

Depression, CNS
American ginseng, Coffee, Ginseng, Guaraná, Kola nut, Maté, Valerian, Wild oats
Depression, mental/emotional
St. John's wort, Wild oats
Insomnia/anxiety
American ginseng, Chamomile, Hops, Kava, Lavender, Lemonbalm, Motherwort, Passionflower, Valerian, Wild lettuce
Memory loss/poor cognition/Alzheimer's
American ginseng, Ginkgo, Ginseng, Rosemary, Sage
Multiple sclerosis
American ginseng, Ginseng
Myasthenia gravis
American ginseng, Astragalus, Rosemary
Neuropathy
Bilberry, Ginkgo
Oxidative stress
American ginseng, Eleuthero, Ginkgo, Ginseng, Gota kola
Raynaud's syndrome
Bilberry, Ginkgo
Seizure activity/Convulsions
Lobelia, Passionflower, Valerian

PAIN

Arthritis, rheumatoid
Creosote bush, Ginger, Turmeric, Yucca
Arthritis with constipation
Cascara sagrada, Yucca
Arthritis–like
Black cohosh
Dental
Clove, Yarrow
Headache, migraine, acute pain
Coffee, Guaraná, Kola nut
Headache, migraine, beginning stages
Black cohosh
Headache, general
Coffee, Peppermint
Headache, stress

Lavender, Lemonbalm

Injury, acute, with pain

Clove, Lavender, Lobelia, Peppermint, Rosemary, White willow

Injury, chronic, with pain

Arnica, Cayenne pepper, Clove, Ginger, Turmeric, White willow

Nerve

Cannabis, Cayenne pepper, Motherwort, St. John's wort

Spasm, general

Cannabis, Lobelia

RENAL/URINARY

Fluid retention

Elder, Horehound, Horsetail

Incontinence/bed wetting from lack of bladder tone

Agrimony, Mullein, Thuja

Inflammation/pain, lower urinary tract, acute

Agrimony, Cannabis, Comfrey, Corn silk, Horsetail, Licorice, Marshmallow, Nettle, Plantain, Red raspberry, Squaw vine

Inflammation/pain, lower urinary tract, chronic

Eucalyptus, Horsetail, Juniper, Kava, Saw palmetto, Squaw vine, Stoneroot, Yerba santa

Inflammation with hematuria

Horsetail, Shepherd's purse, Yarrow

Infection, alkaline urine

Cranberry, Uva-ursi,

Infection, general

Eucalyptus, Grindelia, Juniper, Myrrh, Thuja, Yerba santa

Kidney stones, general

Corn silk, Marshmallow, Shepherd's purse

Kidney stones, passage

Lobelia, Wild yam

Kidney stones, preventative

Corn silk, Marshmallow

Kidney stones, uric acid

Burdock, Dandelion

Nephritis, acute

Corn silk, Marshmallow

Nephritis, chronic

Agrimony, Corn silk, Myrrh

Urine, low-specific gravity

Bilberry

RESPIRATORY (LOWER)

Asthma, copious phlegm

Ephedra, Horehound, Yerba santa

Asthma, dry, non-spasmodic

Ligusticum, Pleurisy root

Asthma, general

Creosote bush, Ephedra, Ginkgo, Grindelia, Horse chestnut, Ligusticum, Lobelia

Bronchitis, chronic, difficult expectoration

Eucalyptus, Grindelia, Ligusticum, Pleurisy root

Bronchitis, chronic, weak cough

Eucalyptus, Grindelia, Ligusticum, Myrrh, Thuja

Bronchitis, copious phlegm

Yerba santa

Bronchitis, dry fever

Ligusticum, Pleurisy root

Bronchitis, general

Echinacea, Horehound, Lobelia, Wild cherry

Cough, spasmodic

Cannabis, Ephedra, Horehound, Mullein, Passionflower, Wild lettuce

Cough, with irritation

Comfrey, Licorice, Marshmallow, Mullein, Plantain, Pleurisy root, Red clover, Slippery elm, Wild cherry

Emphysema

Ligusticum

Hemorrhaging, passive

Horsetail, Yarrow

Pleurisy

Cayenne pepper, Lobelia, Pleurisy root

RESPIRATORY (UPPER)/EYES/EARS

Conjunctivitis

Oregongrape, Calendula, Goldenseal

Earache

Garlic, Mullein

Glaucoma

Black cohosh

Irritation, optic nerve

Kava

Night vision, to improve

Bilberry

Ocular disorders, antioxidant

Bilberry

Rhinitis

Ginkgo, Nettle, Yerba santa

Sinusitis

Barberry, Cayenne pepper, Echinacea, Ephedra, Goldenseal, Myrrh, Oregongrape, Wild indigo, Witch hazel, Yerba santa

Styes

Thuja

SKIN

Abscess

Calendula, Echinacea, Marshmallow, Thuja, Wild indigo

Bedsores

Chamomile, Gota kola, Myrrh, Thuja,

Bites, venomous snake

Echinacea, Turmeric

Bites, venomous spider

Creosote bush, Turmeric

Bites/Stings

Creosote bush, Plantain, Turmeric

Boils

Burdock, Echinacea, Yellowdock

Burns form heat and sunburn

Aloe, Gota kola, Lavender, Marshmallow, Milk thistle, Sage, St. John's wort, Tea, Witch hazel

Candida infections

Oregongrape, Garlic, Thuja

Chicken pox

See Herpes virus group under Skin section

Cuts, scrapes, abrasions

Cayenne pepper, Clove, Creosote bush, Eucalyptus, Hops, Rosemary, Tea, Witch hazel

Dermatitis, dry scabby

Barberry, Oregongrape, Slippery elm

Eczema

Burdock, Creosote bush, Barberry, Oregongrape, Grindelia, Juniper, Turmeric

Herpes virus group

Creosote bush, Clove, Echinacea, Garlic, Lemonbalm, Licorice, Mugwort, Peppermint, St. John's wort, Tea tree, Wormwood

Hives, Rashes

Plantain, Yellowdock

HPV (Human papillomavirus)

Creosote bush, Tea tree, Thuja

Infections, bacterial

Aloe, Barberry, Eucalyptus, Garlic, Oregongrape, Tea tree, Turmeric

Infections, fungal

Aloe, Barberry, Clove, Eucalyptus, Garlic, Oregongrape, Tea tree, Thuja, Turmeric

Poison ivy reaction, local

Grindelia, Lobelia

Poorly healing skin

Oregongrape, Burdock, Horsetail, Echinacea, Pleurisy root

Poorly healing skin with tendency towards ulceration

Burdock, Echinacea

Psoriasis

Oregongrape, Burdock, Gota kola, Juniper, Turmeric

Shingles

See Herpes virus group under Skin section

Scar formation, to lessen

Calendula

Sun damaged skin/Actinic keratosis

Creosote bush, Milk thistle

Ulcers, poorly healing

Arnica, Burdock, Calendula, Comfrey, Eucalyptus, Gota kola, Grindelia, Myrrh, St. John's wort, Thuja

Warts, common and genital

See HPV under Skin section

Wounds

Aloe, Arnica, Bilberry, Calendula, Chamomile, Comfrey, Elder, Eucalyptus, Gota kola, Horsetail, St. John's wort, Thuja, Yarrow

TISSUE/STRUCTURE

Bursitis
Echinacea

Broken bones/Fractures
Comfrey

Connective/Soft tissue damage
Comfrey

Connective tissues, hair, nails, skin, and bones, weakened
Horsetail

Injuries, chronic
Echinacea

Tendinitis
Echinacea

WOMEN

Amenorrhea
Black cohosh, Blue cohosh, Catnip, Chamomile, Fennel, Motherwort, Mugwort, Myrrh, Pennyroyal, Rosemary, Wormwood

Anovulatory cycles
Chaste tree

Cervicitis
Calendula, Red raspberry, Squaw vine

Cervicitis, chronic
Blue cohosh, Calendula

Depression, hormonal fluctuation
Black cohosh

Dysmenorrhea
Black cohosh, Blue cohosh, Cannabis, Chamomile, Fennel, Ginger, Lobelia, Motherwort, Rosemary, Squaw vine, Wild yam

Dysplasia, cervical
Calendula, Echinacea
Also see HPV in Skin section

Endometriosis
Blue cohosh, Myrrh

Fibroids, uterine, subserous
Chaste tree

Hemorrhaging, postpartum
Shepherd's purse, Yarrow

Herpes virus group
See Skin section

Lactation, insufficient
Chaste tree, Fennel

Lactation, to lessen
Sage

Libido, decreased
American ginseng, Ginseng

Mastitis
Red root

Menopause
Black cohosh, Hawthorn

Menstruation, heavy
Agrimony, Chaste tree, Red raspberry, Shepherd's purse, Yarrow

Menstruation, slowed
Catnip, Pennyroyal

Miscarriage, threatened, with cramps
Wild yam

Miscarriage, threatened, with spotting
Shepherd's purse, Squaw vine

Morning sickness
Ginger

Ovarian irritation
Saw palmetto

Pelvic inflammatory disease
Blue cohosh

Perimenopause
Black cohosh, Chaste tree

Premenstrual discomfort with breast tenderness
Chaste tree

Uterine laxity
Saw palmetto, Stoneroot

Uterine tonic, pregnancy
Agrimony, Red raspberry

Uterine tonic, postpartum
Agrimony, Red raspberry, Uva–ursi

Vaginitis
Agrimony, Calendula, Eucalyptus, Red raspberry, Uva–ursi, Witch hazel

Vaginitis, chronic
Blue cohosh, Eucalyptus, Goldenseal, Yarrow

Warts, genital
See HPV in Skin section

MISCELLANEOUS

Cancer, as a preventative

American ginseng, Garlic, Ginger, Maté, Milk thistle, Turmeric

Cerebral spinal fluid pressure, elevated

Black cohosh, Cannabis

Fatigue

American ginseng, Coffee, Eleuthero, Ginseng

Fever, dry, low–moderate temperature

Elder, Catnip, Cayenne pepper, Chamomile, Mugwort, Ginger, Pennyroyal, Peppermint, Pleurisy root, Rosemary, Sage, Spearmint, White willow, Wormwood, Yarrow

Fever, dry, moderate–high

Pleurisy root, White willow

Fever, general

Barberry, Oregongrape

Sweating, colliquative

Sage

Valley fever

Thuja

Weakness/Debility from old–age/sickness

American ginseng, Astragalus, Eleuthero, Ginseng

**APPENDIX B
REPOSITORY**

Abies [Pitch]
DPT (95% alcohol): 5–10 drops bid–tid; Ointment/Salve: as needed.

Acacia (Southwest varieties) [Leaf]
Infusion: 4–6 oz. bid–tid.

Acacia senegal [Gum]
Prepared as a mucilage: 1–2 teaspoons 2–3 timed daily.

Acalypha [Herb]
Oil/Salve/Poultice: use as needed.

Achillea [Leaf/Flower/Root]
FPT/DPT of leaf/flower (50% alcohol): 30–60 drops bid–tid; Herbal infusion: 3–6 oz. bid–tid; external preparations: as needed; douche: qd–bid.

Aconitum [Herb/Root]
FPT (1:4)/DPT (1:10–70% alcohol) of herb: 5–10 drops qd–bid or externally as a liniment; DPT of root (1:10–70% alcohol): 1–5 drops qd–bid or externally bid–tid. Use with care.

Acorus calamus [Root]
FPT/DPT: (60% alcohol): 30–60 drops bid–tid.

Actaea arguta
(See Actaea racemosa)

Actaea racemosa [Root/Leaf]
FPT/DPT (80% alcohol) of root: 20–30 drops bid–tid; FPT/DPT (70% alcohol) of leaf: 30–50 drops bid–tid; Fluidextract of root: 10–20 drops bid–tid; Capsule (00) of root: 1–2 bid–tid; Leaf infusion: 2–4 oz. bid–tid.

Adiantum [Herb]
Infusion: 2–4 oz. bid–tid or topically as needed.

Aesculus californica
(See Aesculus hippocastanum)

Aesculus glabra
(See Aesculus hippocastanum)

Aesculus hippocastanum [Fruit/Bark]
DPT (50% alcohol): 5–15 drops bid–tid; Ointment/Oil/Salve: as needed.

Agar [Seaweed mucilage]
1–2 tablespoons in water or juice as needed.

Agathosma [Leaf]
Cold infusion: 2–4 oz. bid–tid; FPT/DPT (80% alcohol): 30–60 drops bid–tid.

Agrimonia [Herb]
Infusion: 4–8 oz. bid–tid; FPT/DPT (50% alcohol): 1 teaspoon bid–tid; Douche/sitz bath: as needed.

Agropyron repens [Rhizome/Creeping stem]
Standard/Cold infusion: 4–6 oz. tid–qid; DPT (50% alcohol): 60–90 drops tid–qid; Fluidextract: 20–30 drops tid–qid.

Ailanthus altissima [Bark]
Cold infusion/decoction: 2–4 oz. bid–tid; FPT/DPT (50% alcohol): 20–30 drops bid–tid; Fluidextract: 10–20 drops bid–tid.

Alchemilla [Whole plant]
Infusion: 4–8 oz. bid–tid.

Aletris farinosa [Root]
DPT (50% alcohol): 30–60 drops bid–tid; Infusion: 2–4 oz. bid–tid.

Allium sativum [Clove]
Fresh clove: 1–2 qd–bid; Fresh clove: topically as needed and as a suppository; FPT/DPT (65% alcohol): ½–1 teaspoon bid–tid; Oil: as needed. May irritate skin.

Alnus [Bark]
Decoction: 2–4 oz. bid–tid or as needed for external use.

Aloe [Exudate/Pulp]
Leaf exudate (fresh): 10–20 drops qd–bid or externally as needed; DPT (50% alcohol) of leaf exudate: 30–60 drops qd–bid; Leaf pulp: 1–2 tablespoons bid–tid or externally as needed.

Aloysia [Herb]
Infusion: 4–8 oz. tid–qid; FPT/DPT (50% alcohol): 30–60 drops tid–qid.

Alpinia [Root]
Infusion: 2–4 oz. bid–tid; FPT/DPT (70% alcohol): 20–50 drops bid–tid; Fluidextract: 5–15 drops bid–tid; Spirit: 20–30 drops bid–tid; Poultice: as needed.

Althaea officinalis [Root]
Infusion: 4–8 oz. as needed; Capsule (00): 2–3 bid–tid; Douche: bid–tid; Moistened powder for poultice.

Amaranthus [Leaf/Seed]
As an edible.

Ambrosia ambrosioides [Leaf/Root]
FPT/DPT (60% alcohol): 20–60 drops bid–tid;

Leaf infusion/root decoction: 2–4 oz. bid–tid.

Ammi majus [Seed]

(See Ammi visnaga)

Ammi visnaga [Seed]

FPT/DPT (60% alcohol): 60–90 drops tid–qid.

Anagallis [Herb]

FPT: 10–30 drops bid–tid.

Anaphalis [Herb]

Infusion: 4–8 oz. bid–tid.

Anemone [Herb]

FPT: 10–20 drops bid–tid; Fresh poultice: apply as needed; Eyewash: tid–qid.

Anemopsis californica [Root/Leaf]

FPT/DPT (60% alcohol): 30–60 drops tid–qid; Standard/Cold infusion: 4–6 oz., tid–qid; Oil/Ointment/Salve: as needed.

Angelica [Root]

FPT/DPT (60% alcohol): 30–60 drops bid–tid; Standard/Cold infusion: 2–4 oz. bid–tid;

Angelica sinensis [Root]

DPT (60% alcohol): 20–40 drops bid–tid; Capsules (00): 1–2 bid–tid.

Antennaria [Herb]

Infusion: 4–6 oz. bid–tid; FPT/DPT (50% alcohol): 30–60 drops bid–tid.

Anthemis [Herb]

Infusion: 4–6 oz. bid–tid.

Apium [Seed]

Infusion: 4–6 oz. bid–tid; DPT (60% alcohol): 30–60 drops bid–tid.

Apocynum [Root]

DPT (50% alcohol): 5–25 drops qd–tid. Use with care.

Aralia nudicaulis [Root]

DPT (60% alcohol): 20–40 drops bid–tid; Fluidextract: 10–20 drops bid–tid.

Aralia racemosa [Root]

FPT/DPT (60% alcohol): 20–40 drops bid–tid.

Arbutus [Leaf]

(Same as Arctostaphylos)

Arctium lappa [Root/Seed]

Standard/Cold infusion of root: 4–8 oz. bid–tid; FPT/DPT (50% alcohol) of root: 45–90 drops bid–tid; Fluidextract of root: 15–45 drops bid–tid; Capsule (00) (root): 2–3 bid–tid; DPT of seeds (50% alcohol): 15–45 drops bid–tid; Capsule (00) (seed): 2 bid–tid.

Arctostaphylos (Manzanita type) [Leaf]

Decoction: 4–6 oz. bid–tid; DPT (40% alcohol, 10% glycerin): 60–90 drops bid–tid; Fluidextract: 30–50 drops bid–tid; Sitz bath: as needed.

Arctostaphylos uva–ursi [Leaf]

Decoction: 4–6 oz. bid–tid; DPT (40% alcohol, 10% glycerin): 60–90 drops bid–tid; Fluidextract: 30–50 drops bid–tid; Sitz bath: as needed.

Argemone [Herb/Fruit]

Infusion: 2–4 oz. bid–tid; DPT (50% alcohol): 20–40 drops bid–tid; Eyewash: tid–qid. Use internally with caution.

Arisaema [Corm]

FPT: 5–10 drops as needed.

Aristolochia [Root]

FPT/DPT (65% alcohol) 10–30 drops qd–tid. Use with care.

Arnica [Whole plant]

FPT/DPT: (65% alcohol): 3–8 drops qd–tid; Liniment/Ointment/Oil/Salve: as needed.

Artemisia absinthium [Herb]

Infusion: 2–6 oz. qd–bid; FPT/DPT (50% alcohol): 20–40 drops qd–bid; Enema: qd before bed.

Artemisia douglasiana [Herb]

(See Artemisia vulgaris)

Artemisia filifolia [Herb]

(See Artemisia ludoviciana)

Artemisia ludoviciana [Herb]

Standard/Cold infusion: 4–6 oz. bid–tid; FPT/DPT (50% alcohol): 20–40 drops bid–tid; DPT (100% vinegar): 20–40 drops bid–tid.

Artemisia tridentata [Herb]

Standard/Cold infusion: 2–4 oz. qd–bid; FPT/DPT (60% alcohol): 10–30 drops qd–bid; DPT (100% vinegar): 10–30 drops qd–bid; Inhaled steam: bid–tid; External preparations: as needed.

Artemisia vulgaris [Herb}

Standard/Cold infusion: 4–6 oz. bid–tid; FPT/DPT (50% alcohol): 30–60 drops bid–tid; DPT (100% vinegar): 30–60 drops bid–tid.

Asafetida (Ferula spp.) [Gum–resin]

DPT (85% alcohol): 10–20 drops bid–tid; Capsules (0): 1–3 bid–tid.

Asarum [Root]

FPT/DPT (60% alcohol): 30–60 drops bid–tid.

Asclepias asperula [Root]

Standard/Cold infusion: 2 oz. bid–tid; DPT (50% alcohol): 5–30 drops bid–tid; Fluidextract: 5–10 drops bid–tid; Latex pellets or Capsules (00): 1–2 bid–tid; Latex: externally as needed.

Asclepias tuberosa [Root]

FPT/DPT (50% alcohol): 20–40 drops bid–tid; Standard/Cold infusion: 4–6 oz. bid–tid; Fluidextract: 10–20 drops bid–tid; Capsule (00): 1–2 bid–tid.

Asclepias subulata [Root]

DPT: (50% alcohol) 10–30 drops bid; Fluidextract: 5–10 drops bid; Latex tincture: (50% alcohol) 5–20 drops bid; Latex pellets or capsule (00): 1–2 bid

Asparagus [Root]

FPT/DPT (50% alcohol): 30–60 drops bid–tid; Infusion: 4–6 oz. bid–tid.

Aspidium [Root]

(Synonym for Dryopteris filix–mas)

Aspidosperma

(Synonym for Iodina rhombifolia)

Astragalus membranaceus [Root]

Decoction/Cold infusion: 4–6 oz. bid–tid; Fluidextract: 10–30 drops bid–tid; DPT (60% alcohol): ½–1 teaspoon bid–tid.

Atropa belladonna [Whole plant]

Liniment: tid–qid; Oil/Salve/Wash: tid–qid; Smoke: several inhalations bid–tid in acute situations; FPT (1:4)/DPT (1:10 60% alcohol): 5–10 drop qd–tid. Use with caution.

Avena [Unripe seed]

FPT: 30–90 drops tid–qid; Oatstraw infusion: 4–8 oz. bid–tid.

Baccharis [Leaf]

Infusion: 4–8 oz. bid–tid; FPT/DPT (60% alcohol): 30–60 drops bid–tid.

Balsamorhiza [Root]

FPT/DPT (65% alcohol): 30–60 drops bid–tid.

Baptisia [Root]

FPT/DPT (60% alcohol): 10–20 drops qd–tid;

Decoction: 2–4 oz. qd–tid; External preparations: use as needed.

Berberis [Root]

Decoction/Cold infusion: 2–4 oz. bid–tid; FPT/DPT (40% alcohol): 30–60 drops bid–tid; Capsule (00): 1–2 bid–tid; Fluidextract: 10–30 drops bid–tid; External preparations: as needed.

Betula [Bark]

Decoction: 2–4 oz. qd–tid; Wash/Fomentation as needed.

Bidens [Herb]

Infusion: 4–8 oz. bid–tid; FPT/DPT (50% alcohol): 30–60 drops bid–tid; Wash/Oil/Salve: as needed.

Brickellia [Herb]

Infusion: 4–6 oz. bid–tid.

Bryonia [Root]

FPT/DPT (50% alcohol): 2–10 drops qd–tid. Use with care.

Bursera microphylla [Gum/Leaf/Twig]

FPT/DPT (80% alcohol) of gum: 10–20 drops bid–tid; FPT/DPT (80% alcohol) of Leaf/Twig: 30–60 drops bid–tid.

Caesalpinia [Leaf/Stem/Flower]

Infusion/Decoction: 4–6 oz. bid–tid; Wash or poultice: as needed.

Cacalia decomposita [Root]

FPT/DPT (70% alcohol): 20–40 drops qd–tid. Use with care.

Coffea arabica [Roasted seed]

Water percolation: 4–8 oz. qd–tid; Fluidextract (25% alcohol, 10% glycerin): 30–60 drops qd–tid.

Cactus grandiflorus

(Synonym for Selenicereus grandiflorus)

Calendula [Flower]

FPT/DPT (80% alcohol): 10–30 drops bid–tid; Fluidextract: 5–10 drops bid–tid; Eyewash: tid–qid; Ointment/Oil/Salve: as needed; Douche/Sitz bath/Wash: as needed; Suppository: bid–tid.

Campsis radicans [Leaf/Flower]

FPT/DPT (50% alcohol): 30–60 drops bid–tid; Infusion: 4–6 oz. bid–tid; Wash/Bath/Fomentation: as needed.

FPT (fresh plant tincture | DPT (dry plant tincture) | qd (once daily) | bid (two times daily) | tid (three times daily) | qid (four times daily)

Cannabis [Female flower/Leaf]

FPT/DPT (80% alcohol) of flower and leaf: 5–30 drops qd–tid; Liniment/Ointment: topically as needed.

Capsella bursa–pastoris [Whole plant]

FPT: 30–60 drops bid–tid.

Capsicum [Fruit]

DPT (80% alcohol): 2–10 drops qd–tid; Capsule (0): 1–2 qd–tid; Plaster/Liniment/Ointment: as needed.

Carduus marianus

(Synonym for Silybum marianum)

Carum [Seed]

Infusion: 2–6 oz. bid–tid; Spirit: 20–30 drops bid–tid; several seeds chewed as needed.

Caryophyllus

(Synonym for Syzygium aromaticum)

Cassia

(Synonym for Senna)

Castela emoryi [Branch ends]

FPT/DPT (50% alcohol): 30–60 drops tid–qid.

Caulophyllum thalictroides [Root]

DPT (60% alcohol): 10–25 drops qd–tid; Fluidextract: 4–8 drops qd–tid.

Ceanothus [Root/Root bark]

FPT/DPT (50% alcohol, 10% glycerin): 30–60 drops bid–tid; Decoction: 4–6 oz. bid–tid.

Centaurium erythraea [Whole plant]

FPT/DPT (50% alcohol): 20–40 drops bid–tid; Cold infusion: 2–4 oz. bid–tid.

Centella asiatica [Whole plant]

Fresh herb: small handful bid–tid; FPT/DPT (50% alcohol): 30–60 drops bid–tid; Infusion: 4–8 oz. bid–tid; Ointment: as needed.

Cephalanthus occidentalis [Leaf/Bark]

Leaf infusion/Bark decoction: 4–6 oz. before meals bid–tid; FPT/DPT (50% alcohol): 30–40 drops before meals bid–tid.

Cereus greggii

(Synonym for Peniocereus greggii)

Cereus grandiflorus

(Synonym for Selenicereus grandiflorus)

Cetraria islandica [Lichen body]

Decoction: 4–8 oz. bid–tid.

Chamomilla recutita

(Synonym for Matricaria recutita)

Chelidonium [Whole plant]

FPT: 15–30 drops qd–tid.

Chelone [Herb]

FPT/DPT (50% alcohol): 30–60 drops bid–tid; Standard/Cold infusion: 2–4 oz. bid–tid.

Chenopodium [Seed]

Capsules (00): 2–4 qd–bid.

Chilopsis linearis [Leaf/Bark]

FPT/DPT (50% alcohol): 30–60 drops bid–tid; Leaf infusion/bark decoction: 4–6 oz. bid–tid; Douche/sitz bath/wash: as needed.

Chimaphila [Herb]

FPT/DPT (50% alcohol): 30–60 drops bid–tid; Infusion: 4–8 oz. bid–tid.

Chionanthus [Bark]

FPT/DPT (55% alcohol): 30–60 drops bid–tid; Fluidextract: 10–20 drops bid–tid; Cold infusion: 2–4 oz. bid–tid.

Chrysanthemum parthenium [Herb]

Infusion: 4–6 oz. bid–tid; FPT/DPT (50% alcohol): 30–60 drops bid–tid.

Chondrus crispus [Whole plant]

Decoction: 4–8 oz. as needed.

Cichorium [Root]

Decoction: 4–8 oz. tid–qid.

Cimicifuga racemosa

(Synonym for Actaea racemosa)

Cinchona [Bark]

DPT (50% alcohol): 20–40 drops qd–bid; Infusion: 2–4 oz. qd–bid. Use as a bitter tonic.

Cineraria maritima [Herb]

Fresh juice/isotonic water (1:10): as an eye drop bid–tid. OTC/Homeopathic preps are available.

Cinnamomum camphora [Non–polar fraction]

Externally as liniment; DPT (95% alcohol): 5–10 drops qd–tid.

Cinnamomum cassia

(See Cinnamomum verum)

Cinnamomum loureiroi

(See Cinnamomum verum)

Cinnamomum verum [Bark]

DPT (60% alcohol, 10% glycerin): 30–60 drops bid–tid; Infusion: 4–6 oz. bid–tid; Spirit: 10–30 drops bid–tid.

Cistus [Resin–Labdanum]

DPT (80% alcohol): 15–30 drops bid–tid.

Citrus aurantium [Rind]
FPT/DPT (60% alcohol): 30–60 drops bid–tid.

Clematis [Leafing vine]
FPT/DPT (50% alcohol): 10–40 drops bid–tid; Infusion: 2–4 oz. bid–tid; Fresh plant poultice: use as needed, remove when skin begins to redden.

Cnicus benedictus [Herb]
Infusion: 4–6 oz. bid–tid.

Cola nitida [Seed]
DPT (60% alcohol, 10% glycerin): 30–60 drops qd–tid; Fluidextract: 5–30 drops qd–tid; Decoction: 4–6 oz. qd–tid.

Collinsonia canadensis [Root]
FPT/DPT (60% alcohol): 30–60 drops bid–tid.

Commiphora habessinica
(See Commiphora myrrha)

Commiphora myrrha [Gum–resin]
DPT (85% alcohol): 15–30 drops bid–tid; Capsule (0): 1–2 bid–tid; External preparations: as needed.

Conopholis [Whole plant]
FPT/DPT (50% alcohol): 30–60 drops bid–tid; Infusion: 4–6 oz. bid–tid.

Convallaria [Root/Leaf]
FPT/DPT (65% alcohol): 5–15 drops qd–tid. Use with care.

Conyza canadensis [Leaf]
Leaf infusion: 4–6 oz. tid–qid; Essential oil: 3–10 drops bid–tid.

Copaifera [Resin]
Resin/Essential oil: 5–10 drops in a capsule qd–tid; Dilute in 1–2 parts carrier oil for topical application.

Coptis [Root]
FPT/DPT (50% alcohol): 30–60 drops bid–tid; Decoction: 2–6 oz. bid–tid; Wash/Fomentation: as needed.

Corallorhiza [Root]
FPT/DPT (60% alcohol): 45–90 drops bid–tid; Standard/Cold infusion: 4–8 oz. bid–tid.

Coriandrum [Seed]
DPT (60% alcohol): 15–30 drops bid–tid.

Cornus [Bark]
Fluidextract (50% alcohol): 15–30 drops bid–

tid; Cold infusion: 4–6 oz. bid–tid.

Corydalis aureus [Herb]
FPT/DPT (50% alcohol): 10–30 drops bid–tid; Infusion: 2–4 oz. bid–tid. Use with care.

Crataegus [Fruit/Flower/Leaf]
FPT/DPT (60% alcohol): 30–60 drops bid–tid; Berry/Leaf/Flower infusion: 4–8 oz. bid–tid.

Crocus sativus [Stigma]
DPT: (75% alcohol): 10–30 drops bid–tid.

Cupressus [Leaf]
FPT: 20–40 drops bid–tid; Infusion: 4–6 oz. bid–tid; Steam inhalation: 5 minutes bid–tid; Oil/Salve/Wash/poultice: as needed.

Curcuma longa [Root]
FPT/DPT (60% alcohol): 30–60 drops bid–tid; Capsule (00): 2–3 bid–tid; Oil/Salve/Ointment: as needed.

Cuscuta [Above ground portion]
DPT (50% alcohol): 20–40 drops bid–tid; Infusion: 2–4 oz. bid–tid.

Cynara [Leaf/Root]
Leaf infusion/Root decoction: 4–6 oz. bid–tid; DPT (60% alcohol): 30–90 drops bid–tid; Fluidextract: 15–25 drops bid–tid.

Datura [Whole plant]
Liniment: bid–qid; Oil/Salve/Wash: bid–qid; Smoke: several inhalations qd–tid in acute situations; FPT (1:4)/DPT (1:10 60% alcohol): 5–10 drop qd–tid. Use with care.

Delphininium [Seed]
DPT (80% alcohol): topically as needed; Dilute if irritation develops.

Dicentra canadensis [Corm–tuber]
FPT/DPT (50% alcohol): 10–30 drops bid–tid; Standard/Cold infusion: 2–4 oz. bid–tid. Use with care.

Dicentra formosa [Root]
FPT/DPT (50% alcohol): 10–30 drops bid–tid; Standard/Cold infusion: 2–4 oz. bid–tid. Use with care.

Dioscorea villosa [Root]
FPT/DPT (65% alcohol): 60–90 drops bid–tid; Fluidextract: 30–60 drops bid–tid; Cold infusion: 3–6 oz. bid–tid.

Dipsacus [Herb]
Infusion: 2–4 oz. bid–tid.

FPT (fresh plant tincture | DPT (dry plant tincture) | qd (once daily) | bid (two times daily) | tid (three times daily) | qid (four times daily)

Dodonaea [Leaf]

   Infusion: 4 oz. bid–tid; FPT/DPT (60% alcohol): 30–60 drops bid–tid; Wash/Fomentation/Poultice/Oil/Salve: apply as needed; Sitz bath/Douche: bid.

Drosera [Herb]

   FPT: 10–30 drops bid–tid.

Dryopteris filix–mas [Root]

   Capsule (000) of powdered root: 4–8 (4–8 gm.) qd before bed. Usually taken with a mineral–based laxative; Oleoresin: 2–4 milliliters qd before bed. Use with care.

Dyssodia [Leaf]

   Leaf infusion: 4–8 oz. tid.

Echinacea angustifolia [Root/Flowerhead]

   FPT/DPT (70% alcohol): 30–90 drops bid–tid (in acute situations, every 1–2 hours); Fluidextract: 10–30 drops bid–tid; Standard/Cold infusion: 4–8 oz. bid–tid; Poultice: apply and change several times a day; Mouthwash/Gargle/Nasal spray: tid–qid

Echinacea pallida

   (See *Echinacea angustifolia*)

Echinacea purpurea

   (See *Echinacea angustifolia*)

Elettaria cardamomum [Seed]

   DPT (50% alcohol): 10–30 drops bid–tid; Infusion: 2–4 oz. bid–tid; several seeds chewed as needed.

Eleutherococcus [Root bark]

   DPT (60% alcohol): 60–90 drops bid–tid; Fluidextract: 20–40 drops bid–tid; Cold infusion: 4–6 oz. bid–tid.

Encelia farinosa [Leaf and stem]

   FPT/DPT (50% alcohol): 30–60 drops bid–tid; Infusion: 4–6 oz. bid–tid; External preparations: as needed.

Ephedra (American varieties) [Stem]

   Decoction: 4–6 oz. qd–tid; DPT (50% alcohol): 30–60 drops qd–tid; Capsules (00): 1–2 qd–bid.

Ephedra sinica [Stem]

   Infusion: 2–4 oz. qd–bid; DPT (50% alcohol): 20–40 drops qd–bid. Use with care.

Epigaea repens [Leaf]

   (See *Arctostaphylos uva–ursi*)

Epipactis gigantea [Whole plant]

   FPT/DPT (60% alcohol): 60–90 drops as needed.

Epilobium [Herb]

   Infusion: 4–8 oz. bid–tid.

Equisetum arvense [Stem]

   Fresh juice: 1 oz. bid–tid; Infusion: 2–4 oz. bid–tid; Poultice: as needed.

Equisetum hiemale, E. laevigatum

   (See *Equisetum arvense*)

Ericameria laricifolia [Leaf]

   Infusion: 4–6 oz. bid–tid; DPT (50% alcohol): 30–60 drops tid; Oil/Salve/Poultice/Powder: as needed.

Erigeron canadensis

   (Synonym for *Conyza canadensis*)

Eriodictyon [Leaf]

   FPT/DPT (70% alcohol): 30–60 drops bid–tid; Fluidextract: 10–30 drops bid–tid; Infusion: 2–4 oz. bid–tid.

Eriogonum [Leaf/Flower]

   Infusion: 4–8 oz. tid.

Erodium [Whole plant]

   Infusion: 4–8 oz. bid–tid; Sitz bath.

Eryngium yuccifolium [Root]

   FPT/DPT (60% alcohol): 20–40 drops bid–tid.

Eschscholtzia [Whole plant]

   FPT/DPT (50% alcohol): 60–90 drops bid–tid; Infusion: 4–8 oz. bid–tid; Topical preparations: as needed.

Eucalyptus globulus [Leaf]

   FPT/DPT (60% alcohol): 20–40 drops bid–tid; Infusion: 4–6 oz. bid–tid; Spirit: 10–20 drops bid–tid; Essential oil: topically as needed; Douche: bid.

Eugenia aromaticum, E. caryophyllata

   (See *Syzygium aromaticum*)

Euonymus [Bark]

   DPT (45% alcohol): 10–30 drops bid–tid; Fluidextract: 5–15 drops bid–tid; Cold infusion: 2–4 oz. bid–tid. Use with care.

Eupatorium perfoliatum [Herb]

   FPT: 30–60 drops bid–tid; Infusion: 4–6 oz. bid–tid.

Eupatorium purpureum [Root]

   Decoction: 4–8 oz. tid–qid; FPT/DPT (60% alcohol): 30–90 drops tid–qid.

Euphrasia [Herb]

FPT/DPT (50% alcohol): 45–90 drops bid–tid; Infusion: 4–6 oz. bid–tid.

Eysenhardtia [Bark/Branch]

Decoction: 4–8 oz. bid–tid.

Ferula moschata [Root]

DPT (85% alcohol): 20–40 drops bid–tid; Capsule (00): 1–2 bid–tid.

Filipendula [Herb]

FPT/DPT (50% alcohol): 60–90 drops bid–tid; Infusion: 4–8 oz. bid–tid.

Flourensia cernua [Leaf]

Leaf infusion: 2–4 oz. before meals; Oil/Salve/Wash: as needed.

Foeniculum vulgare [Seed]

Infusion: 4–8 oz. bid–tid; FPT/DPT (50% alcohol): 30–60 drops bid–tid.

Fouquieria splendens [Bark/Root]

FPT/DPT (70% alcohol): 30–60 drops bid–tid; Decoction: 4–6 oz. bid–tid.

Fragaria [Herb]

Infusion: 4–8 oz. as needed.

Frangula alnus [Bark]

DPT (30% alcohol): 1 teaspoon qd–bid; Fluidextract: 10–15 drops qd–bid; Decoction/Cold infusion: 2–4 oz. qd–bid.

Fremontia californica [Bark]

(See Ulmus fulva)

Fraxinus [Bark]

Decoction: 4–6 oz. bid–tid; Poultice/Oil/Salve: externally as needed.

Fucus [Whole plant]

Capsules (00): 2–3 bid–tid.

Fumaria [Herb]

FPT/DPT (50% alcohol): 10–30 drops bid–tid; Infusion: 2–4 oz. bid–tid. Use with care.

Galega officinalis [Herb]

Infusion: 4–6 oz. bid–tid.

Galium aparine [Whole plant]

Fresh juice: 60–90 drops bid–tid.

Ganoderma lucidum [Fruiting body]

Capsules: 1–2 bid–tid.

Garrya [Leaf/Root bark]

DPT (50% alcohol) of leaf: 30–60 drops bid–tid; DPT (50% alcohol) of root bark: 15–30

drops bid–tid. Use with care.

Gaultheria [Herb]

Essential oil: externally in a carrier oil or internal use of the spirit: 20–30 drops bid–tid; Infusion: 2–4 oz. bid–tid.

Gelsemium [Root]

FPT (1:4)/DPT (1:10 70% alcohol): 5–20 drops qd–qid. Use with care.

Gentiana [Root] Gentian

FPT/DPT (50% alcohol): 15–30 drops before meals.

Geranium [Root]

Decoction: 4–6 oz. bid–tid; FPT/DPT (50% alcohol 10% glycerin): 30–60 drops bid–tid; Wash/Fomentation/Douche: as needed.

Geum [Root]

Decoction: 4–6 oz. bid–tid.

Ginkgo biloba [Leaf]

Standardized extract: 100–300 mg. daily, taken in divided doses; DPT (60% alcohol): 30–60 drops bid–tid; Infusion: 2–4 oz. bid–tid.

Glechoma hederacea [Herb]

FPT/DPT (50% alcohol): 20–40 drops bid–tid; Infusion: 2–4 oz. bid–tid.

Glycyrrhiza glabra [Root]

DPT (50% alcohol): 10–50 drops qd–tid; Fluidextract: 5–10 drops qd–tid; Decoction: 2–4 oz. qd–tid; Capsule (00): 1–2 qd–tid; Ointment: as needed.

Glycyrrhiza lepidota [Root]

DPT (50% alcohol): 40–60 drops bid–tid; Fluidextract: 10–20 drops bid–tid; Decoction: 4–6 oz. bid–tid.

Gnaphalium [Herb]

Infusion: 4–8 oz. tid–qid.

Gossypium [Root bark]

FPT: 20–40 drops tid.

Grindelia [Flower/Leaf]

FPT/DPT (70% alcohol): 20–50 drops bid–tid; Fluidextract: 15–30 drops bid–tid; Ointment/Poultice: externally as needed.

Guaiacum officinale [Resin]

DPT (95% alcohol): 5–10 drops bid–tid.

Gutierrezia [Herb]

Infusion: add to bath water; Internally, 1 cup daily; Oil/Salve/Liniment: as needed.

FPT (fresh plant tincture | DPT (dry plant tincture) | qd (once daily) | bid (two times daily) | tid (three times daily) | qid (four times daily)

Gymnema silvestre [leaf]
Infusion: 4–6 oz. qd–bid.

Haematoxylon campechianum [Heartwood]
Decoction: 4–6 oz. bid–tid.

Hamamelis virginiana [Bark/Twig/Leaf]
FPT/DPT (50% alcohol, 10% glycerin): 30–60 drops bid–tid, or used externally; Fluidextract: 10–30 drops bid–tid; Douche: bid–tid; Nasal wash: as needed; Other external preparations: as needed.

Haplopappus laricifolius
(See *Ericameria laricifolia*)

Harpagophytum procumbens [Root]
DPT (60% alcohol): 30–60 drops bid–tid; Capsules (00): 1–2 bid–tid. Use substitutes, wild populations are threatened.

Hedeoma [Herb]
FPT/DPT (50% alcohol): 30–60 drops bid–tid; Infusion: 2–4 oz. bid–tid.

Hedera helix [Leaf/Gum]
FPT of leaf: 20–40 drops bid–tid; DPT (70% alcohol) of gum: 10–20 drops qd–bid.

Helenium hoopesii [Root]
FPT/DPT (60% alcohol) as a liniment: apply as needed.

Hepatica [Herb]
Infusion: 4–8 oz. bid–qid.

Heracleum [Root/Seed]
FPT/DPT (60% alcohol) of root: 30–60 drops bid–tid, topically as needed; FPT/DPT (60% alcohol) of seed: 30–60 drops bid–tid, topically as needed.

Heterotheca [Herb]
Infusion/Liniment/Oil: topically as needed.

Heuchera [Whole plant]
Decoction: 4–6 oz. bid–tid; FPT/DPT (50% alcohol 10% glycerin): 30–60 drops bid–tid; Wash/Fomentation/Douche: as needed.

Hibiscus [Flower/Whole plant]
Standard/Cold infusion: 4–8 oz. as needed; Emollient poultice: as needed.

Humulus [Flower/Leaf]
FPT/DPT (60% alcohol): 30–60 drops bid–tid; Fluidextract: 10–30 drops bid–tid; Infusion: 3–6 oz. bid–tid; DPT (70% alcohol) of resin glands, 20–40 drops bid–tid.

Hydrangea arborescens [Root]
Decoction: 4–8 oz. bid–tid; FPT/DPT (50% alcohol): 45–90 drops bid–tid.

Hydrastis canadensis [Root]
FPT/DPT (60% alcohol): 30–60 drops bid–tid; Fluidextract: 10–20 drops bid–tid; Capsule (00): 2–3, bid–tid; Leaf infusion: 2–4 oz. bid–tid. Endangered, use cultivated stock.

Hydrocotyle asiatica
(See *Centella asiatica*)

Hymenoclea [Leaf]
FPT/DPT (60% alcohol): 20–60 drops bid–tid; Infusion: 2–4 oz. bid–tid.

Hyocyamus niger [Herb]
FPT/DPT (75% alcohol): 5–15 drops bid–tid, or topically as needed. Use with care.

Hypericum [Bud/Flower/Leaf]
FPT/DPT (60% alcohol): 30–60 drops bid–tid; Infusion: 3–6 oz. bid–tid; Oil/Ointment/Salve: as needed.

Hyptis [Herb]
Infusion: 4–8 oz. bid–tid; FPT/DPT (60% alcohol): 30–60 drops bid–tid.

Hyssop [Herb]
Infusion 4–8 oz. bid–tid; FPT/DPT (50% alcohol): 30–60 drops bid–tid.

Ilex paraguayensis [Herb]
Infusion: 6–8 oz. bid–tid.

Ilex verticillata [Bark]
Decoction: 2–4 oz. bid–tid.

Illicium anisatum [Seed]
Infusion: 2–4 oz. qd–bid; Essential oil: 2–4 drops qd–bid; Spirit: 20–40 drops qd–bid.

Impatiens capensis [Whole plant]
Fresh juice/Poultice: topically as needed.

Inula helenium [Root]
FPT/DPT (60% alcohol): 30–60 drops bid–tid; Decoction: 4–6 oz. bid–tid; Capsules (00): 2–3 bid–tid.

Iodina rhombifolia [Bark]
FPT/DPT (50% alcohol): 20–40 drops bid–tid; Fluidextract: 5–15 drops bid–tid.

Iris florentina, I. germanica, I. pallida [Rhizome]
Powder for perfume/cosmetic uses.

Iris versicolor, I. virginica, I. missouriensis [Rhizome]

DPT (80% alcohol): 5–20 drops bid–tid.

Jateorhiza palmata [Root]
DPT (60% alcohol): 20–40 drops bid–tid; Fluidextract: 10–15 drops bid–tid; Cold infusion: 1–2 oz. bid–tid.

Jatropha (Limberbush type) [Stem]
Decoction: 2–4 oz. bid–tid; Sap/Stem poultice: externally as needed.

Jeffersonia diphylla [Rhizome]
FPT/DPT (40% alcohol): 30–60 drops bid–tid; Cold infusion: 4–6 oz. bid–tid.

Juglans [Leaf/Bark/Rind]
FPT/DPT (50% alcohol): 30–60 drops bid–tid; Infusion: 4–6 oz. bid–tid.

Juniperus [Fruit/Leaf]
Infusion: 4–6 oz. bid–tid; FPT/DPT (75% alcohol): 30–40 drops bid–tid; Spirit: 20–30 drops bid–tid; Ointment/Oil/Salve: as needed.

Kallstroemia [Whole plant]
Infusion: 4 oz. bid–tid; Eyewash: bid–tid.

Kalmia latifolia [Leaf]
FPT/DPT (50% alcohol): 5–15 drops bid–tid. Use with care.

Krameria [Root/Herb]
FPT/DPT (50% alcohol, 10% glycerin): 30–60 drops bid–tid; Cold infusion: 2–6 oz. bid–tid, topically as needed; Suppository: 1–2 daily (one before bed).

Lactuca [Herb]
DPT of lactucarium (80% alcohol): 30–60 drops bid–tid; FPT/DPT (60% alcohol): 60–90 drops bid–tid; Leaf infusion: 4–8 oz. bid–tid.

Larrea [Leaf]
DPT (75% alcohol): 20–40 drops qd–tid; Standard/Cold infusion: 2–4 oz. qd–tid (1 teaspoon of herb to 1 cup of water); Ointment/Oil/Salve: as needed; Douche: qd–bid.

Lavandula [Flower]
Essential oil: topical use as needed; Ointment: as needed; Spirit: 10–30 drops bid–tid.

Ledum [Leaf]
Infusion: as a beverage tea; Topically as a wash.

Lentinula edodes [Fruiting body]
Capsules: 2–3 bid–tid.

Leonurus cardiaca [Herb]

FPT/DPT (50% alcohol): 30–60 drops bid–tid; Infusion: 4–6 oz. bid–tid.

Lepidium [Fruit]
FPT/DPT (60% alcohol): 30–40 drops bid–tid; Infusion: 2–4 oz. bid–tid; Poultice/Plaster: as needed.

Liatris [Root]
Decoction: 4–6 oz. bid–qid.

Ligusticum porteri [Root]
FPT/DPT (70% alcohol): 30–60 drops bid–tid; Standard/Cold infusion: 4–6 oz. bid–tid; Syrup: 1 tablespoon tid–qid.

Ligustrum vulgare [Bark]
Decoction: 2–4 oz. bid–tid.

Lilium tigrinum [Whole plant]
FPT: 5–20 drops qd–bid.

Linaria [Herb]
DPT (50% alcohol): 20–40 drops bid–tid; Infusion: 2–4 oz. bid–tid; Poultice/Fomentation: as needed.

Linum [Seed]
1–2 tablespoons soaked in water: qd–bid. Ground seed as a poultice: as needed.

Liquidambar [Balsam]
DPT (95% alcohol): 10–30 drops bid–tid; Topically applied mixed with 2 parts olive oil.

Lithospermum [Root]
Decoction: topically as needed; DPT (50% alcohol): topically as needed; Oil/Salve/Poultice: as needed.

Lobaria pulmonaria [Whole lichen]
DPT (60%): 20–40 drops bid–tid; Infusion: 2–4 oz. bid–tid.

Lobelia inflata [Whole plant]
FPT of whole plant (1:4)/DPT (1:10 50% alcohol) of seed: 20–30 drops bid–tid (full dose); FPT of whole plant (1:4)/DPT (1:10 50% alcohol) of seed: 5–10 drops bid–tid (lesser dose); External preparations: apply as needed.

Lomatium dissectum [Root]
FPT/DPT (70% alcohol): 20–60 drops bid–tid; Standard/Cold infusion: 2–4 oz. bid–tid.

Lycium pallidum [Leaf]
FPT/DPT (50% alcohol): 20–30 drops qd–tid; Infusion: 2–4 oz. qd–tid; Poultice/Liniment: as needed.

FPT (fresh plant tincture | DPT (dry plant tincture) | qd (once daily) | bid (two times daily) | tid (three times daily) | qid (four times daily)

Lycopus [Herb]
FPT: 30–60 drops bid–tid.

Lysichiton americanus
(*See Symplocarpus foetidus*)

Lythrum [Herb]
Standard/Cold infusion: 4–8 bid–tid; Externally as needed.

Mahonia [Root]
Decoction/Cold infusion: 2–4 oz. bid–tid; FPT/DPT (40% alcohol): 30–60 drops bid–tid; Capsule (00): 1–2 bid–tid; Fluidextract: 10–30 drops bid–tid; External preparations: as needed.

Malva [Whole plant]
Leaf infusion/root decoction: 4–8 oz. bid–tid.

Marrubium [Herb]
Infusion: 4–6 oz. bid–tid; FPT/DPT (50% alcohol): 30–60 drops bid–tid; Syrup: 1 teaspoon tid–qid.

Matricaria recutita [Flower]
Infusion: 4–8 oz. as needed; External preparations: as needed.

Matricaria matricariodes [Flower]
Infusion: 4–8 oz. as needed.

Medicago sativa [Herb]
Infusion: 4–8 oz. bid–tid.

Melilotus [Herb]
Infusion: 4–6 oz. qd–bid; Topically as needed.

Melaleuca alternifolia [Leaf]
Essential oil, externally applied: as needed; Ointment/Oil/Salve: as needed; Suppository: bid (one before bed); Spirit: 10–20 drops bid–tid.

Melaleuca cajuputi [Leaf]
Essential oil, externally applied: as needed; Ointment/Oil/Salve: as needed.

Melaleuca quinquenervia [Leaf]
Essential oil, externally applied: as needed; Ointment/Oil/Salve: as needed.

Melissa officinalis [Herb]
Infusion: 4–8 oz. bid–tid; Spirit: 20–40 drops bid–tid; Encapsulated essential oil: 2–4 drops bid–tid; Essential oil: topically as needed.

Menispermum canadense [Root]
DPT (70% alcohol): 20–40 drops bid–tid; Flui-dextract: 5–15 drops bid–tid.

Mentha piperita [Herb]
Infusion: 4–8 oz. bid–tid; FPT/DPT (60% alcohol): 30–60 drops bid–tid; Essential oil: 2–3 drops taken in a capsule bid–tid, or applied topically as needed; Spirit: 20–30 drops bid–tid.

Mentha pulegium [Herb]
FPT: 30–60 drops qd–tid; Infusion: 4–6 oz. qd–tid.

Mentha spicata [Herb]
Infusion: 4–8 oz. as needed; Essential oil: 2–3 drops in a capsule bid–tid; Spirit: 20–30 drops bid–tid.

Menyanthes [Leaf/Root]
FPT/DPT (50% alcohol): 20–40 drops bid–tid; Standard/Cold infusion: 2–4 oz. bid–tid.

Mimosa [Leaf]
Wash/Powder/Poultice: apply as needed; Infusion: gargle as needed.

Mitchella repens [Herb]
FPT/DPT (50% alcohol): 30–60 drops bid–tid; Infusion: 4–8 oz. bid–tid.

Monarda [Herb]
FPT/DPT: 20–40 drops bid–tid; Infusion: 2–6 oz. bid–tid; Spirit: 10–20 drops bid–tid; Steam inhalation: bid–tid; Essential oil (diluted with carrier oil): topically as needed; Ointment/Oil/Salve: as needed.

Myrica [Root bark]
FPT/DPT (60% alcohol): 30–60 drops bid–tid; Cold infusion: 2–4 oz. bid–tid; Gargle: as needed; Nasal wash: as needed.

Myristica [Seed]
DPT (75% alcohol): 5–10 drops bid–tid; Spirit: 5–20 drops bid–tid. Use small doses in formula.

Myroxylon pereirae [Resin/Balsam]
5–15 drops, diluted, qd–tid (internal); Externally as a dressing, mixed with a carrier oil (1 or 2 parts).

Myroxylon toluifera [Resin/Balsam]
Tincture 1:5 (80% alcohol): 15–30 drops bid–tid; steam inhalation: as needed.

Nepeta [Herb]
Infusion: 4–8 oz. bid–tid; FPT/DPT (50% alco-

hol): 30–60 drops bid–tid.

Nicotiana [Herb]

Liniment/Poultice/Salve/Oil/Bath: topically as needed.

Nolina [Leaf]

Oil/salve: as needed; Decoction: 2–4 oz. bid–tid; Capsules (00): 2–3 bid–tid.

Nuphar luteum/lutea [Root/Seed]

FPT/DPT (60% alcohol): 20–40 drops bid–tid; Decoction: 4–6 oz. bid–tid.

Nymphaea odorata [Root]

FPT/DPT (60% alcohol): 20–40 drops bid–tid; Decoction: 2–4 oz. bid–tid or externally as needed.

Nymphaea alba [Root]

(*See Nymphaea odorata*)

Oenothera [Herb]

Infusion: 4–6 oz. bid–tid.

Olea europaea [Leaf]

Infusion: 2–4 oz. 2–3 times daily.

Oplopanax horridum [Root bark]

FPT/DPT (60% alcohol): 30–60 drops bid–tid.

Opuntia (Cholla type) [Root/Gum]

Root/gum tea: 4–8 oz. bid–tid; Gum tea: apply as needed.

Opuntia (Prickly pear type)

Pulp slurry/cooked pad: 1–2 oz. before meals; External pulp/flower infusion/salve: apply as needed; Flower infusion: 4–8 oz. bid–tid.

Orobanche [Whole plant]

FPT/DPT (50% alcohol): 30–60 drops bid–tid; Infusion: 4–6 oz. bid–tid.

Osmorhiza [Root]

FPT/DPT (60% alcohol): 60–90 drops bid–tid.

Oxydendrum arboreum [Leaf]

Decoction: 4–6 oz. bit–tid

Paeonia [Root]

FPT/DPT (60%): 30–60 drops qd–tid; Standard/Cold infusion: 4–6 oz. qd–tid; Capsules (00): 1–2 bid–tid.

Panax ginseng [Root]

Capsule (00): 1–2 qd–tid; DPT (70% alcohol): 15–30 drops qd–tid; Dried whole root: 1–3 small pieces daily.

Panax quinquefolius [Root/Leaf]

Capsule (00): 1–2 qd–tid; DPT (70% alcohol):

15–30 drops qd–tid; Dried whole root: 2–3 small pieces daily; Cold infusion of leaf: 4–6 oz. bid–tid.

Parietaria [Herb]

Infusion: 4–6 oz. bid–tid; expressed juice: 1 oz. bid–tid.

Parthenium incanum [Leaf]

Leaf infusion: 2–4 oz. bid–tid

Passiflora [Leaf/Vine/Flower]

FPT/DPT (50% alcohol): 60–90 drops bid–tid; Fluidextract: 20–40 drops bid–tid; Infusion: 4–8 oz. bid–tid.

Paullinia [Seed]

DPT (65% alcohol, 10% glycerin): 30–90 drops, qd–tid; Fluidextract: 20–30 drops qd–tid; Capsule (00): 2–3 qd–tid.

Pausinystalia yohimbe [Bark]

DPT (65% alcohol): 10–30 drops qd–tid.

Pectis [Herb]

Infusion: 4–6 oz. bid–tid; FPT/DPT (60% alcohol): 30–60 drops bid–tid.

Peganum harmala [Seed]

DPT (60% alcohol): 30–60 drops tid; Poultice/Powder/Oil/Salve: topically as needed.

Pedicularis [Herb]

FPT/DPT (50% alcohol): 60–90 drops bid–tid; Infusion: 4–8 oz. bid–tid.

Peniocereus greggii [Stem]

FPT: 10–25 drops qd–qid. Use cultivated stock – scare in some areas.

Penstemon [Herb]

Oil/Salve/Poultice: as needed.

Petasites [Herb]

Infusion: 2–4 oz. bid–tid. Use low/free PA stock/preparations.

Petroselinum crispum [Root]

DPT (60% alcohol): 30–60 drops bid–tid; Infusion: 4–6 oz. bid–tid.

Peumus boldus [Leaf]

DPT (60% alcohol): 15–30 drop qd–tid; Fluidextract: 5–10 drops qd–tid.

Pfaffia paniculata [Root]

DPT (60% alcohol): 30–60 drops bid–tid; Capsules (00): 1–2 bid–tid.

Phytolacca [Root] Poke root

FPT/DPT (50% alcohol): 5–10 drops qd–

bid; Poultice (fresh or dry root): apply until "lymph" fluid appears on skin.

Picrasma [Wood]
Cold infusion: 2–4 oz. bid–tid; DPT (40% alcohol): 30–60 drops bid–tid; Enema qd.

Pilocarpus [Leaf]
DPT (75% alcohol): 15–30 drops qd–bid; Externally as scalp treatment.

Pimenta racemosa [Leaf]
Spirit: 10–30 drops qd–tid; Externally as needed.

Pimenta dioica [Fruit]
Spirit: 10–30 drops qd–tid; Externally as needed.

Pimpinella anisum [Seed]
Infusion: 2–4 oz. qd–bid; Essential oil: 3–5 drops qd–bid; Spirit: 30–50 drops qd–bid.

Pinus [Pitch/Resin]
DPT (95% alcohol): 5–10 drops bid–tid; Small piece as an expectorant; Ointment/Salve: as needed; Needle infusion: 4–6 oz. bid–tid.

Pinus alba [Bark]
DPT (75% alcohol): 30–60 drops bid–tid.

Piper aduncum [Leaf]
DPT (60% alcohol): 30–60 drops bid–tid; Poultice as needed.

Piper angustifolia
(Synonym for Piper aduncum)

Piper cubeba [Immature fruit]
DPT (75% alcohol): 10–30 drops bid–tid; Capsule (00): 2–4 bid–tid.

Piper Methysticum [Root]
Standard/Cold infusion: 4–6 oz. bid–tid; FPT/DPT (60% alcohol): 30–60 drops bid–tid; Fluidextract: 10–20 drops bid–tid.

Piper nigrum [Immature fruit]
DPT (65% alcohol): 10–20 drops bid–tid.

Piscidia piscipula [Root bark/Bark]
DPT (60% alcohol): 30–60 drops bid–tid.

Plantago major [Herb]
Fresh plant poultice/Oil/Ointment/Salve: as needed; Standard/Cold infusion: 4–8 oz. bid–tid; Fresh juice: 1–2 oz. bid–tid or topically as needed.

Plantago ovata [Seed/Seed husk]
1–2 tablespoons in water qd–bid.

Plantago psyllium
(See Plantago ovata)

Pluchea camphorata [Herb]
FPT/DPT (60% alcohol): 30–60 drops tid; Leaf/Root infusion: 4–6 oz. bid–tid; External preparations: as needed.

Pluchea purpurascens
(See Pluchea camphorata)

Pluchea sericea [Root]
FPT/DPT (60% alcohol): 30–60 drops bid–tid; Leaf/Root tea: 4–6 oz. bid–tid; External preparations: as needed.

Plumbago [Herb]
Herb poultice/Fomentation/Salve/Oil: topically as needed.

Podophyllum peltatum [Root]
DPT (95% alcohol): 10–20 drops qd–bid. Use with care.

Polygala senega [Root]
FPT/DPT (60% alcohol): 20–40 drops bid–tid; Fluidextract: 10–20 bid–tid.

Polygonatum [Root]
Decoction: 2–4 oz. bid–tid.

Polygonum aviculare [Herb]
Infusion: 2–4 oz. qd–tid.

Polygonum bistorta [Root]
Decoction: 2–4 oz. bid–tid; DPT (30% alcohol, 10% glycerin): 60–90 drops bid–tid.

Polygonum hydropiper [Herb]
Infusion: 2–4 oz. qd–tid.

Polypodium glycyrrhiza [Root]
Decoction: 2–4 oz. bid–tid.

Populus candicans [Immature leaf bud]
FPT/DPT (75% alcohol): 20–40 drops bid–tid; Oil/Ointment/Salve: as needed.

Populus [Bark/Leaf bud]
Decoction: 4 oz. bid–tid, externally as needed; External applications of leaf bud: as needed.

Potentilla [Herb]
Infusion: 4–6 oz. bid–tid.

Primula [Root]
Decoction: 2–4 oz. bid–tid.

Prosopis [Leaf/Gum/Pod]
Infusion, topically or as a gargle: as needed; Eyewash: bid–tid for 2–3 days, then rotate to a tannin free solution; Gum: bid–tid.

Porophyllum [Herb]

Fresh leaves and flowers: eaten as needed; Infusion: 4–8 oz. bid–tid.

Prunella vulgaris [Herb]

FPT: 60–90 drops bid–qid; Infusion: bid–qid.

Prunus [Bark]

Cold infusion: 4–6 oz. bid–tid; DPT (40% alcohol, 10% glycerin): 60–90 drops bid–tid; Fluidextract: 20–40 drops bid–tid; Syrup: 1–2 teaspoons qd–tid.

Ptelea [Leaf]

FPT/DPT (65% alcohol): 20–40 drops bid–tid; Infusion: 2–4 oz. bid–tid.

Pterocarpus marsupium [Gum]

DPT (65% alcohol/15% glycerin): 30–60 drops in water qd–bid; Infusion: 2–4 oz. qd–bid.

Punica granatum [Root bark]

Decoction: 2–4 oz. bid–tid.

Ptychopetalum olacoides [Root/Bark]

DPT (70% alcohol): 30–60 drops qd–tid; Infusion: 2–4 oz. qd–tid.

Pulmonaria officinalis [Herb]

Infusion: 4–6 oz. bid–tid.

Pygeum africanum [Bark]

Capsules (00) 2–4 bid–tid. Use substitutes, wild populations are threatened.

Pyrola [Herb]

FPT/DPT (50% alcohol): 30–60 drops bid–tid; Infusion: 4–8 oz. bid–tid.

Quercus [Bark]

Decoction: 2–4 oz. bid or topically as needed.

Rhamnus californica [Aged bark]

Cold infusion: 2–4 oz. qd–bid; DPT (30% alcohol): 30–60 drops qd–bid; Fluidextract: 15–30 drops qd–bid.

Rhamnus fragula [Bark]

(*See Frangula alnus*)

Rhamnus purshiana [Bark]

DPT (30% alcohol): 1–2 teaspoon qd–bid; Fluidextract: 10–30 drops qd–bid; Bark decoction/Cold infusion: 2–6 oz. qd–bid.

Rheum officinale [Root]

DPT (45% alcohol, 10% glycerin): 20–50 drops bid–tid; Fluidextract: 5–15 drops bid–tid; Decoction: 2–4 oz. bid–tid; Syrup: 1 teaspoon bid–tid.

Rheum palmatum

(*See Rheum officinale*)

Rhus (Lemonade–berry type) [Leaf]

Infusion: 2–4 oz. bid–tid; Wash/Powder/Poultice/Oil/Salve: as needed; Beverage from fruit.

Rosa [Bud–petal]

Infusion: 2–4 oz. as needed, or as an eyewash.

Rosa [Fruit]

Infusion: 4–6 oz. bid–tid; Capsules (00): 2–4 bid–tid.

Rosa [Leaf]

Infusion: 4–6 oz. bid–tid.

Rosmarinus [Herb]

Infusion: 3–6 oz. bid–tid; FPT/DPT (60% alcohol): 20–40 drops bid–tid; Spirit: 20–40 drops bid–tid; External preparations: as needed.

Rubia tinctorium [Root]

Decoction: 4–8 oz. bid–tid.

Rubus idaeus [Leaf]

Herb infusion: 4–8 oz. qd–tid; Douche/Sitz bath: qd–bid.

Rubus villosus [Root]

Decoction: 4–6 oz. tid–qid.

Rumex crispus [Root]

FPT/DPT (50% alcohol): 30–60 drops bid–tid; Fluidextract: 10–20 drops bid–tid; Decoction: 4–6 oz. bid–tid.

Rumex hymenosepalus [Root]

Juice/Powder/Decoction: externally as needed.

Ruscus aculeatus [Roots]

FPT/DPT (60% alcohol): 30–60 drops bid–tid; Fluidextract: 15–30 drops bid–tid; Ointment/Oil: as needed.

Ruta graveolens [Herb]

Poultice as a counterirritant.

Salix alba [Bark]

Decoction: 2–6 oz. bid–tid

Salix nigra [Leaf bud]

FPT: 30–60 drops tid–qid.

Salvia [Herb]

Infusion: 4–8 oz. bid–tid; FPT/DPT (50% alcohol): 30–60 drops bid–tid; Spirit: 20–30 drops

---

FPT (fresh plant tincture | DPT (dry plant tincture) | qd (once daily) | bid (two times daily) | tid (three times daily) | qid (four times daily)

bid–tid; Essential oil: topically as needed;
Ointment/Oil/Salve: as needed; Steam inhalation: bid–tid.

Sambucus [Flower/Leaf]
Infusion: 2–4 oz. bid–tid.

Sanguinaria [Root]
DPT (60% alcohol): 10–15 drops in water bid.

Sanicula marilandica [Root]
Decoction: 4–6 oz. bid–tid; DPT (60% alcohol):
30–90 drops bid–tid.

Santalum [Wood]
Essential oil: 3–9 drops qd–tid; Spirit: 30–90
drops qd–tid.

Sapindus saponaria [Leaf/Fruit]
Leaf infusion: 2–4 oz. qd–tid; Fruit decoction:
1–2 oz. qd–tid; Capsules (00) powdered leaf:
2–4 qd–tid; Capsules (00) powdered fruit: 1–2
qd–tid.

Sassafras [Root bark]
Decoction: 4–6 oz. bid–tid.

Scrophularia [Root]
Decoction: 4–8 oz. bid–tid.

Scutellaria [Herb]
FPT/DPT (50% alcohol): 30–60 drops tid–qid.

Senecio aureus [Herb]
Infusion: 2–4 oz. bid–tid; DPT (50% alcohol):
30–60 drops bid–tid.

Selenicereus grandiflorus [Stem]
FPT: 5–15 drops qd–qid.

Senna [Pod/Leaf]
Cold infusion: 1–2 grams of whole pods to 1
cup of water taken before bed; Fluidextract
(40% alcohol): 5–20 drops before bed.

Serenoa repens [Fruit]
FPT/DPT (75% alcohol): 30–60 drops bid–tid;
Fluidextract: 10–30 drops bid–tid; Berry infusion: 4–6 oz. bid–tid; Capsule (00): 2–3 bid–
tid.

Silybum marianum [Seed]
Capsule (00): 2–3 bid–tid; Powdered seed:
1–2 teaspoons bid–tid; Fluidextract (60% alcohol): 20–40 drops bid–tid; Liniment/Oint-
ment: as needed.

Simmondsia [Leaf]
Decoction: 4–6 oz. bid–tid; Topical preparations: as needed; Oil: topically as needed.

Sinapis [Seed]
Plaster (1 part mustard powder, one part
binder, enough water to form a paste): apply until skin turns pink. Remove and wash
skin.

Smilacina racemosa [Whole plant]
Infusion: 4–8 oz. bid–tid; Field poultice: as
needed.

Smilax [Root]
Fluidextract (50% alcohol): 20–40 drops bid–
tid.

Solanum dulcamara [Stem]
FPT/DPT (60% alcohol): 15–30 drops bid–tid.

Solidago [Herb]
Infusion: 4–6 oz. 3–4 times daily.

Sphaeralcea [Herb]
Infusion: 4–8 oz. tid; Poultice: as needed.

Spigelia [Root]
Capsules (00): 4–8 bid for several days. A
number of species are listed as threatened,
use substitutes when able.

Spiraea [Herb]
FPT/DPT (50% alcohol): 60–90 drops bid–tid;
Infusion: 4–8 oz. bid–tid.

Stachys [Herb]
FPT/DPT (50% alcohol): 30–60 drops bid–tid;
Infusion: 4–8 oz. bid–tid.

Stellaria [Herb]
Poultice/Wash/Oil/Salve/Juice: as needed; Infusion: 4–8 oz. bid–tid.

Stillingia sylvatica [Root]
FPT/DPT (50% alcohol): 10–30 drops bid–tid.

Styrax [Resin]
DPT (95% alcohol): 15–30 drops bid–tid.

Swertia radiata [Leaf/Root]
FPT/DPT of leaf: 20–40 drops qd–tid; DPT
(50% alcohol) of root: 15–30 drops qd–tid.

Symphytum [Root and Herb]
Herb infusion: 4–6 oz. bid–tid; Root decoction: 2–4 oz. bid–tid; FPT/DPT (50% alcohol)
of herb/root: 20–40 drops bid–tid; Fresh root/
herb poultice: as needed; Oil/Salve/Ointment
(root): as needed. Use non–American strains
with caution.

Symplocarpus foetidus [Root]
FPT/DPT (50% alcohol): 20–60 drops bid–tid.

Syzygium aromaticum [Bud]

DPT (70% alcohol): 10–20 drops bid–tid; Spirit: 10–20 drops bid–tid; Capsule (00): 1–2 bid–tid; Liniment: topically as needed; Essential oil: topically as needed.

Tabebuia [Bark]

Decoction: 4–6 oz. bid–tid; DPT (50% alcohol): 30–60 drops bid–tid; Fluidextract: 20–30 drops bid–tid.

Tagetes [Herb]

FPT: 30–60 drops tid–qid; Infusion: 4–8 oz. tid–qid; Oil or salve made from the flowers: topically as needed.

Tamarix [Leaf/Bark]

External preparations: as needed.

Taraxacum officinale [Root/Leaf]

Root decoction: 2–6 oz. bid–tid; Leaf infusion: 4–8 oz. bid–tid; FPT/DPT (40% alcohol) of root: 60–90 drops bid–tid; Fluidextract of root: 20–40 drops bid–tid; Capsule of root (00): 2–3 bid–tid.

Tecoma stans [Leaf/Bark/Root]

Herb infusion/Bark/Root decoction: 4–8 oz. bid–tid; Sitz bath: bid–tid.

Thelesperma [Herb]

Herb infusion: as desired.

Thuja occidentalis [Leaf]

FPT/DPT (60% alcohol): 20–40 drops bid–tid; Infusion: 4–6 oz. bid–tid; Inhaled steam from the infusion or essential oil: 5 minutes bid–tid; Spirit: 10–20 drops bid–tid; Essential oil, topically applied: as needed; Oil/Salve/Ointment/Poultice: as needed; Suppository: bid, one before bed; Eye wash: bid–tid.

Thymus [Herb]

Infusion: 4–6 oz. bid–tid; FPT/DPT (60% alcohol): 20–50 drops bid–tid; Spirit: 20–40 drops bid–tid; Essential oil/Ointment/Oil/Salve: as needed.

Tribulus terrestris [Seed/Herb]

Infusion: 2–4 oz. bid–tid; FPT/DPT (60% alcohol): 30–40 drops bid–tid; Topical preparations: as needed.

Trifolium pratense [Herb]

Herb infusion: 4–8 oz. bid–tid.

Trillium [Root]

FPT/DPT (60% alcohol): 20–40 drops bid–tid.

Turnera diffusa [Herb]

FPT/DPT (60% alcohol): 30–60 drops bid–tid; Infusion: 4–6 oz. bid–tid.

Tussilago farfara [Herb]

Infusion: 4–6 oz. qd–bid.

Ulmus fulva [Bark]

Cold infusion (shredded bark): 4–8 oz. as needed; Capsule (00): 2–3 bid–tid; Gruel: 2–3 tablespoons bid–tid; Poultice (powdered bark): as needed.

Ulmus rubra

(See *Ulmus fulva*)

Umbellularia californica [Leaf]

FPT/DPT (60% alcohol): 20–30 drops bid–tid; Spirit: 15–30 drops bid–tid; Steam inhalation bid–tid; Essential oil: topically as needed.

Uncaria gambir [Leaf/Twigs]

Infusion: 4–6 oz. bid–tid.

Uncaria tomentosa [Bark/Root bark]

DPT (60% alcohol): 30–60 drops bid–tid.

Urtica [Leaf/Root]

Leaf infusion/Root decoction: 4–8 oz. bid–tid; FPT/DPT (50% alcohol): of root: 30–60 drops bid–tid; Fluidextract of root: 15–30 drops bid–tid.

Usnea [Whole lichen]

DPT (65% alcohol): 30–60 drops bid–tid; Decoction: 4–6 oz. bid–tid.

Ustilago [Whole fungus]

FPT/DPT (60% alcohol): 20–40 drops bid–tid.

Vaccinium [Leaf/Fruit]

Infusion: 4–8 oz. bid–tid; FPT/DPT (50% alcohol) of leaf: ½–1 teaspoon bid–tid; Fluidextract of fruit: 30–60 drops bid–tid; Capsule (00) of powdered fruit: 2–4 bid–tid.

Vaccinium macrocarpon [Fruit]

Juice: 3–4 oz. bid–tid; Fresh or frozen fruit: 1–2 oz. bid–tid.

Valeriana [Root/Whole plant]

Infusion: 3–6 oz. qd–tid; FPT/DPT (70% alcohol): 45–90 drops qd–tid; Fluidextract: 20–40 drops bid–tid; Capsule (00): 2–3 qd–tid.

Veratrum [Root]

DPT (1:10 80% alcohol): 5–10 drops qd–tid. Use with caution.

FPT (fresh plant tincture | DPT (dry plant tincture) | qd (once daily) | bid (two times daily) | tid (three times daily) | qid (four times daily)

Verbascum thapsus [Leaf/Root/Flower]

Leaf infusion/Root decoction: 4–6 oz. bid–tid; FPT/DPT (50% alcohol): 30–60 drops bid–tid; Flower oil/Tincture: 1–2 drops tid–qid.

Verbesina encelioides [Herb]

Infusion: 2–4 oz. bid–tid; External applications: as needed.

Verbena [Herb]

FPT/DPT (60% alcohol): 30–60 drops bid–tid; Infusion: 4–6 oz. bid–tid.

Veronicastrum virginicum [Root]

DPT (60% alcohol): 10–30 drops bid–tid.

Viburnum opulus [Root bark]

DPT (50% alcohol): 30–90 drops bid–tid; Decoction: 4–6 oz. bid–tid.

Viburnum prunifolium [Root bark]

DPT (50% alcohol): 30–90 drops bid–tid; Decoction: 4–6 oz. bid–tid.

Vinca major [Herb]

FPT/DPT (50% alcohol): 20–40 drops qd–tid.

Vinca minor

(See Vinca major)

Viola [Herb]

Infusion: 4–6 oz. bid–tid.

Viscum album [Herb]

DPT (50% alcohol): 20–40 drops bid–tid; Infusion: 2–4 oz. bid–tid.

Vitex agnus–castus [Fruit]

DPT (60% alcohol): 30–40 drops bid–tid; Fluidextract: 10–25 drops bid–tid; Capsule (00): 2–3, bid–tid.

Withania [Root]

FPT/DPT (65% alcohol): 20–40 drops bid–tid.

Xanthium [Herb/Bur]

Herb infusion/Bur decoction: 2–3 oz. bid–tid; DPT (60% alcohol): 20–30 drops bid–tid; Oil/Salve/Wash: topically as needed.

Xanthoxylum [Bark/Fruit]

DPT (65% alcohol): 20–40 drops bid–tid.

Yucca [Root]

Decoction: 4–6 oz. bid–tid; DPT (50% alcohol): 30–60 drops bid–tid; Fluidextract: 10–30 drops bid–tid; Capsule (00): 2–3 bid–tid.

Zea mays [Silk or flower styles]

Infusion: 4–8 oz. bid–tid; Fluidextract (40% alcohol): 30–40 drops bid–tid.

Zingiber [Root]

Infusion: 2–4 oz. bid–tid; FPT/DPT (70% alcohol): 20–50 drops bid–tid; Fluidextract: 5–15 drops bid–tid; Spirit: 20–30 drops bid–tid; Poultice: as needed.

APPENDIX C
FAMILY GROUPING

Anacardiaceae (Sumac Family)
Mangifera (Mango)
Rhus (Sumac)
Toxicodendron (Poison Ivy–Oak)

Agavaceae (Agave Family)
Agave (Century plant)
Yucca (Soaptree)

Apiaceae/Umbelliferae (Carrot Family)
Angelica
Cicuta (Water hemlock)
Conium (Poison hemlock)
Daucus (Carrot, Queen ann's lace)
Eryngium (Rattlesnake master)
Heracleum (Cow parsnip)
Ligusticum (Mountain lovage)
Lomatium (Biscuit root)
Pimpinella (Burnet–Saxifrage)

Apocynaceae (Dogbane Family)
Apocynum (Dog bane)
Nerium (Oleander)
Vinca (Periwinkle)

Aristolochiaceae (Birthwort Family)
Aristolochia (Pipevine)
Asarum (Wild ginger)

Asteraceae (Sunflower Family)
Achillea (Yarrow)
Ambrosia (Bursage)
Anaphalis (Everlasting)
Arctium (Burdock)
Arnica
Artemisia (Mugwort, Wormwood, Sage-brush)
Baccharis (Seepwillow, Yerba del pasmo)
Balsamorhiza (Balsam root)
Bidens (Spanish needles)
Brickellia (Bricklebush)
Calendula
Chrysanthemum
Cichorium (Chicory)
Cirsium (Thistle)
Cnicus (Blessed Thistle)
Conyza/Erigeron (Canadian fleabane)
Cynara (Artichoke)
Echinacea
Encelia (Brittlebush)
Ericameria (Turpentine bush)

Eupatorium (Boneset, Gravel root)
Gnaphalium (Cudweed)
Grindelia (Gumweed)
Gutierrezia (Snakeweed)
Helenium (Sneezeweed)
Heterotheca (Camphorweed)
Inula (Elecampane)
Lactuca (Wild lettuce)
Liatris (Gayfeather)
Matricaria (Chamomile)
Petasites (Western coltsfoot)
Pluchea (Marsh fleabane)
Rudbeckia (Coneflower)
Senecio (Life root)
Silybum (Milk thistle)
Solidago (Goldenrod)
Stevia
Tanacetum (Feverfew, Tansy)
Taraxacum (Dandelion)
Thelesperma (Greenthread)
Tussilago (Coltsfoot)
Verbesina (Crownbeard)
Xanthium (Cocklebur)

Berberidaceae (Barberry Family)
Berberis (Barberry)
Caulophyllum (Blue Cohosh)
Mahonia (Oregongrape)
Podophyllum (American Mandrake)

Bignoniaceae (Bignonia Family)
Chilopsis (Desert willow)
Tabebuia Pau d' arco)
Tecoma (Yellowbells)

Boraginaceae (Borage Family)
Borago (Borage)
Lithospermum (Groomwell)
Pulmonaria (Lungwort)
Symphytum (Comfrey)

Burseraceae (Torchwood Family)
Bursera (Elephant tree)
Commiphora (Myrrh, Guggul)
Boswellia (Frankincense)

Campanulaceae (Bellflower/Bluebell Family)
Lobelia

Cannabaceae (Hemp Family)
Cannabis (Marijuana)
Humulus (Hops)

Caprifoliaceae (Honeysuckle Family)
    Sambucus (Elder)
    Viburnum (Cramp bark)
Caryophyllaceae (Pink Family)
    Stellaria (Chickweed)
    Saponaria (Soapwort)
Clusiaceae (St. John's Wort Family)
    Garcinia (Gambooge)
    Hypericum (St. john's wort)
Cucurbitaceae (Cucumber Family)
    Bryonia
Cupressaceae (Cypress Family)
    Cupressus (Cypress)
    Juniperus (Juniper)
    Thuja (Cedar)
Ericaceae (Heath Family)
    Arbutus (Madrone)
    Arctostaphylos (Uva–ursi)
    Gaultheria (Winterberry)
    Ledum (Labrador tea)
    Vaccinium (Bilberry, Blueberry, Cranberry)
Euphorbiaceae (Spurge Family)
    Acalypha (Copperleaf)
    Jatropha (Limberbush)
    Ricinus (Castor bean)
    Stillingia
Fabaceae (Pea Family)
    Acacia (Gum acacia)
    Amorpha (False indigo))
    Arachis (Peanut)
    Astragalus
    Baptisia (Wild indigo)
    Caesalpinia (Bird of paradise)
    Cassia (Senna)
    Eysenhardtia (Kidneywood)
    Glycine (Soybean)
    Glycyrrhiza (Licorice)
    Medicago (Alfalfa)
    Melilotus (Yellow clover)
    Phaseolus (Bean)
    Prosopis (Mesquite)
    Sophora
    Trifolium (Red clover)
    Trigonella (Fenugreek)
Fagaceae (Beech Family)
    Quercus (Oak)

Fumariaceae (Fumitory Family)
    Corydalis (Golden smoke)
    Dicentra (Bleeding heart)
    Fumaria (Fumitory)
Gentianaceae (Gentian Family)
    Gentiana (Gentian)
    Swertia (Green gentian)
Geraniaceae (Geranium Family)
    Erodium (Stork's bill)
    Geranium
Hydrophyllaceae (Waterleaf Family)
    Eriodictyon (Yerba santa)
Iridaceae (Iris Family)
    Iris
    Crocus sativus (Saffron)
Juglandaceae (Walnut Family)
    Juglans (Walnut, Butternut)
Lamiaceae (Mint Family)
    Collinsonia (Stoneroot)
    Hedeoma (Western pennyroyal)
    Hyptis (Desert lavender)
    Hyssopus (Hyssop)
    Lavandula (Lavender)
    Leonurus (Motherwort)
    Lycopus (Bugleweed)
    Marrubium (Horehound)
    Mellissa (Lemonbalm)
    Mentha (Mint)
    Monarda (Wild oregano)
    Nepeta (Catnip)
    Ocimum (Basil)
    Poliomintha (Rosemary mint)
    Prunella (Self heal)
    Rosmarinus (Rosemary)
    Salvia (Sage)
    Scutellaria (Skullcap)
    Stachys (Betony)
    Teucrium (Germander)
    Thymus (Thyme)
Lauraceae (Laurel Family)
    Cinnamomum (Cinnamon)
    Sassafras
    Laurus (Laurel)
Liliaceae (Lily Family)
    Aletris (False unicorn root)
    Allium (Garlic, Onion)

Asparagus
Convallaria (Lily of the valley)
Polygonatum (Solomon's seal)
Scilla (Squill)
Trillium (Beth root)
Veratrum (Hellebore)
Loganiaceae (Pink Root Family)
Gelsemium
Spigelia (Pinkroot)
Lycopodiaceae (Clubmoss Family)
Huperzia (Clubmoss)
Lycopodium (Clubmoss)
Malvaceae (Mallow Family)
Althaea (Marshmallow)
Alcea (Hollyhock)
Gossypium (Cotton)
Hibiscus
Malva (Mallow)
Sida (Fanpetals)
Sidalcea (Checker mallow)
Sphaeralcea (Globemallow)
Myricaceae (Bayberry Family)
Myrica (Bayberry)
Myrtaceae (Myrtle Family)
Eucalyptus
Melaleuca (Tee tree)
Pimenta (All spice)
Psidium (Guava)
Nyctaginaceae (Four O'clock Family)
Mirabilis (Four o' clock)
Nymphaeaceae (Waterlily Family)
Nuphar (Yellow pond lily)
Nymphaea (Water lily)
Oleaceae (Olive Family)
Chionanthus (Fringetree)
Fraxinus (Ash)
Ligustrum (Privet)
Olea (Olive)
Onagraceae (Evening Primrose Family)
Epilobium (Fireweed)
Oenothera (Evening primrose)
Orchidaceae (Orchid Family)
Calypso (Fairy slipper)
Corallorhiza (Coral root)
Cypripedium (Lady's slipper)
Epipactis (Stream orchid)

Vanilla
Orobanchaceae (Broom–Rape Family)
Conopholis (Cancer root)
Orobanche (Broomrape)
Paeoniaceae (Peony Family)
Paeonia (Peony)
Papaveraceae (Poppy Family)
Argemone (Prickly poppy)
Chelidonium (Celandine)
Eschscholzia (California poppy)
Papaver (Poppy)
Sanguinaria (Blood root)
Pinaceae (Pine Family)
Abies (Fir)
Cedrus (Cedar)
Picea (Spruce)
Pinus (Pine)
Tsuga (Hemlock)
Piperaceae (Pepper Family)
Piper (Pepper, Kava)
Polygonaceae (Buckwheat Family)
Eriogonum (Desert buckwheat)
Polygonum (Knotweed, Smartweed)
Rheum (Rhubarb)
Rumex (Yellowdock)
Portulacaceae (Purslane Family)
Lewisia (Bitter root)
Portulaca (Purslane)
Primulaceae (Primrose Family)
Anagallis (Scarlet pimpernel)
Primula (Primrose)
Pteridaceae (Maidenhair Fern Family)
Adiantum (Maidenhair fern)
Pyrolaceae (Wintergreen Family)
Chimaphila (Pipsissewa)
Pyrola (Wintergreen)
Ranunculaceae (Buttercup Family)
Aconitum (Aconite)
Actaea (Cohosh)
Anemone
Caltha (Marsh marigold)
Clematis Virgin's bower)
Coptis (Goldthread)
Delphinium (Larkspur)
Hepatica (Liverwort)
Hydrastis (Goldenseal)

Pulsatilla

Rhamnaceae (Buckthorn Family)
Ceanothus (Reed root)
Frangula (Alder buckthorn)
Rhamnus (Cascara, Buckthorn)

Rosaceae (Rose Family)
Agrimonia (Agrimony)
Alchemilla (Lady's mantle)
Crataegus (Hawthorn)
Eriobotrya (Loquat)
Fallugia (Apache plume)
Filipendula (Meadowsweet)
Fragaria (Strawberry)
Geum (Avens)
Potentilla (Cinquifoil)
Purshia (Cliffrose)
Rosa (Rose)
Rubus (Raspberry)

Rubiaceae (Madder Family)
Asperula (Woodruff)
Cephalanthus (Buttonbush)
Cinchona (Quinine bark)
Coffea (Coffee)
Galium (Cleavers)
Mitchella (Squaw vine)
Rubia (Madder)

Rutaceae (Rue Family)
Citrus (Orange, Lime, Lemon, Grapefruit)
Fortunella (Kumquat)
Pilocarpus (Jaborandi)
Ptelea (Waferash)
Ruta (Rue)
Zanthoxylum (Prickly ash bark)

Salicaceae (Willow Family)
Populus (Popular, Cottonwood)
Salix (Willow)

Sapindaceae (Soapberry Family)
Dodonaea (Hopbush)
Sapindus (Soapberry)

Saururaceae (Lizard's Tail Family)
Anemopsis (Yerba mansa)
Saururus (Lizard's tail)

Saxifragaceae (Saxifrage Family)
Heuchera (Alum root)
Saxifraga (Saxifrage)

Scrophulariaceae (Figwort Family)

Chelone (Turtle head)
Digitalis (Foxglove)
Euphrasia (Eyebright)
Leucophyllum (Texas sage)
Linaria (Toadflax)
Pedicularis (Elephant head)
Penstemon
Scrophularia (Figwort)
Verbascum (Mullein)
Veronica (Speedwell)

Simaroubaceae (Quassia Wood Family)
Ailanthus (Tree or heaven)
Castela (Crucifixion thorn)
Quassia

Smilacaceae (Green Brier Family)
Smilax (Sarsaparilla)

Solanaceae (Nightshade Family)
Atropa (Belladonna)
Capsicum (Cayenne)
Datura (Jimson weed)
Lycium (Wolfberry)
Nicotiana (Tobacco)
Solanum (Nightshade)

Taxaceae (Yew Family)
Taxus (Yew)

Tiliaceae (Linden Family)
Tilia (Linden)

Ulmaceae (Elm Family)
Ulmus (Slippery Elm)

Urticaceae (Nettle Family)
Urtica (Nettle)

Valerianaceae (Valerian Family)
Valeriana (Valerian)

Verbenaceae (Verbena Family)
Aloysia (Lemon verbena)
Lantana
Lippia (Wild oregano)
Verbena (Vervain)
Vitex (Chaste tree)

Violacea (Violet Family)
Viola (Violet)

Viscaceae (Mistletoe Family)
Phoradendron (Mistletoe)
Viscum (Mistletoe)

Zingiberaceae (Ginger Family)
Curcuma (Turmeric)

Zingiber (Ginger)
Zygophyllaceae (Caltrop Family)
Guiacum (Lignum vitae)
Kallstroemia (Caltrop)
Larrea (Creosote bush, Chaparral)
Peganum (Syrian rue)
Tribulus (Goathead)

APPENDIX D
WORKSHEETS

PERCOLATION WORKSHEET

Plant Name:_____ | Date:_____

Part Used:_____ | Weight of Powdered Plant:_____oz. | Vol. of Lightly Compressed Powder:_____oz.

Ratio of strength (ex. 1:5):_____ | FTV (Final Tincture Volume):_____oz.

Calculating the Base Menstruum

1. FTV_____oz. + Volume of Lightly Compressed Powder_____oz. = Base Menstruum_____oz.

2. If Base Menstruum is _____oz. then its Specific Composition is:

        _____% of Water =_____oz. of Menstruum

        _____% of Alcohol =_____oz. of Menstruum

        _____% of Glycerin =_____oz. of Menstruum

        _____% of Vinegar =_____oz. of Menstruum

> The sum of the menstruum parts should equal the volume of the base menstruum

        TOTAL_____

Procedure

1. Moisten, pack, and digest as explained in Preparations.

2. Percolate and Catch Drip.

Notes:

FLUIDEXTRACT WORKSHEET
(Alcohol content 50% or less)

Plant Name:_____ | Date:_____

Part Used:_____ | Weight of Powdered Plant:____oz. | Vol. of Lightly Compressed Powder:____oz.

Ratio of strength: 1:1 | FFV (Final Fluidextract Volume):____oz.

Calculating the Base Menstruum

1. FFV x 5 =_____oz. + Volume of compressed herb_____oz. = Base Menstruum_____oz.

2. If Base Menstruum is_____oz. then its Specific Composition is:

_____% of Water =_____oz. of Menstruum

_____% of Alcohol =_____oz. of Menstruum

_____% of Glycerin =_____oz. of Menstruum

_____% of Vinegar =_____oz. of Menstruum

The sum of the menstruum parts should equal the volume of the base menstruum

TOTAL_____

Procedure

3. Moisten, pack, and digest as explained in Preparations.

4. Drip and catch ¾ of FFV (if FFV is 8oz. then catch 6oz.).

5. Remove first catch and set aside/Drip and catch the remainder of the Base Menstruum (second catch).

6. With a double boiler, slowly heat the second catch and reduce volume to the remaining ¼ of FFV.

7. Combine the first and second catches/Should total FFV.

Notes:

FLUIDEXTRACT WORKSHEET

(Alcohol content 51% or more)

Plant Name:_____ | Date:_____

Part Used:_____ | Weight of Powdered Plant:____oz. | Vol. of Lightly Compressed Powder:____oz.

Ratio of strength: 1:1 | FFV (Final Fluidextract Volume):____oz.

Calculating the Base Menstruum

1. FFV x 5 =_____oz. + Volume of compressed herb_____oz. = Base Menstruum_____oz.

2. Base Menstruum is composed of:_____oz. of HAM (volume of compressed herb + 75% of FFV) and _____oz. of LAM (remaining amount of Base menstruum)

	HAM			LAM
_____% of Water =_____oz. of Menstruum	The sum of the menstruum parts should equal the volume of the HAM	_____% of Water =_____oz. of Menstruum		The sum of the menstruum parts should equal the volume of the LAM
_____% of Alcohol =_____oz. of Menstruum		_____% of Alcohol =_____oz. of Menstruum		
_____% of Glycerin =_____oz. of Menstruum		_____% of Glycerin =_____oz. of Menstruum		
_____% of Vinegar =_____oz. of Menstruum		_____% of Vinegar =_____oz. of Menstruum		

TOTAL_____   TOTAL_____

Procedure

1. Moisten, pack, and digest with HAM as explained in Preparations.

2. Drip and catch ¾ of FFV using HAM.

3. Remove first catch and set aside.

4. Drip and catch the remaining HAM. If you have not already done so add and drip LAM.

4. With a double boiler, slowly heat the second catch and reduce volume to the remaining ¼ of FFV.

5. Combine the first and second catches/Should total FFV.

Notes:

**APPENDIX E
WEIGHTS AND MEASURES**

LIQUID VOLUME (APOTHECARY)

20 minims (min or ℳ) = 1 fluid scruple (ƒӬ)

60 minims (min or ℳ) = 1 fluid dram (fl dr or ƒӠ)

8 fluid drams = 1 fluid ounce (fl oz or ƒӠ̵)

16 fluid ounces = 1 pint (pt) = 128 fluid drams

2 pints = 1 quart (qt) = 32 fluid ounces = 256 fluid drams

4 quarts = 1 gallon (gal) = 128 fluid ounces = 1024 fluid drams

LIQUID VOLUME (STANDARD/COOKING)

1 teaspoon = 100 drops

1 tablespoon = 3 teaspoons = 300 drops

1 fluid ounce = 2 tablespoons = 600 drops

8 fluid ounces = 1 cup = 16 tablespoons = 4800 drops

LIQUID VOLUME (METRIC)

10 milliliters (ml) = 1 centiliter (cl)

10 centiliters = 1 deciliter (dl) = 100 milliliters

10 deciliters = 1 liter (l) = 1000 milliliters

LIQUID VOLUME (MISCELLANEOUS)

1 cc = 20 drops

1 cc = 1 ml

1 fluid ounce = 29.57 milliliters

MASS (STANDARD)

27.34375 grains = 1 dram

16 drams = 1 ounce (oz) = 437.5 grains

16 ounces = 1 pound (lb) = 256 drams = 7000 grains

MASS (METRIC)

1000 micrograms (mcg) = 1 milligram (mg)

10 milligrams = 1 centigram (cg)

10 centigrams = 1 decigram (dg) = 100 milligrams

10 decigrams = 1 gram (g) = 1000 milligrams

10 grams = 1 dekagram (dag)

MASS (MISCELLANEOUS)

1 grain = 64.79891 milligrams

1 gram = 15.432 grains

1 ounce = 28.35 grams

LENGTH (STANDARD)

12 inches (in) = 1 foot (ft)

3 feet = 1 yard (yd)

LENGTH (METRIC)

10 millimeters (mm) = 1 centimeter (cm)
10 centimeters = 1 decimeter (dm) = 100 millimeters
10 decimeters = 1 meter (m) = 1000 millimeters

BIBLIOGRAPHY

AGRIMONY

Copland, A., L. Nahar, C.T.M. Tomlinson, V. Hamilton, M.Middleton, Y.Kumarasamy, and S.D. Sarker. "Antibacterial and Free Radical Scavenging Activity of the Seeds of Agrimonia Eupatoria." *Fitoterapia* 74 (2003): 133–135.

Venskutonis, P.R., M. Škėmaitė, and B. Sivik. "Assessment of Radical Scavenging Capacity of Agrimonia Extracts Isolated by Supercritical Carbon Dioxide." *J. of Supercritical Fluids* 45 (2008): 231–237.

Venskutonis, P.R., M. Škėmaitė, and O. Ragažinskienė. "Radical Scavenging Capacity of Agrimonia Eupatoria and Agrimonia Procera." *Fitoterapia* 78 (2007): 166–168.

ALOE

Chithra, P., G.B. Sajithlal, and Gowri Chandrakasan. "Influence of Aloe Vera on the Glycosaminoglycans in the Matrix of Healing Dermal Wounds in Rats." *Journal of Ethnopharmacology* 59 (1998): 179–186.

Femenia, Antoni, Emma S. Sánchez, Susana Simal, and Carmen Rosselló. "Compositional Features of Polysaccharides from Aloe Vera (Aloe Barbadensis Miller) Plant Tissues." *Carbohydrate Polymers* 39 (1999): 109–117.

Grover, J.K., S. Yadav, and V. Vats. "Medicinal Plants of India with Anti–dDiabetic Potential." *Journal of Ethnopharmacology* 81 (2002): 81–100.

Herndon, D.N. and J.P. Heggers. "Retardation of Wound Healing by Silver Sulfadiazine is Reversed by Aloe Vera and Nystatin." *Burns* 29 (2003): 834–836.

Kent, Carol Miller. *Aloe Vera.* Arlington: Carol Miller Kent, 1980.

Muller, M.J., M.A. Hollyoak, Z. Moaveni, Tim La H. Brown, T. Reynolds, A.C. Dweck. "Aloe Vera Leaf Gel: A Review Update." *Journal of Ethnopharmacology* 68 (1999): 3–37.

Rodríguez, D. Jasso de, D. Hernández–Castillo, R. Rodríguez–García, and J.L. Angulo–Sánchez. "Antifungal Activity In Vitro of Aloe Vera Pulp and Liquid Fraction Against Plant Pathogenic Fungi." *Industrial Crops and Products* xxx (2004): xxx–xxx (Article in Press).

Sadiq, Yusuf, Agunu Abdulkarim, and Diana Mshelia. "The Effect of Aloe Vera A. Berger (Liliaceae) on Gastric Acid Secretion and Acute Gastric Mucosal Injury in Rats." *Journal of Ethnopharmacology* 93 (2004): 33–37.

Seyger, M.M.B., P.C.M. van de Kerkhof, I.M.J.J. van Vlijmen–Willems, E.S.M. de Bakker, F. Zwiers, and E.M.G.J. de Jong. "The Efficacy of a New Topical Treatment for Psoriasis: Mirak." *Journal of the European Academy of Dermatology and Venereology* 11 (1998): 13–18.

Váquez, Beatriz, Guillermo Avila, David Segura, and Bruno Escalante. "Antiinflammatory Activity of Extracts from Aloe Vera Gel." *Journal of Ethnopharmacology* 55 (1996): 69–75.

Verlag, Gustav Fischer. "Antidiabetic Activity of Aloe Vera L. Juice. I. Clinical Trial in New Cases of Diabetes Mellitus." *Phytomedicine* 3, 3 (1996): 241–243.

AMERICAN GINSENG

Assinewe, V. A., J. T. Arnason, A. Aubry, J. Mullin, and I. Lemaire. "Extractable Polysaccharides of Panax Quinquefolius L. (North American Ginseng) Root Stimulate TNF± Production by Alveolar Macrophages." *Phytomedicine* 9 (2002): 398–404.

Fujimoto, Yasuo, Hongcheng Wang, Mitsuru Satoh, and Naoki Takeuchi. Polyacetylenes from Panax Quinquefolium." *Phytochemistry* 35, 5 (1994): 1255–1257.

Kang, Ki Sung, Noriko Yamabe, Hyun Young Kim, Takuya Okamoto, Yasuo Sei, Takako Yokozawa. "Increase in the Free Radical Scavenging Activities of American Ginseng by Heat Processing and its Safety Evaluation." *Journal of Ethnopharmacology* 113 (2007): 225–232.

Liu, Dong, Bei Li, Yi Liu, Anoja S. Attele, John W. Kyle, and Chun–Su Yuan. "Voltage–Dependent Inhibition of Brain Na Channels by American Ginseng." *European Journal of Phar-*

macology 413 (2001): 47–54.

Nocerino, Emilia, Marianna Amato, and Angelo A. Izzo. "The Aphrodisiac and Adaptogenic Properties of Ginseng." *Fitoterapia* 71 (2000): S1–S5.

Schlag, Erin M. and Marla S. McIntosh. "Ginsenoside Content and Variation Among and Within American Ginseng (Panax Quinquefolius L.) Populations." *Phytochemistry* 67 (2006): 1510–1519.

Yuan, C.-S., X. Wang, J.A. Wu, A.S. Attele, J.-T. Xie, and M. Gu. "Effects of Panax Quinquefolius L. on Brainstem Neuronal Activities: Comparison Between Wisconsin–Cultivated and Illinois–Cultivated Roots." *Phytomedicine* 8, 3 (2001): 178–183.

ARNICA

Gertsch, Jurg, O. Sticher, T. Schmidt, and J. Heilmann. "Influence of Helenanolide–Type Sesquiterpene Lactones on Gene Transcription Profiles in Jurkat T Cells and Human Peripheral Blood Cells: Anti–Inflammatory and Cytotoxic Effects". *Biochemical Pharmacology* 66 (2003): 2141–2153.

Kennedy, J.F., D.L. Stevenson, and C.A. White. "Analysis of the Oligosaccharides from the Roots of Arnica Montana L., Artemisia Absinthium L., and Artemisia Dracunculus L." *Carbohydrate Polymers* 9 (1988): 277–285.

Koo, H., B.P.F.A. Gomes, P.L. Rosalen, G.M.B. Ambrosano, Y.K. Park, and J.A. Cur. "In Vitro Antimicrobial Activity of Propolis and Arnica Montana Against Oral Pathogens." *Archives of Oral Biology* 45 (2000): 141–148.

Merfort, I. and D. Wendisch. "Sesquiterpene Lactones of Arnica Cordifolia, Subgenus Austromotana." *Phytochemistry* 34, 5 (1993): 1436–1437.

Puhlmann, J., M.H. Zenk, and H. Wagner. "Immunologically Active Polysaccharides of Arnica Montana Cell Cultures." *Phytochemistry* 30, 4 (1991): 1141–1145.

Wagner, Steffen and I. Merfort. "Skin Penetration Behavior of Sesquiterpene Lactones from Different Arnica Preparations Using a Validated GC–MSD Method." *Journal of Pharmaceutical and Biomedical Analysis* 43 (2007): 32–38.

ARTICHOKE

Fratianni, Florinda, Marina Tucci, Monica De Palma, Rosa Pepe, and Filomena Nazzaro. "Polyphenolic Composition in Different Parts of Some Cultivars of Globe Artichoke (Cynara Cardunculus L. var. Scolymus (L.) Fiori)." *Food Chemistry* 104 (2007): 1282–1286.

Lopez–Molina, Dorotea, Maria Dolores Navarro–Martinez, Francisco Rojas Melgarejo, Alexander N.P. Hiner, Soledad Chazarra, and Jose Neptuno Rodriguez–Lopez. "Molecular Properties and Prebiotic Effect of Inulin Obtained from Artichoke (Cynara Scolymus L.). *Phytochemistry* 66 (2005): 1476–1484.

Falleh, Hanen, Riadh Ksouri, Kamel Chaieb, Najoua Karray–Bouraoui, Najla Trabelsi, Mondher Boulaaba, and Chedly Abdelly. "Phenolic Composition of Cynara Cardunculus L. Organs, and their Biological Activities." *C. R. Biologies* 331 (2008): 372–379.

Speroni, E., R. Cervellati, P. Govoni, S. Guizzardi, C. Renzulli, and M.C. Guerra. "Efficacy of Different Cynara Scolymus Preparations on Liver Complaints." *Journal of Ethnopharmacology* 86 (2003): 203–211.

ASTRAGALUS

Choa, William Chi Shing and Kwok Nam Leung. "In Vitro and In Vivo Immunomodulating and Immunorestorative Effects of Astragalus Membranaceus." *Journal of Ethnopharmacology* 113 (2007): 132–141.

Chor, S.Y., A.Y. Hui, K.F. To, K.K. Chana, Y.Y. Go, H.L.Y. Chan, W.K. Leung, and J.J.Y. Sung. "Anti–Proliferative and Pro–Apoptotic Effects of Herbal Medicine on Hepatic Stellate Cell." *Journal of Ethnopharmacology* 100 (2005): 180–186.

Ko, Han–Chieh, Bai–Luh Wei, and Wen–Fei Chiou. "The Effect of Medicinal Plants Used in Chinese Folk Medicine on RANTES Excretion by Virus–Infected Human Epithelial Cells." *Journal of Ethnopharmacology* 107 (2006): 205–210.

Lee, Kun Yeong and Young Jin Jeon. "Macrophage Activation by Polysaccharide Isolated from Astragalus Membranaceus." *International Immunopharmacology* 5 (2005): 1225–1233.

Liu, Wei, Jing Chen, Wen Jian Zuo, Xian Li, and Jin Hui Wang. "A New Isoflavane from Processed Astragalus Membranaceus." *Chinese Chemical Letters* 18 (2007): 1092–1094.

Molyneux, Russell J., S.T. Lee, D.R. Gardner, K.E. Panter, and L.F. James. "Phytochemicals: The Good, the Bad and the Ugly?" *Phytochemistry* 68 (2007): 2973–2985.

Shao, Bao–Mei, Wen Xu, Hui Dai, Pengfei Tu, Zhongjun Li, and Xiao–Ming Gao. "A Study on the Immune Receptors for Polysaccharides from the Roots of Astragalus Membranaceus, a Chinese Medicinal Herb." *Biochemical and Biophysical Research Communications* 320 (2004): 1103–1111.

Song, Jing–Zheng, Hillary H.W. Yiu, Chun–Feng Qiao, Quan–Bin Han, and Hong–Xi Xu. "Chemical Comparison and Classification of Radix Astragali by Determination of Isoflavonoids and Astragalosides." *Journal of Pharmaceutical and Biomedical Analysis* 47 (2008): 399–406.

Toda, Shizuo and Yoshiaki Shirataki. "Inhibitory Effects of Astragali Radix, a Crude Drug in Oriental Medicines, on Lipid Peroxidation and Protein Oxidative Modification by Copper." *Journal of Ethnopharmacology* 68 (1999): 331–333.

Yesilada, Erdem, Erdal Bedir, Ihsan Calıs, Yoshihisa Takaishi, and Yasukazu Ohmoto. "Effects of Triterpene Saponins from Astragalus Species on In Vitro Cytokine Release." *Journal of Ethnopharmacology* 96 (2005): 71–77.

Yu, Qing Tao, Ping Li, Zhi Ming Bi, Jun Luo, and Xiao Dan Gao. "Two New Saponins from the Aerial Part of Astragalus Membranaceus Var. Mongholicus." *Chinese Chemical Letters* 18 (2007): 554–556.

Zhang, Bi–Qi, Shen–Jiang Hu, Li–Hong Qiu, Jian–hua Zhu, Xian–Ji Xie, Jian Sun, Zhao–Hui Zhu, Qiang Xia, and Ka Bian. "Effects of Astragalus Membranaceus and its Main Components on the Acute Phase Endothelial Dysfunction Induced by Homocysteine." *Vascular Pharmacology* 46 (2007): 278–285.

Zhang, Zhen–Lun, Qi–Zhen Wen, and Chand–Xiao Liu. "Hepatoprotective Effects of Astragalus Root." *Journal of Ethnopharmacology* 30 (1990): 145– 149.

BARBERRY

Ivanovska, N. and S. Philipov. "Study on the Anti–Inflammatory Action of Berberis Vulgaris Root Extract, Alkaloid Fractions and Pure Alkaloids." *International Journal Of Immunopharmacology* 18,10 (1996): 553–561.

Janbaz, K.H. and A.H. Gilani. "Studies on Preventive and Curative Effects of Berberine on Chemical–Induced Hepatotoxicity in Rodents." *Fitoterapia* 71 (2000): 25–33.

Ji, Xiuhong, Yi Li, Huwei Liu, Yuning Yan, and Jiashi Li. "Determination of the Alkaloid Content in Different Parts of some Mahonia Plants by HPCE." *Pharmaceutica Acta Helvetiae* 74 (2000): 387–391.

Kostalova, D., A. Kardosova, and V. Hajnicka. "Effect of Mahonia Aquifolium Stem Bark Crude Extract and One of its Polysaccharide Components on Production of IL–8." *Fitoterapia* 72 (2001): 802–806.

Maung–U, Khin and Nwe–Nwe–Wai. "Effect of Berberine on Enterotoxin–Induced Intestinal Fluid Accumulation in Rats." *J Diarrhoeal Dis Res* 10, 4 (1992): 201–204.

Sack, R.B. and J.L. Froehlich. "Berberine Inhibits Intestinal Secretory Response of Vibrio Cholerae and Escherichia Coli Enterotoxins." *Infect Immun* 35, 2 (1982): 471–475.

Shamsa, F., A. Ahmadiani, and R. Khosrokhavar. "Antihistaminic and Anticholinergic Activity of Barberry Fruit (Berberis Vulgaris) in the Guinea–Pig Ileum." *Journal of Ethnopharmacology* 64 (1999): 161–166

Sohni, Y.R., P. Kaimal, and R.M. Bhatt. "The Antiamoebic Effect of a Crude Drug Formulation of Herbal Extracts Against Entamoeba Histolytica In Vitro and in Vivo." *Journal of Ethnopharmacology* 45, 1 (1995): 43–52.

Sohni, Youvraj R. and Ranjan M. Bhatt. "Activity of a Crude Extract Formulation in Experimental Hepatic Amoebiasis and in Immunomodulation Studies." *Journal of Ethnopharmacology* 54 (1996): 119–124.

Stermitz, F.R., J. Tawara–Matsuda, P. Lorenz, P. Mueller, L. Zenewicz, and K. Lewis. "5'–Methoxyhydnocarpin–D and Pheophorbide A: Berberis Species Components that Potentiate Berberine Growth Inhibition of Resistant Staphylococcus Aureus." *Journal of Natural Products* 63, 8 (2000): 1146–1149.

Stermitz, Frank R., Teresa D. Beeson, Paul J. Mueller, Jen–Fang Hsiang, and Kim Lewis. "Staphylococcus Aureus MDR Efflux Pump Inhibitors from a Berberis and a Mahonia (Sensu Strictu) Species." *Biochemical Systematics and Ecology* 29 (2001): 793–798.

Yesilada, Erdem and Esra Küpeli. "Berberis Crataegina DC. Root Exhibits Potent Anti–Inflammatory, Analgesic and Febrifuge Effects in Mice and Rats." *Journal of Ethnopharmacology* 79 (2002): 237–248.

BAYBERRY

Chistokhodova, Natalya, Chi Nguyen, Tony Calvino, Ioulia Kachirskaia, Glenn Cunningham, and D. Howard Miles. "Antithrombin Activity of Medicinal Plants from Central Florida." *Journal of Ethnopharmacology* 81 (2002): 277–280.

Fujimoto, Masafumi, Shin–ichi Mihara, Shigeyuki Nakajima, Motohiko Ueda, Miharu Nakamura and Ken–suke Sakurai. "A Novel Non–Peptide Endothelin Antagonist Isolated from Bayberry, Myrica Cerifera." *Federation of European Biochemical Societies* 305, 1 (1992): 41–44.

Halim, Ahmed F. and Ralph P. Collins. "Essential Oil Analysis of the Myricaceae of the Eastern United States." *Phytochemistry* 12 (1973): 1077–1083.

BILBERRY

Canter, Peter H. and Edzard Ernst. "Anthocyanosides of Vaccinium Myrtillus (Bilberry) for Night Vision—A Systematic Review of Placebo–Controlled Trials." *Survey of Ophthalmology* 49, 1 (2004): 38–50.

Seeram, N. P., R. A. Momin, M. G. Nair and L. D. Bourquin. "Cyclooxygenase Inhibitory and Antioxidant Cyanidin Glycosides in Cherries and Berries." *Phytomedicine* 8, 5 (2001): 362–369.

Yao, Yu and Amandio Vieira. "Protective Activities of Vaccinium Antioxidants with Potential Relevance to Mitochondrial Dysfunction and Neurotoxicity." *NeuroToxicology* 28 (2007): 93–100.

BLACK COHOSH

Frei–Kleinera, S., W. Schaffnera, V.W. Rahlfsb, Ch. Bodmerc, and M. Birkhauser. "Cimicifuga Racemosa Dried Ethanolic Extract in Menopausal Disorders: A Double–Blind Placebo–Controlled Clinical Trial." *Maturitas* 51 (2005): 397–404.

Jarry, H., P. Thelen, V. Christoffel, B. Spengler, W. Wuttke. "Cimicifuga Racemosa Extract BNO 1055 Inhibits Proliferation of the Human Prostate Cancer Cell Line LNCaP." *Phytomedicine* 12 (2005): 178–182.

Jiang, B., H. Yang, P. Nuntanakorn, M.J. Balick, F. Kronenberg, and E.J. Kennelly. "The Value of Plant Collections in Ethnopharmacology: A Case Study of an 85–Year–Old Black Cohosh (Actaea racemosa L.) Sample." *Journal of Ethnopharmacology* 96 (2005): 521–528.

Kretzschmar, Georg, Thomas Nisslein, Oliver Zierau, and Gunter Vollmer. "Estrogen–Like Effects of an Isopropanolic Extract of Rhizoma Cimicifugae Racemosae on Uterus and Vena Cava of Rats After 17 Day Treatment." *Journal of Steroid Biochemistry & Molecular Biology* 97

(2005): 271–277.

Seidlova–Wuttke, D., L. Pitzel, P. Thelen, and W. Wuttke. "Inhibition of 5–Reductase in the Rat Prostate by Cimicifuga Racemosa." *Maturitas* 55S (2006): S75–S82.

Wuttke, Wolfgang, Guillermo Rimoldi, Julie Christoffel, and Dana Seidlova–Wuttke. "Plant Extracts for the Treatment of Menopausal Women: Safe?" *Maturitas* 55S (2006): S92–S100.

BLACK WALNUT

Biancoa, M. A., A. Handajia, and H. Savolainenb. "Quantitative Analysis of Ellagic Acid in Hardwood Samples." *The Science of the Total Environment* 222 (1998): 123–126.

Boelkins, James N., Lloyd K. Everson, and Theodore K. Auyong. "Effects of Intravenous Juglone in the Dog." *Toxicon* 6, 2 (1968): 99–102.

Guarrera, Paolo Maria. "Traditional Antihelmintic, Antiparasitic and Repellent Uses of Plants in Central Italy." *Journal of Ethnopharmacology* 68 (1999): 183–192.

Lopez, A., J.B. Hudson, and G.H.N. Towers. "Antiviral and Antimicrobial Activities of Colombian Medicinal Plants." *Journal of Ethnopharmacology* 77 (2001): 189–196.

Omar, S., B. Lemonnier, N. Jones, C. Ficker, M.L. Smith, C. Neema, Towers, G.H.N., K. Goel, and J.T. Arnason. "Antimicrobial Activity of Extracts of Eastern North American Hardwood Trees and Relation to Traditional Medicine." *Journal of Ethnopharmacology* 73 (2000): 161–170.

BLUE COHOSH

Ali, Zulfiqar and Ikhlas A. Khan. "Alkaloids and Saponins from Blue Cohosh." *Phytochemistry* 69 (2008): 1037–1042.

Jones, Thomas K. and Barry M. Lawson. "Profound Neonatal Congestive Heart Failure Caused by Maternal Consumption of Blue Cohosh Herbal Medication." *J Pediatr* 132 (1998): 550–552.

Woldemariam, Tibebe Z., Joseph M. Betz, and Peter J. Houghton. "Analysis of Aporphine and Quinolizidine Alkaloids from Caulophyllum Thalictroides by Densitometry and HPLC." *Journal of Pharmaceutical and Biomedical Analysis* 15 (1997): 839–843.

BURDOCK

Cho, Min Kyung, Y.P. Janga, Y.C. Kima, and S.G. Kim. "Arctigenin, a Phenylpropanoid Dibenzylbutyrolactone Lignan, Inhibits MAP Kinases and AP–1 Activation Via Potent MKK Inhibition: The Role in TNF–a Inhibition." *International Immunopharmacology* 4 (2004): 1419–1429.

Hirose, Masao, T. Yamaguchi, C. Lin, N. Kimoto, M. Futakuchi, T. Kono, S. Nishibe, and T. Shirai. "Effects of Arctiin on PhIP–Induced Mammary, Colon and Pancreatic Carcinogenesis in Female Sprague–Dawley Rats and MeIQx–Induced Hepatocarcinogenesis in Male F344 Rats." *Cancer Letters* 155 (2000): 79–88.

Kardošová, A., A. Ebringerová, J. Alföldi, G. Nosálová, S. Franová, and V. Hribalová. "A Biologically Active Fructan From the Roots of Arctium Lappa L., var. Herkules." *International Journal of Biological Macromolecules* 33 (2003): 135–140.

Kardošová, A. and E. Machová. "Antioxidant Activity of Medicinal Plant Polysaccharides." *Fitoterapia* 77 (2006): 367–373.

Morita, Kazuyoshi, T. Kada, and M. Namiki. "A Desmutagenic Factor Isolated from Burdock (Arctium Lappa Linne)." *Mutation Research* 129 (1984): 25–31.

Wang, Bor–Sen, G–C. Yen, L–W. Chang, W–J. Yen, and P–D. Duh. "Protective Effects of Burdock (Arctium Lappa Linne) on Oxidation of Low–Density Lipoprotein and Oxidative Stress in RAW 264.7 Macrophages." *Food Chemistry* 101 (2006): 729–738.

BUTCHER'S BROOM

Combarieu, E. de, M. Falzoni, N. Fuzzati, F. Gattesco, A. Giori, M. Lovati, and R. Pace. "Identification of Ruscus Steroidal Saponins by HPLC–MS Analysis." *Fitoterapia* 73 (2002): 583–596.

Guarrera, Paolo Maria. "Traditional Phytotherapy in Central Italy (Marche, Abruzzo, and Latium)." *Fitoterapia* 76 (2005): 1–25.

Kite, Geoffrey C., Porter, Elaine A., and Simmonds, Monique S.J. "Chromatographic Behaviour of Steroidal Saponins Studied by High–Performance Liquid Chromatography–Mass Spectrometry." *Journal of Chromatography A* 1148 (2007): 177–183.

Lascasas–Porto, Carmen Lucia, Milhomens, Ana Letícia M., Virgini–Magalhães, Carlos Eduardo, Fernandes, Fabiano F.A., Sicuro, Fernando L., and Bouskela, Eliete. "Use of Microcirculatory Parameters to Evaluate Clinical Treatments of Chronic Venous Disorder (CVD)." *Microvascular Research* xxx (2008): xxx–xxx (Article in Press)

Rubanyi, G., G. Marcelon, and P.M. Vanhoutte. "Effect of Temperature on the Responsiveness of Cutaneous Veins to the Extract of Ruscus Aculeatus." *Gen. Pharmac.* 15, 5 (1984): 431–434.

CALENDULA

Bako, Eszter, J. Deli, and G. Toth. "HPLC Study on the Carotenoid Composition of Calendula Products." *J. Biochem. Biophys. Methods* 53 (2002): 241–250.

Cetkovic, Gordana S., S.M. Djilas, J.M. Canadanovic–Brunet, and V.T. Tumbas. "Antioxidant Properties of Marigold Extracts." *Food Research International* 37 (2004): 643–650.

Lavagna, Silvio M., D. Secci, P. Chimenti, L. Bonsignore, A. Ottaviani, and B. Bizzarri. "Efficacy of Hypericum and Calendula Oils in the Epithelial Reconstruction of Surgical Wounds in Childbirth with Caesarean Section." *Il Farmaco* 56 (2001): 451–453.

Miliauskasa, G., P.R. Venskutonisa, and T.A. Van Beekb. "Screening of Radical Scavenging Activity of Some Medicinal and Aromatic Plant Extracts." *Food Chemistry* 85 (2004): 231–237.

Wilkomirski, Boguslaw. "Pentacyclic Triterpene Triols from Calendula Officinalis Flowers." *Phytochemistry* 24, 12 (1985): 3066–3067.

CANNABIS

Amar, Mohamed Ben. "Cannabinoids in Medicine: A Review of their Therapeutic Potential." *Journal of Ethnopharmacology* 105 (2006): 1–25.

Baker, David, Gareth Pryce, Gavin Giovannoni, and Alan J Thompson. "The Therapeutic Potential of Cannabis." *Lancet Neurology* 2 (2003): 291–98.

Brady, C. M., R. Dasgupta, C. Dalton, O. J. Wiseman, K. J. Berkley, and C. J. Fowler. "Voiding Function and Dysfunction, Bladder Physiology and Pharmacology, and Female Urology; An Open–Label Pilot Study of Cannabis–Based Extracts for Bladder Dysfunction in Advanced Multiple Sclerosis" *The Journal of Urology* 173 (2005): 1262–1267.

Brooks, J.W. "Cannabinoids and Analgesia." *Current Anaesthesia & Critical Care* 13 (2002): 215–220.

Engels, Frederike K., Floris A. de Jong, Ron H.J. Mathijssen, Joelle A. Erkens, Ron M. Herings, and Jaap Verweij. "Medicinal Cannabis in Oncology." *European Journal of Cancer* 43 (2007): 2638–2644.

Grant, Igor and B. Rael Cahn. "Cannabis and Endocannabinoid Modulators: Therapeutic Promises and Challenges." *Clinical Neuroscience Research* 5 (2005): 185–199.

Iversen, Leslie and Victoria Chapman. "Cannabinoids: a Real Prospect for Pain Relief?" *Current Opinion in Pharmacology* 2 (2002): 50–55.

Lynch, Mary E., Judee Young, and Alexander J. Clark. "A Case Series of Patients Using Medicinal Marihuana for Management of Chronic Pain Under the Canadian Marihuana Medical Access Regulations." *Journal of Pain and Symptom Management* 32, 5 (2006): 497–501.

Mackie, Ken. "Signaling Via CNS Cannabinoid

Receptors." *Molecular and Cellular Endocrinology* 286S (2008): S60–S65.

Martin, Billy R. and Aron H. Lichtman. "Cannabinoid Transmission and Pain Perception." *Neurobiology of Disease* 5 (1998): 447–461.

Ware, Mark A., Crystal R. Doyle, Ryan Woods, Mary E. Lynch, and Alexander J. Clark. "Cannabis Use for Chronic Non–Cancer Pain: Results of a Prospective Survey." *Pain* 102 (2003): 211–216.

CAYENNE PEPPER

Careaga, Monica, Elizabeth Fernandez, Lidia Dorantes, Lydia Mota, Maria Eugenia Jaramillo, Humberto Hernandez–Sanchez. "Antibacterial Activity of Capsicum Extract Against Salmonella Typhimurium and Pseudomonas Aeruginosa Inoculated in Raw Beef Meat" *International Journal of Food Microbiology* 83 (2003): 331–335.

Cichewicz, Robert H. and Patrick A. Thorpe. "The Antimicrobial Properties of Chile Peppers (Capsicum Species) and their Uses in Mayan Medicine." *Journal of Ethnopharmacology* 52 (1996): 61–70.

Materska, Magorzata, Sonia Piacente, Anna Stochmal, Cosimo Pizza, Wiesaw Oleszek, and Irena Perucka. "Isolation and Structure Elucidation of Flavonoid and Phenolic Acid Glycosides from Pericarp of Hot Pepper Fruit Capsicum Annuum L." *Phytochemistry* 63 (2003): 893–898.

Singh, Tripti and Colleen Chittenden. "In–Vitro Antifungal Activity of Chilli Extracts in Combination with Lactobacillus Casei Against Common Sapstain Fungi." *International Biodeterioration & Biodegradation* xxx (2008): 1–4.

Tsuchiya, Hironori. "Biphasic Membrane Effects of Capsaicin, an Active Component in Capsicum Species." *Journal of Ethnopharmacology* 75 (2001): 295–299.

CHAMOMILE

Kobayashi, Y., Y. Nakano, K. Inayama, A. Sakai,

and T. Kamiya. "Dietary Intake of the Flower Extracts of German Chamomile (Matricaria Recutita L.) Inhibited Compound 48/80–Induced Itch–Scratch Responses in Mice." *Phytomedicine* 10 (2003): 657–664.

Kobayashi, Yoshinori, R. Takahashi, and F. Ogino. "Antipruritic Effect of the Single Oral Administration of German Chamomile Flower Extract and its Combined Effect with Antiallergic Agents in ddY Mice." *Journal of Ethnopharmacology* 101 (2005): 308–312.

Loggia, Roberto Della, U. Traversa, V. Scarcia, and A. Tubaro. "Depressive Effects of Chamomilla Recutita (L.) Rausch, Tubular Flowers, on Central Nervous System in Mice." *Pharmacological Research Communications* 14, 2 (1982): 153–162.

Mazokopakis, E.E., G.E. Vrentzos, J.A. Papadakis, D.E. Babalis, and E.S. Ganotakis. "Wild Chamomile (Matricaria Recutita L.) Mouthwashes in Methotrexate–Induced Oral Mucositis." *Phytomedicine* 12 (2005): 25–27.

Svenlikova, Vanda and M. Repcak. "Apigenin Chemotypes of Matricaria Chamomilla L." *Biochemical Systematics and Ecology* 34 (2006): 654–657.

Zaiter, Lahcene, M. Bouheroum, S. Benayache, F. Benayache, F. Leon, I. Brouard, J. Quintana, F. Estevez, and J. Bermejo. "Sesquiterpene Lactones and Other Constituents from Matricaria Chamomilla L." *Biochemical Systematics and Ecology* 35 (2007): 533–538.

CHASTE TREE

Böhnert, K. J. "The Use of Vitex Agnus Castus for Hyperprolactinemia." *Quarterly Review of Natural Medicine*, spring (1997): 19–21.

Brown, Donald J. "Vitex Agnus Castus Clinical Monograph from Quarterly Review of Natural Medicine." *Herbal Research Review*, Summer (1994)

Halaška, M., P. Beles, C. Gorkow, and C. Sieder. "Treatment of Cyclical Mastalgia with a Solution Containing a Vitex Agnus Castus Extract: Results of a Placebo–Controlled Double–Blind Study." *The Breast* 8 (1999): 175–181.

Lauritzen, CH., H.D. Reuter, R. Repges, K.J. Böhnert, and U. Schmidt. "Treatment of Premenstrual Tension Syndrome with Vitex Agnus Castus Controlled, Double–Blind Study Versus Pyridoxine." *Phytomedicine* 4, 3 (1997): 183–189.

Lucks, Barbara Chopin. "Vitex Agnus Castus Essential Oil and Menopausal Balance: A Research Update." *Complementary Therapies in Nursing and Midwifery* 8 (2003): 148–154.

Schellenberg, R. "Treatment for the Premenstrual Syndrome with Agnus Castus Fruit Extract: Prospective, Randomized, Placebo Controlled Study." *British Medical Journal* 322 (2001): 134–137.

CINNAMON

Babu, P. Subash, S. Prabuseenivasan, and S. Ignacimuthu. "Cinnamaldehyde—A Potential Antidiabetic Agent." *Phytomedicine* 14 (2007): 15–22.

Hersch–Martınez, P., B.E. Leanos–Miranda, and F. Solorzano–Santos. "Antibacterial Effects of Commercial Essential Oils over Locally Prevalent Pathogenic Strains in Mexico." *Fitoterapia* 76 (2005): 453– 457.

Mathew, Sindhu and T. Emilia Abraham. "Studies on the Antioxidant Activities of Cinnamon (Cinnamomum Verum) Bark Extracts, through Various In Vitro Models." *Food Chemistry* 94 (2006): 520–528.

McCarty, Mark F. "Nutraceutical Resources for Diabetes Prevention – An Update." *Medical Hypotheses* 64 (2005): 151–158.

Singh, Gurdip, Sumitra Maurya, M.P. deLampasona, and Cesar A.N. Catalan. "A Comparison of Chemical, Antioxidant and Antimicrobial Studies of Cinnamon Leaf and Bark Volatile Oils, Oleoresins and their Constituents." *Food and Chemical Toxicology* 45 (2007): 1650–1661.

CLOVE

Ghelardini, C., N. Galeotti, L. Di Cesare Mannelli, G. Mazzanti, and A. Bartolini. "Local Anaesthetic Activity of β–Caryophyllene." *Il Farmaco* 56 (2001): 387–389.

Kurokawa, Masahiko, Kazuhiko Nagasaka, Tatsuji Hirabayashi, Shin–ichi Uyama, Hideki Sato, Takashi Kageyama, Shigetoshi Kadota, Haruo Ohyama, Toyoharu Hozumi, Tsuneo Namba, and Kimiyasu Shiraki. "Efficacy of Traditional Herbal Medicines in Combination with Acyclovir Against Herpes Simplex Virus Type 1 Infection In Vitro and In Vivo." *Antiviral Research* 27 (1995): 19–37.

Lee, Kwang–Geun and Takayuki Shibamoto. "Antioxidant Property of Aroma Extract Isolated from Clove Buds [Syzygium Aromaticum (L.) Merr. et Perry]." *Food Chemistry* 74 (2001): 443–448.

Moreira, M.R., A.G Ponce, C.E. del Valle, and S.I. Roura. "Inhibitory Parameters of Essential Oils to Reduce a Foodborne Pathogen." *LWT* 38 (2005): 565–570.

Nassar, Mahmoud I. "Flavonoid Triglycosides from the Seeds of Syzygium Aromaticum." *Carbohydrate Research* 341 (2006): 160–163.

Srivastava, K. C. and N. Malhotra. "Acetyl Eugenol, a Component of Oil of Cloves (Syzygium Aromaticum Z,.) Inhibits Aggregation and Alters Arachidonic Acid Metabolism in Human Blood Platelets." *Prostaglandins Leukotrienes and Essential Fatty Acids* (1991): 42 73–81.

Steenkamp, V., A.C. Fernandes, and C.E.J. Van Rensburg. "Screening of Venda Medicinal Plants for Antifungal Activity Against Candida Albicans." *South African Journal of Botany* 73 (2007): 256–258.

COFFEE

Ashihara, Hiroshi, Hiroshi Sano, and Alan Crozier. "Caffeine and Related Purine Alkaloids: Biosynthesis, Catabolism, Function and Genetic Engineering." *Phytochemistry* 69 (2008): 841–856.

Nagasampago, B. A. and J. W. Rowe. "Sterols of

Coffee." *Phytochemistry* 10 (1971): 1101–1107.

Perrone, Daniel, Adriana Farah, Carmen M. Donangelo, Tomas de Paulis, Peter R. Martin. "Comprehensive Analysis of Major and Minor Chlorogenic Acids and Lactones in Economically Relevant Brazilian Coffee Cultivars." *Food Chemistry* 106 (2008): 859–867.

CRANBERRY

Bailey, David T., Carol Dalton, F. Joseph Daugherty, and Michael S. Tempesta. "Can a Concentrated Cranberry Extract Prevent Recurrent Urinary Tract Infections in Women? A Pilot Study." *Phytomedicine* 14 (2007): 237–241.

Celik, Huseyin, Mustafa Ozgen, Sedat Serce, and Cemal Kaya. "Phytochemical Accumulation and Antioxidant Capacity at Four Maturity Stages of Cranberry Fruit." *Scientia Horticulturae* 117 (2008): 345–348.

Croteau, Rodney and Irving S. Fagerson. "Seed Lipids of the American Cranberry (Vaccinium Marcocarpon)." *Phytochemistry* 8 (1969): 2219–2222.

Foo, Lai Yeap, Yinrong Lu, Amy B. Howell, and Nicholi Vors. "The Structure of Cranberry Proanthocyanidins which Inhibit Adherence of Uropathogenic P–Fimmbriated Escherichia Coli In Vitro." *Phytochemistry* 54 (2000): 173–181.

Howell, Amy B., Jess D. Reed, Christian G. Krueger, Ranee Winterbottom, David G. Cunningham, and Marge Leahy. "A–Type Cranberry Proanthocyanidins and Uropathogenic Bacterial Anti–Adhesion Activity". *Phytochemistry* 66 (2005): 2281–2291.

Seeram, N. P., R. A. Momin, M. G. Nair, and L. D. Bourquin. "Cyclooxygenase Inhibitory and Antioxidant Cyanidin Glycosides in Cherries and Berries." *Phytomedicine* 8, 5 (2001): 362–369.

Vvedenskaya, Irina O. and Nicholi Vorsa. "Flavonoid Composition Over Fruit Development and Maturation in American Cranberry, Vaccinium Macrocarpon Ait." *Plant Science* 167 (2004): 1043–1054.

CREOSOTE BUSH

Anesini, Claudia and Cristina Perez. "Screening of Plants Used in Argentine Folk Medicine for Antimicrobial Activity." *Journal of Ethnopharmacology* 39 (1993): 119–128.

Craigo, Jodi, Michelle Callahan, Ru Chih C. Huang, and Angelo L. DeLucia. "Inhibition of Human Papillomavirus Type 16 Gene Expression by Nordihydroguaiaretic Acid Plant Lignan Derivatives." *Antiviral Research* 47 (2000): 19–28.

Grant, Kathryn L., Leslie V. Boyer, and Boyd E. Erdman. "Chaparral Induced Hepatotoxicity." *Integrative Medicine* 1, 2 (1998): 83–87.

Hyder, Paul W., E.L. Fredrickson, Rick E. Estell, Mario Tellez, and Robert P. Gibbens. "Distribution and Concentration of Total Phenolics, Condensed Tannins, and Nordihydroguaiaretic Acid (NDGA) in Creosotebush (Larrea Tridentata)." *Biochemical Systematics and Ecology* 30 (2002): 905–912.

Quiroga, Emma Nelly, Antonio Rodolfo Sampietro, and Marta Amelia Vattuone. "Screening Antifungal Activities of Selected Medicinal Plants." *Journal of Ethnopharmacology* 74 (2001): 89–96.

Verástegui, M. Angeles, César A. Sánchez, Norma L. Heredia, and J. Santos García–Alvarado. "Antimicrobial Activity of Extracts of Three Chihuahuan Desert Major Plants from the Chihuahuan Desert." *Journal of Ethnopharmacology* 52 (1996): 175–177.

DANDELION

Grases, F., G. Melero, A. Costa–Bauza, R. Prieto, and J.G. March. "Urolithiasis and Phytotherapy." *International Urology and Nephrology* 26, 5 (1994): 507–511.

Kisiel, W. and B. Barszcz. Further Sesquiterpenoids and Phenolics from Taraxacum Officinale. *Fitoterapia* 71 (2000): 269–273.

Rauwald, Hans–Willi and Jai–Tung Huang. "Taraxacoside, A Type of Acylated Gamma–.

Butyrolactone Glycoside from Taraxacum officinale." *Photochemistry* 24, 7 (1985): 1557–1559.

Williams, Christine A., Fiona Goldstone, and Jenny Greenham. "Flavonoids, Cinnamic Acids, and Coumarins from the Different Tissues and Medicinal Preparations of Taraxacum Officinale." *Phytochemistry* 42, 1 (1996): 121–127.

ECHINACEA

Arroll, B. "Non–Antibiotic Treatments for Upper–Respiratory Tract Infections (Common Cold)." *Respiratory Medicine* 99 (2005): 1477–1484.

Barrett, B. "Medicinal Properties of Echinacea: A Critical Review." *Phytomedicine* 10 (2003): 66–86.

Chicca, A., B. Adinolfi, E. Martinotti, S. Fogli, M.C. Breschi, F. Pellati, S. Benvenuti, and P. Nieri. "Cytotoxic Effects of Echinacea Root Hexanic Extracts on Human Cancer Cell Lines." *Journal of Ethnopharmacology* 110 (2007): 148–153.

Classena, B., S. Thude, W. Blaschek, M. Wack, and C. Bodinet. "Immunomodulatory Effects of Arabinogalactan–Proteins from Baptisia and Echinacea." *Phytomedicine* 13 (2006): 688–694.

Gan, Xiao–Hu, Ling Zhang, David Heber, and Benjamin Bonavida. "Mechanism of Activation of Human Peripheral Blood NK Cells at the Single Cell Level by Echinacea Water Soluble Extracts: Recruitment of Lymphocyte–Target Conjugates and Killer Cells and Activation of Programming for Lysis." *International Immunopharmacology* 3 (2003): 811–824.

He, Xian–guo, Long–ze Lin, Matthew W. Bernart, and Li–zhi Lian. "Analysis of Alkamides in Roots and Achenes of Echinacea Purpurea by Liquid Chromatography–Electrospray Mass Spectrometry." *Journal of Chromatography A* 815 (1998): 205–211.

Hinz, Burkhard, Karin Woelkart, and Rudolf Bauer. "Alkamides from Echinacea Inhibit Cyclooxygenase–2 Activity in Human Neuroglioma Cells." *Biochemical and Biophysical Research Communications* 360 (2007): 441–446.

Matthias, A., R.S. Addison, L.L. Agnew, K.M. Bone, K. Watson, and R.P. Lehmann. "Comparison of Echinacea Alkylamide Pharmacokinetics Between Liquid and Tablet Preparations." *Phytomedicine* 14 (2007): 587–590.

Matthias, Anita, Linda Banbury, Kerry M. Bone, David N. Leach, and Reg P. Lehmann. "Echinacea Alkylamides Modulate Induced Immune Responses in T–Cells." *Fitoterapia* 79 (2008): 53–58.

Morazzoni, P., A. Cristoni, F. Di Pierro, C. Avanzini, D. Ravarino, S. Stornello, M. Zucca, and T. Musso. "In Vitro and In Vivo Immune Stimulating Effects of a New Standardized Echinacea Angustifolia Root Extract (Polinacea)." *Fitoterapia* 76 (2005): 401–411.

Naser, B., B. Lund, H.–H. Henneicke–von Zepelin, G. Kohler, W. Lehmacher, and F. Scaglione. "A Randomized, Double–Blind, Placebo–Controlled, Clinical Dose–Response Trial of an Extract of Baptisia, Echinacea and Thuja for the Treatment of Patients with Common Cold." *Phytomedicine* 12 (2005): 715–722.

Pellati, Federica, Stefania Benvenuti, Lara Magro, Michele Melegari, and Fabrizia Soragni. "Analysis of Phenolic Compounds and Radical Scavenging Activity of Echinacea Spp." *Journal of Pharmaceutical and Biomedical Analysis* 35 (2004): 289–301.

Rehman, Jalees, Jennifer M. Dillow, Steve M. Carter, James Chou, Brian Le, and Alan S. Maisel. "Increased Production of Antigen–Specific Immunoglobulins G and M Following in Vivo Treatment with the Medicinal Plants Echinacea Angustifolia and Hydrastis Canadensis." *Immunology Letters* 68 (1999): 391–395.

Rousseau, Bernard, Ichiro Tateya, XinHong Lim, Alejandro Munoz–del–Rio, and Diane M. Bless. "Investigation of Anti–Hyaluronidase Treatment on Vocal Fold Wound Healing." *Journal of Voice* 20, 3 (2006): 443–451.

Schoop, Roland, Peter Klein, Andy Suter, and Sebastian L. Johnston. "Echinacea in the Prevention of Induced Rhinovirus Colds: A

Meta–Analysis." *Clinical Therapeutics/Volume* 28, 2 (2006): 174–183.

Schwarz, E., A. Parlesak, H.–H. Henneicke–von Zepelin, J.C. Bode, and C. Bode. "Effect of Oral Administration of Freshly Pressed Juice of Echinacea Purpurea on the Number of Various Subpopulations of B– and T–Lymphocytes in Healthy Volunteers: Results of a Double–Blind, Placebo–Controlled Cross–Over Study." *Phytomedicine* 12 (2005): 625–631.

Speroni, E., P. Govoni, S. Guizzardi, C. Renzulli, and M.C. Guerra. "Anti–Inflammatory and Cicatrizing Activity of Echinacea Pallida Nutt. Root Extract." *Journal of Ethnopharmacology* 79 (2002): 265–272.

Thompson, Kenneth D. "Antiviral Activity of Viracea® Against Acyclovir Susceptible and Acyclovir Resistant Strains of Herpes Simplex Virus." *Antiviral Research* 39 (1998): 55–61.

Thude, S., B. Classen, W. Blaschek, D. Barz, and H. Thude. "Binding Studies of an Arabinogalactan–Protein from Echinacea Purpurea to Leucocytes." *Phytomedicine* 13 (2006): 425–427.

Thygesen, Line, Johanna Thulin, Alan Mortensen, Leif H. Skibsted, and Per Molgaard. "Antioxidant Activity of Cichoric Acid and Alkamides from Echinacea Purpurea, Alone and in Combination." *Food Chemistry* 101 (2007): 74–81.

ELDER

Ahmadiani, A., M. Fereidoni, S. Semnanian, M. Kamalinejad, and S. Saremi. "Antinociceptive and Anti–inflammatory Effects of Sambucus Ebulus Rhizome Extract in Rats." *Journal of Ethnopharmacology* 61 (1998): 229–235.

Bergner, Paul. "Elderberry (Sambucus Nigra, Canadensis)." *Medical Herbalism* 8, 4 (1996–1997).

Buhrmester, Rex A., John E. Ebinger, and David S. Seigler. "Sambunigrin and Cyanogenic Variability in Populations of Sambucus Canadensis L. (Caprifoliaceae)." *Biochemical Systemat-*

ics and Ecology 28 (2000): 689–695.

Caceres, Armando, Brenda R. Lopez, Melba A. Giron, and Heidi Logemann. "Plants Used in Guatemala for the Treatment of Dermatophytic Infections. 1. Screening for Antimycotic Activity of 44 Plant Extracts." *Journal of Ethnopharmacology* 31 (1991): 263–276.

Caceres, Armando, Orlando Cano, Blanca Samayoa and Leila Aguilar. "Plants Used in Guatemala for the Treatment of Gastrointestinal Disorders. 1. Screening of 84 Plants Against Enterobacteria." *Journal of Ethnopharmacology* 30 (1990): 55–73.

Dawidowicza, Andrzej L., Dorota Wianowska, and Barbara Baraniak. "The Antioxidant Properties of Alcoholic Extracts from Sambucus Nigra L. (Antioxidant Properties of Extracts)." *LWT* 39 (2006): 308–315.

Hernández, Nancy E., M.L. Tereschuk, and L.R. Abdala. "Antimicrobial Activity of Flavonoids in Medicinal Plants from Tafí del Valle (Tucumán, Argentina)." *Journal of Ethnopharmacology* 73 (2000): 317–322.

Jordheim, Monica, Nils Harald Giske, and Øyvind M. Andersen. "Anthocyanins in Caprifoliaceae." *Biochemical Systematics and Ecology* 35 (2007): 153–159.

Losey, Robert J., Nancy Stenholm, Patty Whereat–Phillips, and Helen Vallianatos. "Exploring the Use of Red Elderberry (Sambucus Racemosa) Fruit on the Southern Northwest Coast of North America." *Journal of Archaeological Science* 30 (2003): 695–707.

McCutcheon, A.R., T.E. Roberts, E. Gibbions, S.M. Ellis, L.A. Babiuk, R.E.W. Hancock, and G.H.N. Towers. "Antiviral Screening of British Columbian Medicinal Plants." *Journal of Ethnopharmacology* 49 (1995): 101–110.

ELEUTHERO

Baranov, A.I. "Medicinal Uses of Ginseng and Related Plants in the Soviet Union: Recent Trends in the Soviet Literature." *Journal of Ethnopharmacology* 6 (1982): 339–353.

Brekhman, I.I. and Kirillov, O.I. "Effect of

Eleutherococcus on Alarm–Phase of Stress." Life Sciences 8 (1989): 113–121.

Carlo, G. Di, Pacilio M., Capasso, R., and Carlo R. Di. "Effect on Prolactin Secretion of Echinacea Purpurea, Hypericum Perforatum and Eleutherococcus Senticosus". *Phytomedicine* 12 (2005): 644–647.

Cicero, A.F.G., Derosa, G., Brillante, R., Bernard, R., Nascett, S., and Gadd, A. "Effects of Siberian Ginseng (Eleutherococcus Maxim.) on Elderly Quality of Life: A Randomized Clinical Trial." *Arch. Gerontol. Geriatr. Suppl.* 9 (2004): 69–73.

Davydov, Marina and Krikorian, A.D. "Eleutherococcus Senticosus (Rupr. & Maxim.) Maxim. (Araliaceae) as an Adaptogen: A Closer Look." *Journal of Ethnopharmacology* 72 (2000): 345–393.

Gaffney, Ben T., Hügel, Helmut M., and Rich, Peter A. "The Effects of Eleutherococcus Senticosus and Panax Ginseng on Steroidal Hormone Indices of Stress and Lymphocyte Subset Numbers in Endurance Athletes." *Life Sciences* 70 (2001): 431–442.

Gaffney, Ben T., Hügel, Helmut M., and Rich, Peter A. "Panax ginseng and Eleutherococcus Senticosus may Exaggerate an Already Existing Biphasic Response to Stress via Inhibition of Enzymes which Limit the Binding of Stress Hormones to their Receptors." *Medical Hypotheses* 56 (2001): 567–572.

Glatthaar–Saalmüller, Bernadette, Sacher, Fritz, and Esperester, Anke. "Antiviral Activity of an Extract Derived from Roots of Eleutherococcus Senticosus." *Antiviral Research* 50 (2001): 223–228.

Kimura, Yoshiyuki and Sumiyoshi, Maho. Effects of Various Eleutherococcus Senticosus Cortex on Swimming Time, Natural Killer Activity and Corticosterone Level in Forced Swimming Stressed Mice." *Journal of Ethnopharmacology* 95 (2004): 447–453.

Yua, C.Y., Kim, S.H., Lim, J.D. Kim, M.J., and Chung, I.M. "Intraspecific Relationship Analysis by DNA Markers and In Vitro Cytotoxic and Antioxidant Activity in Eleutherococ-

cus Senticosus." *Toxicology in Vitro* 17 (2003): 229–236.

EPHEDRA

Carlini, E.A. "Plants and the Central Nervous System." *Pharmacology, Biochemistry and Behavior* 75 (2003): 501–512.

Dong, Xiangchao, Wei Wang, Shujuan Ma, Hui Sun, Yan Li, and Jingqiang Guo. "Molecularly Imprinted Solid–Phase Extraction of Ephedrine from Chinese Ephedra." *Journal of Chromatography A*, 1070 (2005): 125–130.

Feresin, Gabriela Egly, Alejandro Tapia, Silvia N. López, and Susana A. Zacchino. "Antimicrobial Activity of Plants Used in Traditional Medicine of San Juan Province, Argentine." *Journal of Ethnopharmacology* 78 (2001): 103–107.

Gurni, A. Alberto and Marcelo L. Wagner. "Proanthocyanidins from some Argentine Species of Ephedra." *Biochemical Systematics and Ecology* 12, 3 (1984): 319–320.

Konno, Chohachi, Takashi Taguchi, Misturu Tamada, and Hiroshi Hikino. "Ephedroxane, Anti–Inflammatory Principle of Ephedra Herbs." *Phytochemistry* 18 (1979): 697–698.

Pellati, Federica and Stefania Benvenuti. "Determination of Ephedrine Alkaloids in Ephedra Natural Products Using HPLC on a Pentafluorophenylpropyl Stationary Phase." *Journal of Pharmaceutical and Biomedical Analysis* xxx (2007): xxx–xxx (Article in Press).

Sulzer, David, Mark S. Sonders, Nathan W. Poulsen, and Aurelio Galli. "Mechanisms of Neurotransmitter Release by Amphetamines: A review." *Progress in Neurobiology* 75 (2005): 406–433.

EUCALYPTUS

Amakura, Yoshiaki, Yukiko Umino, Sumiko Tsuji, Hideyuki Ito, Tsutomu Hatano, Takashi Yoshida, and Yasuhide Tonogai. "Constituents and their Antioxidative Effects in Eucalyptus Leaf Extract Used as a Natural Food

Additive." *Food Chemistry* 77 (2002): 47–56.

Hasegawa, Tatsuya, Fumihide Takano, Takano-bu Takata, Masato Niiyama, and Tomihisa Ohta. "Bioactive Monoterpene Glycosides Conjugated with Gallic Acid from the Leaves of Eucalyptus Globulus." *Phytochemistry* 69 (2008): 747–753.

Silva, Jeane, Worku Abebe, S.M. Sousa, V.G. Duarte, M.I.L. Machado, F.J.A. Matos. "Analgesic and Anti–inflammatory Effects of Essential Oils of Eucalyptus." *Journal of Ethnopharmacology* 89 (2003): 277–283.

FENNEL

Damjanovic, Biljana, Zika Lepojevic, Vladimir Zivkovic, and Aleksandar Tolic. "Extraction of Fennel (Foeniculum Vulgare Mill.) Seeds with Supercritical CO_2: Comparison with Hydrodistillation." *Food Chemistry* 92 (2005): 143–149

Choi, Eun–Mi and Jae–Kwan Hwang. "Antiinflammatory, Analgesic, and Antioxidant Activities of the Fruit of Foeniculum Vulgare." *Fitoterapia* 75 (2004): 557– 565

Singh, Gurdip, Sumitra Maurya, M.P. de Lampasona, and C. Catalan. "Chemical Constituents, Antifungal and Antioxidative Potential of Foeniculum Vulgare Volatile Oil and its Acetone Extract." *Food Control* 17 (2006): 745–752.

GARLIC

Arnault, Ingrid and Jacques Auger. "Seleno–Compounds in Garlic and Onion." *Journal of Chromatography A* 1112 (2006): 23–30.

Bakri, I.M. and C.W.I. Douglas. "Inhibitory Effect of Garlic Extract on Oral Bacteria." *Archives of Oral Biology* 50 (2005): 645–651.

Bozin, Biljana, Neda Mimica–Dukic, Isidora Samojlik, Anackov Goran, and Ruzica Igic. "Phenolics as Antioxidants in Garlic (Allium Sativum L., Alliaceae)." *Food Chemistry* 111 (2008): 925–929.

Koscielny, J., D. Klubendorf, R. Latza, R. Schmitt, H. Radtke, G. Siegel, and H. Kiesewetter. "The Antiatherosclerotic Effect of Allium Sativum." *Atherosclerosis* 144 (1999): 237–249.

Lanzotti, Virginia. "The Analysis of Onion and Garlic." *Journal of Chromatography A* 1112 (2006): 3–22.

Nuutila, Anna Maria, Riitta Puupponen–Pimia, Marjukka Aarni, and Kirsi–Marja Oksman–Caldentey. "Comparison of Antioxidant Activities of Onion and Garlic Extracts by Inhibition of Lipid Peroxidation and Radical Scavenging Activity." *Food Chemistry* 81 (2003): 485–493.

Suby, Oommen, Ruby John Anto, Gopal Srinivas, and Devarajan Karunagaran. "Allicin (from Garlic) Induces Caspase–Mediated Apoptosis in Cancer Cells." *European Journal of Pharmacology* 485 (2004): 97– 103.

Powolny, Anna A. and Shivendra V. Singh. "Multitargeted Prevention and Therapy of Cancer by Diallyl Trisulfide and Related Allium Vegetable–Derived Organosulfur Compounds." *Cancer Letters* xxx (2008): xxx–xxx (Article in Press).

Shams–Ghahfarokhi, Masoomeh, Mohammad–Reza Shokoohamiri, Nasrin Amirrajab, Behnaz Moghadasi, Ali Ghajari, Farideh Zeini, Golnar Sadeghi, and Mehdi Razzaghi–Abyaneh. "In Vitro Antifungal Activities of Allium Cepa, Allium Sativum and Ketoconazole Against Some Pathogenic Yeasts and Dermatophytes." *Fitoterapia* 77 (2006): 321–323.

Shukla, Yogeshwer and Pankaj Taneja. "Antimutagenic Effects of Garlic Extract on Chromosomal Aberrations." *Cancer Letters* 176 (2002): 31–36.

GINGER

Ajith, T.A., U. Hema, and M.S. Aswathy. "Zingiber Officinale Roscoe Prevents Acetaminophen–Induced Acute Hepatotoxicity by Enhancing Hepatic Antioxidant Status." *Food and Chemical Toxicology* 45 (2007): 2267–2272.

Ajith, T.A., V. Nivitha, and S. Usha. "Zingiber Officinale Roscoe Alone and in Combination with a–Tocopherol Protect the Kidney Against Cisplatin–Induced Acute Renal Failure." *Food and Chemical Toxicology* 45 (2007): 921–927.

Chaiyakunapruk, Nathorn, N. Kitikannakorn, S. Nathisuwan, K. Leeprakobboon, and C. Leelasettagoolc. "The Efficacy of Ginger for the Prevention of Postoperative Nausea and Vomiting: A Meta–Analysis." *American Journal of Obstetrics and Gynecology* 194 (2006): 95–99.

Fischer–Rasmussen, Wiggo, S.K. Kjser, C. Dahl, and Ulla Asping. "Ginger Treatment of Hyperemesis Gravidarum." *European Journat of Obstetrics & Gynecology and Reproductive Biology* 38 (1990): 19–24.

Goyal, Ramesh K. and Sanjay V. Kadnur. "Beneficial Effects of Zingiber Officinale on Goldthioglucose Induced Obesity." *Fitoterapia* 77 (2006): 160–163.

Jantan, I., I.A.A. Rafi, and J. Jalil. "Platelet–Activating Factor (PAF) Receptor–Binding Antagonist Activity of Malaysian Medicinal Plants." *Phytomedicine* 12 (2005): 88–92.

Kim, Eok–Cheon, J.–K. Min, T.–Y. Kim, S.–J. Lee, H.–O. Yang, S. Han, Y.–M. Kim, and Y.–G. Kwon. "[6]–Gingerol, a Pungent Ingredient of Ginger, Inhibits Angiogenesis In Vitro and In Vivo." *Biochemical and Biophysical Research Communications* 335 (2005): 300–308.

Kim, Misook, S.E. Hamilton, L.W. Guddat, and C.M. Overall. "Plant Collagenase: Unique Collagenolytic Activity of Cysteine Proteases from Ginger." *Biochimica et Biophysica Acta* 1770 (2007): 1627–1635.

Koo, Karen L.K., A.J. Ammit, V.H. Tran, C.C. Duke, and B.D. Roufogalis. "Gingerols and Related Analogues Inhibit Arachidonic Acid–Induced Human Platelet Serotonin Release and Aggregation. *Thrombosis Research* 103 (2001): 387–397.

Lantz, R.C., G.J. Chen, M. Sarihan, A.M. Solyom, S.D. Jolad, and B.N. Timmermann. "The Effect of Extracts from Ginger Rhizome on Inflammatory Mediator Production." *Phytomedicine* 14 (2007): 123–128.

Lee, Hyun Sook, E.Y. Seo, N.E. Kang, and W.K. Kim. "[6]–Gingerol Inhibits Metastasis of MDA–MB–231 Human Breast Cancer Cells." *Journal of Nutritional Biochemistry* xx (2007): xxx–xxx (Article in press).

Miyoshi, Noriyuki, Y. Nakamura, Y. Ueda, M. Abe, Y. Ozawa, K. Uchida, and T. Osawa. "Dietary Ginger Constituents, Galanals A and B, are Potent ApoptosisInducers in Human T Lymphoma Jurkat Cells. *Cancer Letters* 199 (2003): 113–119.

Naveena, B.M., S.K. Mendiratta, A.S.R. Anjaneyulu. "Tenderization of Buffalo Meat Using Plant Proteases from Cucumis Trigonus Roxb (Kachri) and Zingiber Officinale Roscoe (Ginger Rhizome). *Meat Science* 68 (2004): 363–369.

Nicoll, Rachel and M.Y. Henein. "Ginger (Zingiber Officinale Roscoe): A Hot Remedy for Cardiovascular Disease?" *International Journal of Cardiology* xx (2007): xxx–xxx (Article in press).

Shukla, Yogeshwer and Madhulika Singh. "Cancer Preventive Properties of Ginger: A Brief Review." *Food and Chemical Toxicology* 45 (2007): 683–690.

Stoilova, I., A. Krastanov, A. Stoyanova, P. Denev, and S. Gargova. "Antioxidant Activity of a Ginger Extract (Zingiber Officinale)." *Food Chemistry* 102 (2007): 764–770.

Surh, Young–Joon. "Anti–Tumor Promoting Potential of Selected Spice Ingredients with Antioxidative and Anti–Inflammatory Activities: a Short Review." *Food and Chemical Toxicology* 40 (2002): 1091–1097.

Thomson, M., K.K. Al–Qattan, S.M. Al–Sawan, M.A. Alnaqeeb, I. Khan, and M. Ali. "The Use of Ginger (Zingiber Officinale Rosc.) as a Potential Anti–Inflammatory and Antithrombotic Agent." *Prostaglandins, Leukotrienes and Essential FattyAcids* 67, 6 (2002): 475–478.

GINKGO

Dongen, Martien van, Erik van Rossum, Alphons Kessels, Hilde Sielhorst, and Paul Knipschild.

"Ginkgo for Elderly People with Dementia and Age–Associated Memory Impairment: A Randomized Clinical Trial." *Journal of Clinical Epidemiology* 56 (2003): 367–376.

Goh, Lena M. and Philip J. Barlow. "Antioxidant Capacity in Ginkgo Biloba." *Food Research International* 35 (2002): 815–820.

Moulton, Patricia L., Leon N. Boyko, Joan L. Fitzpatrick, and Thomas V. Petros. "The Effect of Ginkgo Biloba on Memory in Healthy Male Volunteers." *Physiology & Behavior* 73 (2001): 659–665.

Smith, Paul F., Karyn Maclennan, and Cynthia L. Darlington. "The Neuroprotective Properties of the Ginkgo Biloba Leaf: A Review of the Possible Relationship to Platelet–Activating Factor (PAF)." *Journal of Ethnopharmacology* 50 (1996): 131–139.

GINSENG

Attele, Anoja S., Ji An Wu, and Chun–Su Yuan. "Ginseng Pharmacology: Multiple Constituents and Multiple Actions." *Biochemical Pharmacology* 58 (1999): 1685–1693.

Lee, Byung–Hwan, Jun–Ho Lee, Sang–Mok Lee, Sang Min Jeong, In–Soo Yoon, Joon–Hee Lee, Sun–Hye Choi, Mi Kyung Pyo, Hyewhon Rhim, Hyoung–Chun Kim, Choon–Gon Jang, Byoung–Cheol Lee, Chul–Seung Park, and Seung–Yeol. "Identification of Ginsenoside Interaction Sites in 5–HT3A Receptors." *Neuropharmacology* 52 (2007): 1139–1150.

Choi, Kyungsun, Myungsun Kim, Jeonghee Ryu, and Chulhee Choi. "Ginsenosides Compound K and Rh2 Inhibit Tumor Necrosis Factor––Induced Activation of the NF–B and JNK Pathways in Human Astroglial Cells." *Neuroscience Letters* 421 (2007): 37–41.

Dey, L., J.T. Xie, A. Wang, J. Wu, S.A. Maleckar, and C.-S. Yuan. "Anti–Hyperglycemic Effects of Ginseng: Comparison Between Root and Berry." *Phytomedicine* 10 (2003): 600–605.

Gaffney, Ben T., Helmut M. Hügel, and Peter A. Rich. "The Effects of Eleutherococcus Senticosus and Panax Ginseng on Steroidal Hormone Indices of Stress and Lymphocyte Subset Numbers in Endurance Athletes." *Life Sciences* 70 (2001): 431–442.

Gaffney, B.T., H.M. Hügel, and P.A. Rich. "Panax Ginseng and Eleutherococcus Senticosus May Exaggerate an Already Existing Biphasic Response to Stress Via Inhibition of Enzymes which Limit the Binding of Stress Hormones to their Receptors." *Medical Hypotheses* 56, 5 (2001): 567–572.

Hong, Bumsik, Toung Hwan Ji, Jun Hyuk Hong, Ki Yeul Nam, and Tai Young Ahn. "A Double–Blind Crossover Study Evaluating the Efficacy of Korean Red Ginseng in Patients with Erectile Dysfunction: A Preliminary Report." *The Journal of Urology* 168 (2002): 2070–2073.

Kim, Seung–Hwan and Kyung–Shin Park. "Effects of Panax Ginseng Extract on Lipid Metabolism in Humans." *Pharmacological Research* 48 (2003): 511–513.

Kennedy, David O. and Andrew B. Scholey. "Ginseng: Potential for the Enhancement of Cognitive Performance and Mood." *Pharmacology, Biochemistry and Behavior* 75 (2003): 687–700.

Kennedy, D.O., A.B. Scholey and, K.A. Wesnes. "Modulation of Cognition and Mood Following Administration of Single Doses of Ginkgo Biloba, Ginseng, and a Ginkgo/Ginseng Combination to Healthy Young Adults." *Physiology & Behavior* 75 (2002): 739–751.

Lee, Sung Pil, Kazuki Honda, Young Ho Rhee, and Shojiro Inoue. "Chronic Intake of Panax Ginseng Extract Stabilizes Sleep and Wakefulness in Food–Deprived Rats." *Neuroscience Letters* 111 (1990): 217–221.

Li, Wei, Kazuo Koike, Yoshihisa Asada, Takafumi Yoshikawa, and Tamotsu Nikaido. "Biotransformation of Umbelliferone by Panax Ginseng Root Cultures." *Tetrahedron Letters Pergamon* 43 (2002): 5633–5635.

Liao, Baisong, Harold Newmark, and Renping Zhou. "Neuroprotective Effects of Ginseng Total Saponin and Ginsenosides Rb1 and Rg1 on Spinal Cord Neurons In Vitro." *Experimental Neurology* 173 (2002): 224–234.

Liu, Juntla, Shu Wang, Hongtao Liu, Liping Yang, and Guozhu Nan. "Stilmulatory Effect of Saponin from Panax Ginseng on Immune Function of Lymphocytes in the Elderly." *Mechanisms of Ageing and Development* 83 (1995): 43–53.

Liu, W.K., S.X. Xu, and C.T. Che. "Anti–Proliferative Effect of Ginseng Saponins on Human Prostate Cancer Cell Line. *Life Sciences* 67 (2000): 1297–1306.

Naval, M.V., M.P. Gomez–Serranillos, M.E. Carretero, and A.M. Villar. "Neuroprotective Effect of a Ginseng (Panax Ginseng) Root Extract on Astrocytes Primary Culture."*Journal of Ethnopharmacology* 112 (2007): 262–270.

Nocerino, Emilia, Marianna Amato, and Angelo A. Izzo. "The Aphrodisiac and Adaptogenic Properties of Ginseng." *Fitoterapia* 71 (2000): S1–S5.

Oliveira, A.C. Cabral de, A.C. Perez, J.G. Prieto, I.D.G. Duarte, and A.I. Alvarez. "Protection of Panax Ginseng in Injured Muscles After Eccentric Exercise." *Journal of Ethnopharmacology* 97 (2005): 211–214.

See, Darryl M., Nikki Broumand, Lisa Sahl, and Jeremiah G. Tilles. "In Vitro Effects of Echinacea and Ginseng on Natural Killer and Antibody–Dependent Cell Cytotoxicity in Healthy Subjects and Chronic Fatigue Syndrome or Acquired Immunodeficiency Syndrome Patients." *Immunopharmacology* 35 (1997): 229–235.

Shah, Zahoor Ahmad, Rabia Afzal Gilani, Pragya Sharma, and Shashi Bharat Vohora. "Cerebroprotective Effect of Korean Ginseng Tea Against Global and Focal Models of Ischemia in Rats." *Journal of Ethnopharmacology* 101 (2005): 299–307.

Shi, Wei, Yutang Wang, Juan Li, Hanqi Zhang, and Lan Ding. "Investigation of Ginsenosides in Different Parts and Ages of Panax Ginseng." *Food Chemistry* 102 (2007): 664–668.

Tachikawa, Eiichi, Kenzo Kudo, Hideo Hasegawa, Takeshi Kashimoto, Kazuhiko Sasaki, Masao Miyazaki, Hideharu Taira, and Jon M. Lindstrom. "In Vitro Inhibition of Adrenal Catecholamine Secretion by Steroidal Metabolites of Ginseng Saponins." *Biochemical Pharmacology* 66 (2003): 2213–2221.

Vuksan, Vladimir and John L. Sievenpiper. "Herbal Remedies in the Management of Diabetes: Lessons Learned from the Study of Ginseng." *Nutrition, Metabolism & Cardiovascular Diseases* 15 (2005): 149–160.

Vuksan, Vladimir, Mi–Kyung Sung, John L. Sievenpiper, P. Mark Stavro, Alexandra L. Jenkins, Marco Di Buono, Kwang–Seung Lee, Lawrence A. Leiter, Ki Yeul Nam, John T. Arnason, Melody Choi, and Asima Naeem. "Korean Red Ginseng (Panax Ginseng) Improves Glucose and Insulin Regulation in Well–Controlled, Type 2 Diabetes: Results of a Randomized, Double–Blind, Placebo–Controlled Study of Efficacy and Safety." *Nutrition, Metabolism & Cardiovascular Diseases* 18 (2008): 46–56.

Xiaoguang, Chen, Liu Hongyan, Lei Xiaohong, Fu Zhaodi, Li Yan, Tao Lihua, and Han Rui. "Cancer Chemopreventive and Therapeutic Activities of Red Ginseng." *Journal of Ethnopharmacology* 60 (1998): 71–78.

Xie, J.T., Y.–P. Zhou, L. Dey, A.S. Attele, J.A. Wu, M. Gu, K.S. Polonsky, and C.–S. Yuan. "Ginseng Berry Reduces Blood Glucose and Body Weight in db/db Mice." *Phytomedicine* 9 (2002): 254–258.

Yu, Lin–Chien, Sung–Ching Chen, Wei–Chun Chang, Ya–Chun Huang, Kurt M. Lin, Po–Hong Lai, and Hsing–Wen Sung. "Stability of Angiogenic Agents, Ginsenoside Rg1 and Re, Isolated from Panax Ginseng: In Vitro and In Vivo Studies." *International Journal of Pharmaceutics* 328 (2007): 168–176.

Yun, Taik–Koo. "Experimental and Epidemiological Evidence on Non–Organ Specific Cancer Preventive Effect of Korean Ginseng and Identification of Active Compounds." *Mutation Research* 523–524 (2003): 63–74.

GOTA KOLA

Asakawa, Y., Matsuda, R., and Takemoto, T.

"Mono– and Sesquiterpenoids from Hydrocotyle and Centella Species." *Phytochemistry* 21, 10 (1982): 2590–2592.

Grimaldi, R., Ponti, F. de, D'Angelo, L.D., Caravaggi, M., Guidi, G., Lecchini, S., Frigo, G.M., and Crema, A. "Pharmacokinetics of the Total Triterpenic Fraction of Centella Asiatica After Single and Multiple Administrations to healthy Volunteers. A New Assay for Asiatic Acid." *Journal of Ethnopharmacology* 28 (1990): 235–241.

Hamid, A. Abdul, Shah, Z.M., Muse, R., and Mohamed, S. "Characterisation of Antioxidative Activities of Various Extracts of Centella Asiatica (L) Urban." *Food Chemistry* 77 (2002): 465–469.

Inamdar, E.K., Yeole, R.D., Ghogare, A.B., Souza, N.J. de. "Determination of Biologically Active Constituents in Centella Asiatica." *Journal of Chromatography A,* 742 (1996): 127–130.

Kimura, Y., Sumiyoshi, M., Samukawa, K., Satake, N., Sakanaka, M. "Facilitating Action of Asiaticoside at Low Doses on Burn Wound Repair and its Mechanism." *European Journal of Pharmacology* 584 (2008): 415–423.

Sampson, J.H., Raman, A., Karlsen, G., Navsaria, H., and Leigh, I. M. "In Vitro Keratinocyte Antiproliferant Effect of Centella Asiatica Extract and Triterpenoid Saponins." *Phytomedicine* 8, 3 (2001): 230–235.

Shukla, A., Rasik, A.M., Jain, G.K., Shankar, R., Kulshrestha, D.K., Dhawan, B.N. "In Vitro and In Vivo Wound Healing Activity of Asiaticoside Isolated from Centella Asiatica." *Journal of Ethnopharmacology* 65 (1999): 1–11.

Subathra, M., Shila, S., Devi, M.A., and Panneerselvam, C. "Emerging Role of Centella Asiatica in Improving Age–Related Neurological Antioxidant Status." *Experimental Gerontology* 40 (2005): 707–715.

Wang, Xue Song, Liu, L., and Fang, Ji Nian. "Immunological Activities and Structure of Pectin from Centella Asiatica" *Carbohydrate Polymers* 60 (2005): 95–101.

Wattanathorn, J., Mator, L., Muchimapura, S., Tongun, T., Pasuriwong, O., Piyawatkul, N., Yimtae, K., Sripanidkulchai, and B., Singkhoraard, J. "Positive Modulation of Cognition and Mood in the Healthy Elderly Volunteer Following the Administration of Centella Asiatica." *Journal of Ethnopharmacology* 116 (2008): 325–332.

Weckerle, Caroline S., Michael A. Stutz, and Thomas W. Baumann. "Purine Alkaloids in Paullinia." *Phytochemistry* 64 (2003): 735–742.

Yu, Quan Lin, Duan, Hong Quan, Gao, Wen Yuan, and Takaishi, Yoshihisa. "A New Triterpene and a Saponin from Centella Asiatica." *Chinese Chemical Letters* 18 (2007): 62–64.

Zainol, M.K., Abd–Hamid, A., Yusof, S., and Muse, R. "Antioxidative Activity and Total Phenolic Compounds of Leaf, Root and Petiole of Four Accessions of Centella Asiatica (L.) Urban." *Food Chemistry* 81 (2003): 575–581.

GRINDELIA

Fraternale, Daniele, Laura Giamperi, Anahi Bucchini,and Donata Ricci. "Essential Oil Composition and Antioxidant Activity of Aerial Parts of Grindelia Robusta from Central Italy." *Fitoterapia* 78 (2007): 443–445.

GUARANÁ

Espinola, E.B., R.F. Dias, R. Mattei, and E.A. Carlini. "Pharmacological Activity of Guarana (Paullinia Cupana Mart.) in Laboratory Animals." *Journal of Ethnopharmacology* 55 (1997): 223–229.

Fukumasu, H., J.L. Avanzo, R. Heidor, T.C. Silva, A. Atroch, F.S. Moreno, and M.L.Z. Dagli. "Protective Effects of Guarana (Paullinia Cupana Mart. var. Sorbilis) Against DEN–Induced DNA Damage on Mouse Liver." *Food and Chemical Toxicology* 44 (2006): 862–867.

Henman, Anthony Richard. "Guarana (Paullinia Cupana var. Sorbilis): Ecological and Social Perspectives on as Economical Plant of the Central Amazon Basin." *Journal of Ethnopharmacology* 6 (1982): 311–338.

Kennedy, D.O., C.F. Haskell, K.A. Wesnes, and

A.B. Scholey. "Improved Cognitive Performance in Human Volunteers Following Administration of Guarana (Paullinia Cupana) Extract: Comparison and Interaction with Panax Ginseng." *Pharmacology, Biochemistry and Behavior* 79 (2004): 401–411.

Majhenic, Lucija, Mojca Skerget, and Zeljko Knez. "Antioxidant and Antimicrobial Activity of Guarana Seed Extracts." *Food Chemistry* 104 (2007): 1258–1268.

HAWTHORN

Degenring, F. H., A. Suter, M. Weber, and R. Saller. "A Randomised Double Blind Placebo Controlled Clinical Trial of a Standardised Extract of Fresh Crataegus Berries (Crataegisan®) in the Treatment of Patients with Congestive Heart Failure NYHA II." *Phytomedicine* 10 (2003): 363–369.

Ozcan, Musa, Haydar Hacıseferogulları, Tamer Marakoglu, and Derya Arslan. "Hawthorn (Crataegus spp.) Fruit: Some Physical and Chemical Properties." *Journal of Food Engineering* 69 (2005): 409–413.

Svedstrom, Ulla, Heikki Vuorela, Risto Kostiainen, Jari Tuominen, Juha Kokkonen, Jussi-Pekka Rauha, Into Laakso, Raimo Hiltunen. "Isolation and Identification of Oligomeric Procyanidins from Crataegus Leaves and Flowers." *Phytochemistry* 60 (2002): 821–825.

Veveris, Maris, Egon Koch, and Shyam S. Chatterjee. "Crataegus Special Extract WSR 1442 Improves Cardiac Function and Reduces Infarct Size in a Rat Model of Prolonged Coronary Ischemia and Reperfusion." *Life Sciences* 74 (2004): 1945–1955.

Zick, Suzanna M., Brenda Gillespie, and Keith D. Aaronson. "The Effect of Crataegus Oxycantha Special Extract WS 1442 on Clinical Progression in Patients with Mild to Moderate Symptoms of Heart Failure." *European Journal of Heart Failure* 10 (2008): 587–593.

HOPS

Chadwick, L.R., G.F. Pauli, and N.R. Farnsworth. "The Pharmacognosy of Humulus Lupulus L. (Hops) with an Emphasis on Estrogenic Properties." *Phytomedicine* 13 (2006): 119–131.

Delmulle, L., A. Bellahcene, W. Dhooge, F. Comhaire, F. Roelens, K. Huvaere, A. Heyerick, V. Castronovo, and D. De Keukeleire. "Anti–Proliferative Properties of Prenylated Flavonoids from Hops (Humulus Lupulus L.) in Human Prostate Cancer Cell Lines." *Phytomedicine* 13 (2006): 732–734.

Gerhauser, Clarissa. "Beer Constituents as Potential Cancer Chemopreventive Agents." *European Journal of Cancer* 41 (2005): 1941–1954.

Heyerick, Arne, Stefaan Vervarcke, Herman Depypere, Marc Bracke, and Denis De Keukeleire. "A First Prospective, Randomized, Double–Blind, Placebo–Controlled Study on the Use of a Standardized Hop Extract to Alleviate Menopausal Discomforts." *Maturitas* 54 (2006): 164–175.

Monteiro, Rosario, Ana Faria, Isabel Azevedo, and Conceicao Calhau. "Modulation of Breast Cancer Cell Survival by Aromatase Inhibiting Hop (Humulus Lupulus L.) Flavonoids." *Journal of Steroid Biochemistry & Molecular Biology* 105 (2007): 124–130.

Overk, Cassia R., Jian Guo, Lucas R. Chadwick, Daniel D. Lantvit, Alberto Minassi, Giovanni Appendino, Shao–Nong Chen, David C. Lankin, Norman R. Farnsworth, Guido F. Pauli, Richard B. van Breemen, and Judy L. Boltona. "In Vivo Estrogenic Comparisons of Trifolium Pratense (Red Clover) Humulus Lupulus (Hops), and the Pure Compounds Isoxanthohumol and 8–Prenylnaringenin." *Chemico–Biological Interactions* xxx (2008): xxx–xxx (Article in Press).

Schiller, H., A. Forster, C. Vonhoff, M. Hegger, A. Biller, and H. Winterhoff. "Sedating Effects of Humulus Lupulus L. Extracts." *Phytomedicine* 13 (2006): 535–541.

Zanoli, Paola and Manuela Zavatti. "Pharmacognostic and Pharmacological Profile of Humulus Lupulus L." *Journal of Ethnopharmacology* 116 (2008): 383–396.

Zanoli, P., M. Zavatti, M. Rivasi, F. Brusiani, G. Losi, G. Puia, R. Avallone, and M. Baraldi. "Evidence that the β–Acids Fraction of Hops Reduces Central GABAergic Neurotransmission." *Journal of Ethnopharmacology* 109 (2007): 87–92.

HOREHOUND

Rey, Jean–Pierre, Joel Levesque, and Jean Louis Pousset. "Extraction and High–Performance Liquid Chroatographic Methods for the A–Lactones Parthenolide (Chrysanthemum Parthenium Bernh.), Marrubiin (Marrubium Vulgare L.) and Artemisinin (Artemisia annua L.)." *Journal of Chromatography* 605 (1992): 124–128.

Roman, Ramos R., F. Alarcon–Aguilar, A. Lara–Lemus, and J.L. Flores–Saenz. "Hypoglycemic Effect of Plants Used in Mexico as Antidiabetics." *Archives of Medical Research* 23, 1 (1992): 59–64.

Sahpaz, Sevser, Nancy Garbacki, Monique Tits, and Francois Bailleul. "Isolation and Pharmacological Activity of Phenylpropanoid Esters from Marrubium Vulgare." *Journal of Ethnopharmacology* 79 (2002): 389–392.

VanderJagt, T.J., R. Ghattas, D.J. VanderJagt, M. Crossey, and R.H Glew. "Comparison of the Total Antioxidant Content of 30 Widely Used Medicinal Plants of New Mexico." *Life Sciences* 70 (2002): 1035–1040.

HORSE CHESTNUT

Carrasco, Omar F. and H. Vidrio. "Endothelium Protectant and Contractile Effects of the Antivaricose Principle Escin in Rat Aorta." *Vascular Pharmacology* 47 (2007): 68–73.

Eastmond, Richard and R.J. Gardener. "Epicatechin and Procyanidins from Seed Hulls of Aesculus Hippocastanum." *Phytochemsitry* 13 (1974): 1477–1478.

Kubo, Isao and B–P. Ying. "Phenolic Constituents of California Buckeye Fruit." *Phytochemistry* 31, 11 (1992): 3793–3794.

Matsuda, Hisashi, Y. Li, T. Murakami, N. Araki, M. Yoshikawa, and J. Yamahara. "Antiinflammatory Effects of Escins Ia, Ib, IIa, and IIb from Horse Chestnut, the Seeds of Aesculus Hippocastanum L." *Bioorganic & Medicinal Chemistry Letters* 7, 13 (1997): 1611–1616.

Santos–Buelga, C., H. Kolodzieij, and D. Treutter. "Procyanidin Trimers Possessing a Doubly Linked Structure from Aesculus Hippocastanum." *Phytochemistry* 38, 2 (1995): 499–504.

Sirtori, Cesare R. "Aescin: Pharmacology, Pharmacokinetics and Theraputic Profile." *Pharmacological Research* 44, 3 (2001): 183–193.

Stankovic, S.K., M.B. Bastic, and J. A. Jovanovic. "Composition of the Triterpene Alcohol Fraction of Horse Chestnut Seed." *Phytochemistry* 24, 1 (1985): 119–121.

HORSETAIL

Amarowicz, R., R.B. Pegg, P. Rahimi–Moghaddam, B. Barl, and J.A. Weil. "Free–Radical Scavenging Capacity and Antioxidant Activity of Selected Plant Species from the Canadian Prairies." *Food Chemistry* 84 (2004): 551–562.

Grases, F., G. Melero, A. Costa–Bauza, R. Prieto, and J.G. March. "Urolithiasis and Phytotherapy." *International Urology and Nephrology* 26, 5 (1994): 507–11.

Gurbuz, Iÿlhan, Osman Ustun, Erdem Yesilada, Ekrem Sezik, and Nalan Akyurek. "In Vivo Gastroprotective Effects of Five Turkish Folk Remedies Against Ethanol–Induced Lesions." *Journal of Ethnopharmacology* 83 (2002): 241–244.

Harrison, C.C. "Evidence for Intramineral Macromolecules Containing Protein from Plant Silicas." *Phytochemistry* 41, 1 (1996): 37–42.

Veit, Markus, Cornelia Beckert, Cornelia Hohne, Katja Bauer, and Hans Geiger. "Interspecific and Intraspecific Variation of Phenolics in the Genus Equisetum Subgenus Equisetum." *Phytochemistry* 38, 4 (1995): 881–891.

JUNIPER

Adams, Robert P. "Systematics of the One Seeded Juniperus of the Eastern Hemisphere Based on Leaf Essential Oils and Random Amplified Polymorphic DNAs (RAPDs)." *Biochemical Systematics and Ecology* 28 (2000): 529–543.

Adams, Robert P., Ernst Von Rudloff, and Lawrence Hogge. "Chemosystematic Studies of the Western North American Junipers Based on their Volatile Oils." *Biochemical Systematics and Ecology* 11, 3 (1983): 189–193.

Adams, Robert P., Thomas A. Zanoni, and Lawrence Hogge. "Analyses of the Volatile Leaf Oils of Juniperus Deppeana and its Infraspecific Taxa: Chemosystematic Implications." *Biochemical Systemics and Ecoclogy* 12, 1 (1984): 23–27.

Adams, Robert P., Thomas A. Zanoni, Ernst Von Rudloff, and Lawrence Hogge. "The South–Western USA and Northern Mexico One–seeded Junipers: their Volatile Oils and Evolution." *Biochemical Systematics and Ecology* 9, 2/3 (1981): 93–96.

Karaman, I., F. Sahin, M. Güllüce, H. Öğütçü, M. Sengül, and A. Adigüzel. "Antimicrobial Activity of Aqueous and Methanol Extracts of Juniperus Oxycedrus L." *Journal of Ethnopharmacology* 85 (2003): 231–235.

San Feliciano, A., M. Gordaliza, J.M. Miguel del Corral, M.A. Castro, M.D. Garcia–Gravalos, and P. Ruiz–Lazaro. "Antineoplastic and Antiviral Activities of some Cyclolignans." *Planta Med* 59, 3 (1993): 246–249.

Tunón, H., C. Olavsdotter, and L. Bohlin. "Evaluation of Anti–Inflammatory Activity of some Swedish Medicinal Plants. Inhibition of Prostaglandin Biosynthesis and PAF–Induced Exocytosis." *Journal of Ethnopharmacology* 48 (1995): 61–76.

LEMONBALM

Allahverdiyev, A., N. Duran, M. Ozguvenc, and S. Koltas. "Antiviral Activity of the Volatile Oils of Melissa Officinalis L. Against Herpes Simplex Virus Type–2." *Phytomedicine* 11 (2004): 657–661.

Carnat, A.P., A. Carnat, D. Fraisse, and J.L. Lamaison. "The Aromatic and Polyphenolic Composition of Lemon Balm (Melissa Officinalis L. Subsp. Officinalis) Tea." *Pharmaceutics Acta Helvetiae* 72 (1998): 301–305.

Dastmalchi, Keyvan, H.J. Damien Dorman, Paivi P. Oinonen, Yusrida Darwis, Into Laakso, and Raimo Hiltunen. "Chemical Composition and In Vitro Antioxidative Activity of a Lemon Balm (Melissa Officinalis L.) Extract." *LWT* 41 (2008): 391–400.

Kennedy, D.O., Andrew B. Scholey, N.T.J. Tildesley, E.K. Perry, and K.A. Wesnes. "Modulation of Mood and Cognitive Performance Following Acute Administration of Melissa Officinalis (Lemon Balm)." *Pharmacology, Biochemistry and Behavior* 72 (2002): 953–964.

Schnitzler, P., A. Schuhmacher, A. Astani, and Jurgen Reichling. "Melissa Officinalis Oil Affects Infectivity of Enveloped Herpesviruses." *Phytomedicine* 15 (2008): 734–740.

LIGUSTICUM

Appelt, Glenn D. "Pharmacological Aspects of Selected Herbs Employed in Hispanic Folk Medicine in the San Luis Valley of Colorado, USA: I. Ligusticum Porteri (Osha) and Matricaria Chamomellia (Manzanilla)." *Journal of Ethnopharmacology* 13 (1985): 51–55.

Linares, Edelmira and Bye, Robert A. "A Study of Four Medicinal Plant Complexes of Mexico and Adjacent United States." *Journal of Ethnopharmacology* 19 (1987): 153–183.

LOBELIA

Felpin, Francois–Xavier and Lebreton, Jacques. "History, Chemistry and Biology of Alkaloids from Lobelia Inflata." *Tetrahedron* 60 (2004): 10127–10153.

Lim, Dong–Yoon, Kim, Yang–Soo, and Miwa, Soichi. "Influence of Lobeline on Catecholamine Release from the Isolated Perfused Rat Adrenal Gland." *Autonomic Neuroscience: Basic and Clinical* 110 (2004): 27–35.

Ma, Yonggang and Wink, Michael. "Lobeline, a Piperidine Alkaloid from Lobelia can Reverse P–gp Dependent Multidrug Resistance in Tumor Cells." *Phytomedicine* xxx (2008): xxx–xxx (Article in Press).

Neugebauer, Nichole M., Harrod, Steven B., Stairs, Dustin J., Crooks, Peter A., Dwoskin, Linda P., and Bardo, Michael T. "Lobelane Decreases Methamphetamine Self–Administration in Rats." *European Journal of Pharmacology* 571 (2007): 33–38.

KAVA

Anke, Jennifer and Iqbal Ramzan. "Pharmacokinetic and Pharmacodynamic Drug Interactions with Kava (Piper Methysticum Forst. f.)." *Journal of Ethnopharmacology* 93 (2004): 153–160.

Bilia, Anna Rita, Luca Scalise, Maria Camilla Bergonzi, and Franco F. Vincieri. "Analysis of Kavalactones from Piper Methysticum (Kava–Kava)." *Journal of Chromatography B,* 812 (2004): 203–214.

Bilia, Anna Rita, Sandra Gallori, and Franco F. Vincieri. "Kava–Kava and Anxiety: Growing Knowledge about the Efficacy and Safety." *Life Sciences* 70 (2002): 2581–2597.

Carlini, E.A. "Plants and the Central Nervous System." *Pharmacology, Biochemistry and Behavior* 75 (2003): 501–512.

Clouatre, Dallas L. "Kava Kava: Examining New Reports of Toxicity." *Toxicology Letters* 150 (2004) 85–96

Cote, Cynthia S., Christine Kor, Jon Cohen, and Karine Auclair. "Composition and Biological Activity of Traditional and Commercial Kava Extracts." *Biochemical and Biophysical Research Communications* 322 (2004): 147–152.

Dragull, Klaus, Wesley Y. Yoshida, and Chung–Shih Tang. "Piperidine Alkaloids from Piper Methysticum." *Phytochemistry* 63 (2003): 193–198.

Ernst, E. "Herbal Remedies for Anxiety – A Systematic Review of Controlled Clinical Trials." *Phytomedicine* 13 (2006): 205–208.

Gruenwald, Joerg and Juergen Skrabal. "Kava Ban Highly Questionable: A Brief Summary of the Main Scientific Findings." *Seminars in Integrative Medicine* 1, 4 (2003): 199–210.

Singh, Yadhu N. "Kava: an overview." *Journal of Ethnopharmacology* 37 (1992): 13–45.

KOLA NUT

Abidoye, R.O. and A.P. Chijioke. "Effect of Kola Nut on the Anthropometric Measurment of Newborn Babies in Nigera." *Nutrition Resaearch* 10 (1990): 1091–1098.

Niemenak, N., P.E. Onomo, Fotso, R. Lieberei, and D.O. Ndoumou. "Purine Alkaloids and Phenolic Compounds in Three Cola Species and Garcinia Kola Grown in Cameroon." *South African Journal of Botany* 74 (2008): 629–638.

Ogunmoyela, O. A. "The Use of Steam Blanching for Preserving the Quality of Kolanuts (Cola Nitida)." *Food Chemistry* 32 (1989): 163–170.

Reid, K.A., A.K. Jager, M.E. Light, D.A. Mulholland, and J. Van Staden. "Phytochemical and Pharmacological Screening of Sterculiaceae Species and Isolation of Antibacterial Compounds." *Journal of Ethnopharmacology* 97 (2005): 285–291.

MILK THISTLE

Alidoost, Fariba, Marjan Gharagozloo, Bahram Bagherpour, Abbas Jafarian, Seyed Ebrahim Sajjadi, Hamid Hourfar, and Behjat Moayedi. "Effects of Silymarin on the Proliferation and Glutathione Levels of Peripheral Blood Mononuclear Cells from β–Thalassemia Major Patients." *International Immunopharmacology* 6 (2006): 1305–1310.

Dvorak, Zdenek, Pavel Kosina, Daniela Walterova, Vilim Simanek, Petr Bachleda, and Jitka Ulrichova. "Primary Cultures of Human Hepatocytes as a Tool in Cytotoxicity Studies: Cell Protection Against Model Toxins by Flavonolignans Obtained from Silybum Marianum." *Toxicology Letters* 137 (2003): 201–212.

Ferenci, P., B. Drapsirs, H. Dittrich, H. Frank, L.

Benda, H. Lochs. S. Meryn, W. Base, and B. Schneider. "Randomized Controlled Trial of Silymarin Treatment in Patients with Cirrhosis of the Liver." *Journal of Hepatology* 9 (1989): 105–113.

Kvasnicka, F., B. Biba, R. Sevcik, M. Voldrich, and J. Kratka. "Analysis of the Active Components of Silymarin." *Journal of Chromatography A* 990 (2003): 239–245.

Ramasamy, Kumaraguruparan and Rajesh Agarwal. "Multitargeted Therapy of Cancer by Silymarin." *Cancer Letters* xxx (2008) xxx–xxx (Article in Press).

Svobodova, Alena, Adela Zdarilova, Daniela Walterova, and Jitka Vostalova. "Flavonolignans from Silybum Marianum Moderate UVA–Induced Oxidative Damage to HaCaT Keratinocytes." *Journal of Dermatological Science* (2007): 48 213–224.

Svobodova, Alena, Adela Zdarilova, Jana Maliskova, Hana Mikulkova, Daniela Walterova, and Jitka Vostalova. "Attenuation of UVA–Induced Damage to Human Keratinocytes by Silymarin." *Journal of Dermatological Science* 46 (2007): 21–30.

Toklu, Hale Z., Tuba Tunali–Akbay, Gozde Erkanli, Meral Yuksel, Feriha Ercan, and Goksel Sener. "Silymarin, the Antioxidant Component of Silybum Marianum, Protects Against Burn–Induced Oxidative Skin Injury." *Burns* 33 (2007): 908–916.

MUGWORT

Carnat, Andree, Annie Heitz, Didier Fraisse, Andre–Paul Carnat, and Jean–Louis Lamaison. "Major Dicaffeoylquinic Acids from Artemisia Vulgaris." *Fitoterapia* 71 (2000): 587–589.

Drake, David and Jorgen Lam. "Polyacetylenes of Artemisia Vulgaris." *Phytochemisttry* 13 (1974): 455–457.

Govindaraj, Sujatha, Bollipo Diana Ranjitha Kumari, Pier Luigi Cioni, and Guido Flamini. "Mass Propagation and Essential Oil Analysis of Artemisia Vulgaris." *Journal of Bioscience and Bioengineering* 105, 3 (2008): 176–183.

Marco, Alberto, J., Juan F. Sanz, and Pilar Del Hierro. "Two Eudesmane Acids from Artemisia Vulgaris." *Pytochemistry* 30, 7 (1991): 2403–2404.

Wallnofer, Bruno, Otmar Hofer, and Harald Greger. "Polyacetylenes from the Artemisia Vulgaris Group." *Phytochemistry* 28, 10 (1989): 2687–2691.

Wang J., F. Zhu, X.M. Zhou, C.Y. Niu, and C.L. Lei. "Repellent and Fumigant Activity of Essential Oil from Artemisia Vulgaris to Tribolium Castaneum (Herbst) (Coleoptera: Tenebrionidae)." *Journal of Stored Products Research* 42 (2006): 339–347.

MULLEIN

Khuroo, M.A., M.A. Qureshi, T.K. Razdan, and P. Nichols. "Sterones, Iridoids and a Sesquiterpene from Verbascum Thapsus." *Phytochemistry* 27, 11 (1988): 3541–3544.

Turker, Arzu Ucar and N.D. Camper. "Biological Activity of Common Mullein, a Medicinal Plant." *Journal of Ethnopharmacology* 82 (2002): 117–125.

Warashina, Tsutomu, Toshio Miyase, and Akira Ueno. "Phenylethanoid and Lignan Glycosides from Verbascum Thapsus." *Phytochemistry* 31, 3 (1992): 961–965.

MYRRH

Assimopoulou, A.N., Zlatanos, S.N., and Papgeorgiou, V.P. "Antioxidant Activity of Natural Resins and Bioactive Triterpenes in Oil Substrates." *Food Chemistry* 92 (2005): 721–727.

Guyatt, Helen L. "Medicinal Merits of Myrrh." *Trends in Parasitology* 18, 5 (2002): 202.

Maradufu, Asafu and Warthen, David J. Jr. "Furanosesquiterpenoids from Commiphora Myrrh Oil." *Plant Science* 57 (1988): 181–184.

Racine, P. and Auffray, B. "Quenching of Singlet Molecular Oxygen by Commiphora Myrrha Extracts and Menthofuran." *Fitoterapia* 76 (2005): 316–323.

NETTLE

Bnouham, Mohamed, Fatima–Zahra Merhfour, Abderrahim Ziyyat, Hassane Mekhfi, Mohammed Aziz, and Abdelkhaleq Legssyer. "Antihyperglycemic Activity of the Aqueous Extract of Urtica Dioica." *Fitoterapia* 74 (2003): 677–681.

Bondarenko, Boris, Carola Walther, Petra Funk, Sandra Schläfke, and Udo Engelmann. "Long–Term Efficacy and Safety of PRO 160/120 (A Combination of Sabal and Urtica Extract) in Patients with Lower Urinary Tract Symptoms (LUTS)." *Phytomedicine* 10 (2003): 53–55.

Guarrera, Paolo Maria. "Traditional Phytotherapy in Central Italy (Marche, Abruzzo, and Latium)." *Fitoterapia* 76 (2005): 1–25.

Guerrero, Guil J.L., M.M. Rebolloso–Fuentes, and M.E. Torija Isasa. "Fatty Acids and Carotenoids from Stinging Nettle (Urtica dioica L.)." *Journal of Food Composition and Analysis* 16 (2003): 111–119.

Gülçin, Ùllhami, O. Irfan Küfrevioglu, Münir Oktay, and Mehmet Emin Büyükokuroglu. "Antioxidant, Antimicrobial, Antiulcer and Analgesic Activities of Nettle (Urtica Dioica L.)." *Journal of Ethnopharmacology* 90 (2004): 205–215.

Lowe, Franklin C. and Elliot Fagelman. "Phytotherapy in the Treatment of Benign Prostatic Hyperplasia: An Update." *Urology* 53 (1999): 671–678.

Madersbacher, Stephan, Anton Ponholzer, Ingrid Berger, and Martin Marszalek. "Medical Management of BPH: Role of Plant Extracts." *Eau–Ebu Update Series* 5 (2007): 197–205.

Ozcan, Mehmet Musa, Ahmet Unver, Tolga Ucar, and Derya Arslan. "Mineral Content of Some Herbs and Herbal Teas by Infusion and Decoction." *Food Chemistry* 106 (2008): 1120–1127.

Sajfrtova, M., H. Sovova, L. Opletal, and M. Bartlova. "Near–Critical Extraction of Sitosterol and Scopoletin from Stinging Nettle Roots." *J. of Supercritical Fluids* 35 (2005): 111–118.

Testai, Lara, Silvio Chericoni, Vincenzo Calderone, Giulia Nencioni, Paola Nieri, Ivano Morelli, and Enrica Martinotti. "Cardiovascular Effects of Urtica Dioica L. (Urticaceae) Roots Extracts: In Vitro and In Vivo Pharmacological Studies." *Journal of Ethnopharmacology* 81 (2002): 105–109.

PASSIONFLOWER

Andersen, Lise, Anne Adsersen and Jerzy W. Jaroszewski. "Cyanogenesis of Passiflora Foetida." *Phytochemistry* 47, 6 (1998): 1049–1050.

Carlini, E.A. "Plants and the Central Nervous System." *Pharmacology, Biochemistry and Behavior* 75 (2003): 501–512.

Dhawan, Kamaldeep and Anupam Sharma. "Antitussive Activity of the Methanol Extract of Passiflora Incarnata Leaves." *Fitoterapia* 73 (2002): 397–399.

Dhawan, Kamaldeep and Anupam Sharma. "Prevention of Chronic Alcohol and Nicotine–Induced Azospermia, Sterility and Decreased Libido, by a Novel Tri–Substituted Benzoflavone Moiety from Passiflora Incarnata Linneus In Healthy Male Rats." *Life Sciences* 71 (2002): 3059–3069.

Dhawan, Kamaldeep, Suresh Kumar, and Anupam Sharma. "Anxiolytic Activity of Aerial and Underground Parts of Passiflora Incarnata." *Fitoterapia* 72 (2001): 922–926.

Dhawan, Kamaldeep, Suresh Kumar, and Anupam Sharma. "Comparative Biological Activity Study on Passiflora Incarnata and P. Edulis." *Fitoterapia* 72 (2001): 698–702.

Dhawan, Kamaldeep, Suresh Kumar, and Anupam Sharma. "Suppression of Alcohol–Cessation–Oriented Hyper–Anxiety by the Benzoflavone Moiety of Passiflora Incarnata Linneus in Mice." *Journal of Ethnopharmacology* 81 (2002): 239–244.

Jaroszewski, Jerzy W., Elin S. Olafsdottir, Petrine Wellendorph, Jette Christensen, Henrik Franzyk, Brinda Somanadhan, Bogdan A. Budnik, Lise Bolt Jørgensen, and Vicki Clausen. "Cyanohydrin Glycosides of Passiflora: Distribution Pattern, a Saturated Cyclopentane Derivative from P. Guatemalensis, and Formation of Pseudocyanogenic a–hydroxyamides as Isolation Artifacts." *Phytochemistry* 59 (2002): 501–511.

Seigler, David S., Guido F. Pauli, Adolf Nahrstedt, and Rosemary Leen. "Cyanogenic Allosides and Glucosides from Passiflora Edulis and Carica Papaya." *Phytochemistry* 60 (2002): 873–882.

Wolfman, Claudia, Hatdee Viola, Alejandro Paladini, Federico Dajas, and Jorge H. Medina. "Possible Anxiolytic Effects of Chrysin, a Central Benzodiazepine Receptor Ligand Isolated from Passiflora Coerulea." *Pharmacology Biochemistry and Behavior* 47 (1994). xx–xx.

PENNYROYAL

Aghel, Nasrin, Yadollah Yamini, Abbas Hadjiakhoondi, and Seied Mahdi Pourmortazavi. "Supercritical Carbon Dioxide Extraction of Mentha Pulegium L. Essential Oil." *Talanta* 62 (2004): 407–411.

Pavela, Roman. "Insecticidal Activity of Some Essential Oils Against Larvae of Spodoptera Littoralis." *Fitoterapia* 76 (2005): 691– 696.

Vian, Maryline Abert, Xavier Fernandez, Franco Visinoni, and Farid Chemat. "Microwave Hydrodiffusion and Gravity, a New Technique for Extraction of Essential Oils." *Journal of Chromatography A,* 1190 (2008): 14–17.

PLANTAIN

Samuelsen, Anne Berit. "The Traditional Uses, Chemical Constituents and Biological Activities of Plantago Major L." *Journal of Ethnopharmacology* 71 (2000): 1–21.

Samuelsen, Anne Berit, Berit Smestad Paulsen, Jens Kristian Wold, Svein H. Knutsen, and Haruki Yamada. "Characterization of a Biologically Active Arabinogalactan from the Leaves of Plantago Major L." *Carbohydrate Polymers* 35 (1998): 145–153.

Taskova, Rilka, Nedjalka Handjieva, Ljubka Evstatieva, Simeon Popov. "Iridoid Glucosides from Plantago Cornuti, Plantago Major and Veronica Cymbalaria." *Phytochemistry* 52 (1999): 1443–1445.

RED CLOVER

Beck, V., E. Unterrieder, L. Krenn, W. Kubelka, and A. Jungbauer. "Comparison of Hormonal Activity (Estrogen, Androgen and Progestin) of Standardized Plant Extracts for Large Scale Use in Hormone Replacement Therapy." *Journal of Steroid Biochemistry & Molecular Biology* 84 (2003): 259–268.

Coon, Joanna Thompson, Max H. Pittler, and Edzard Ernst. "Trifolium Pratense Isoflavones in the Treatment of Menopausal Hot Flushes: A Systematic Review and Meta–Analysis." *Phytomedicine* 14 (2007): 153–159.

Low Dog, Tieraona. "Menopause: A Review of Botanical Dietary Supplements." *The American Journal of Medicine* 118, 12B (2005): 98S–108S.

RED ROOT

Li, Xing–Cong, Cai, Lining, and Wu, D. "ANtimicrobial Compounds from Ceanothus Americanus against Oral Pathogens." *Phytochemisty,* 40, 1 (1997): 97–102.

Baig, Mizra A. and Banthorpe, Derek V. "Accumulation of Tetrapeptide Precursors of Macrocyclic Alkaloids by Callus of Ceanothus Americanus." *Phytochemisty,* 34, 1 (1993): 171–174.

ROSEMARY

Celiktas, O. Yesil, E.E. Hames Kocabas, E. Bedir, F. Vardar Sukan, T. Ozek, and K.H.C. Baser. "Antimicrobial Activities of Methanol Extracts and Essential Oils of Rosmarinus Officinalis, Depending on Location and Seasonal Variations." *Food Chemistry* 100 (2007): 553–559.

Orhan, Ilkay, Sinem Aslan, Murat Kartal, Bilge Sener, and K. Husnu Can Baser. "Inhibitory Effect of Turkish Rosmarinus Officinalis L. on Acetylcholinesterase and Butyrylcholinesterase Enzymes." *Food Chemistry* 108 (2008): 663–668.

Wang, W., N. Wu, Y.G. Zu, and Y.J. Fu. "Antioxidative Activity of Rosmarinus Officinalis L. Essential Oil Compared to its Main Components." *Food Chemistry* 108 (2008): 1019–1022.

SAGE

Al–Yousuf, M.H., A.K. Bashir, B.H. Ali, M.O.M. Tanira, and G. Blunden. "Some Effects of Salvia Aegyptiaca L. on the Central Nervous System in Mice." *Journal of Ethnopharmacology* 81 (2002): 121–127.

Aleksovski, S.A. and H. Sovova. "Supercritical CO_2 Extraction of Salvia Officinalis L." *J. of Supercritical Fluids* 40 (2007): 239–245.

Baricevic, D., S. Sosa, R. Della Loggia, A. Tubaro, B. Simonovska, A. Krasna, and A. Zupancic. "Topical Anti–Inflammatory Activity of Salvia Officinalis L. Leaves: The Relevance of Ursolic Acid." *Journal of Ethnopharmacology* 75 (2001): 125–132.

Gali–Muhtasib, Hala, Christo Hilan, and Carla Khater. "Traditional Uses of Salvia Libanotica (East Mediterranean Sage) and the Effects of its Essential Oils." *Journal of Ethnopharmacology* 71 (2000): 513–520.

Lu, Yinrong and L. Yeap Foo. "Polyphenolics of Salvia—A Review." *Phytochemistry* 59 (2002): 117–140.

Miliauskas, G., P.R. Venskutonis, and T.A. van Beek. "Screening of Radical Scavenging Activity of some Medicinal and Aromatic Plant Extracts." *Food Chemistry* 85 (2004) 231–237.

Perry, Nicolette S.L., Chloe Bollen, Elaine K. Perry, and Clive Ballard. "Salvia for Dementia Therapy: Review of Pharmacological Activity and Pilot Tolerability Clinical Trial." *Pharmacology, Biochemistry and Behavior* 75 (2003): 651–659.

Radulescu, Valeria, Silvia Chiliment, and Eliza Oprea. "Capillary Gas Chromatography–Mass Spectrometry of Volatile and Semi–Volatile Compounds of Salvia Officinalis." *Journal of Chromatography A*, 1027 (2004): 121–126.

Savelev, S., E. Okello, N.S.L. Perry, R.M. Wilkins, and E.K. Perry. "Synergistic and Antagonistic Interactions of Anticholinesterase Terpenoids in Salvia Lavandulaefolia Essential Oil." *Pharmacology, Biochemistry and Behavior* 75 (2003): 661–668.

Tepe, Bektas, Dimitra Daferera, Atalay Sokmen, Munevver Sokmen, and Moschos Polissiou. "Antimicrobial and Antioxidant Activities of the Essential Oil and Various Extracts of Salvia Tomentosa Miller (Lamiaceae)." *Food Chemistry* (2003).

Tepe, Bektas, Erol Donmez, Mehmet Unlu, Ferda Candan, Dimitra Daferera, N.T.J. Tildesley, D.O. Kennedy, E.K. Perry, C.G. Ballard, S. Savelev, K.A. Wesnes, and A.B. Scholey. "Salvia Lavandulaefolia (Spanish Sage) Enhances Memory in Healthy Young Volunteers." *Pharmacology, Biochemistry and Behavior* 75 (2003): 669–674.

Vardar–Unlu, Gülhan, Moschos Polissiou, and Atalay Sokmen. "Antimicrobial and Antioxidative Activities of the Essential Oils and Methanol Extracts of Salvia Cryptantha (Montbret et Aucher ex Benth.) and Salvia Multicaulis (Vahl)." *Food Chemistry* 84 (2004): 519–525.

Wake, George, Jennifer Court, Anne Pickering, Rhiannon Lewis, Richard Wilkins, and Elaine Perry. "CNS Acetylcholine Receptor Activity in European Medicinal Plants Traditionally Used to Improve Failing Memory." *Journal of Ethnopharmacology* 69 (2000): 105–114.

SENNA

Barbosa, Francisco G., Maria da Conceicao F. de Oliveira, Raimundo Braz–Filho, and Edilberto R. Silveira. "Anthraquinones and Naphthopyrones from Senna Rugosa." *Biochemical Systematics and Ecology* 32 (2004): 363–365.

Djozan, DJ and Y. Assadi. "Determination of

Anthraquinones in Rhubarb Roots, Dock Flowers and Senna Leaves by Normal–Phase High Performance Liquid Chromatography." *Talanta* 42, 6 (1995): 861–865.

Fairbairn, J. W. and A.B. Shrestha. "The Distribution of Anthraquinone Glycosides in Cassia Senna L." *Phytochemistry* 6 (1967): 1203–1207.

SHEPARD'S PURSE

Kurode, Keiko and Tenmin Kaku. "Pharmacological and Chemical Studies on the Alcohol Extract of Capsella Bursa–Pastoris." *Life Sciences* 8 (1989): 151–155.

Mukherjee, Kumar D., I. Kiewitt and H. Hurka. "Lipid Content and Fatty Acid Composition of Seeds of Capsella Species from Different Geographical Locations." *Phytochemistry* 23, 1 (1984): 117–119.

SLIPPERY ELM

Lans, Cheryl, N. Turner, T. Khan, and G. Brauer. "Ethnoveterinary Medicines Used to Treat Endoparasites and Stomach Problems in Pigs and Pets in British Columbia, Canada." *Veterinary Parasitology* 148 (2007): 325–340.

SPEARMINT

Arumugam, P., N. Gayatri Priya, M. Subathra, and A. Ramesh. "Anti–Inflammatory Activity of Four Solvent Fractions of Ethanol Extract of Mentha Spicata L. Investigated on Acute and Chronic Inflammation Induced Rats." *Environmental Toxicology and Pharmacology* 26 (2008): 92–95.

Choudhury, R. Paul, A. Kumar, and A.N. Garg. "Analysis of Indian Mint (Mentha Spicata) for Essential, Trace and Toxic Elements and its Antioxidant Behaviour." *Journal of Pharmaceutical and Biomedical Analysis* 41 (2006): 825–832.

Vian, Maryline Abert, Xavier Fernandez, Franco Visinoni, and Farid Chemat. "Microwave Hydrodiffusion and Gravity, a New Technique for Extraction of Essential Oils." *Journal of Chromatography A* 1190 (2008): 14–17.

ST. JOHN'S WORT

Fritz, Daniela, Caroline Rita Venturi, Simone Cargnin, Jan Schripsema, Paulo Michel Roehe, Jarbas Alves Montanha, and Gilsane Lino von Poser. "Herpes Virus Inhibitory Substances from Hypericum Connatum Lam., a Plant Used in Southern Brazil to Treat Oral Lesions." *Journal of Ethnopharmacology* 113 (2007): 517–520.

Linde, K. and L. Knuppel. "Large–Scale Observational Studies of Hypericum Extracts in Patients with Depressive Disorders—A Systematic Review." *Phytomedicine* 12 (2005): 148–157.

Piovan, Anna, Raffaella Filippini, Rosy Caniato, Anna Borsarini, Laura Bini Maleci, and Elsa Mariella Cappellettia. "Detection of Hypericins in the "Red Glands" of Hypericum Elodes by ESI–MS/MS." *Phytochemistry* 65 (2004): 411–414.

Sanchez, C.C. Mateo, B. Prado, and R.M. Rabanal. "Antidepressant Effects of the Methanol Extract of several Hypericum Species from the Canary Islands." *Journal of Ethnopharmacology* 79 (2002): 119–127.

TEA

Ferrara, Lydia, Domenico Montesano, and Alfonso Senatore. "The Distribution of Minerals and Flavonoids in the Tea Plant (Camellia Sinensis)." *Il Farmaco* 56 (2001): 397–401.

Chen, Haixia, Min Zhang, Zhishuang Qu, and Bijun Xie. "Antioxidant Activities of Different Fractions of Polysaccharide Conjugates from Green Tea (Camellia Sinensis)." *Food Chemistry* 106 (2008): 559–563.

Ikigai, Hajime, Taiji Nakae, Yukihiko Hara, and Tadakatsu Shimamura. "Bactericidal Catechins Damage the Lipid Bilayer." *Biochimica et Biophysica Acta* 1147 (1993): 132–136.

Ishihara, N., D.–C. Chu, S. Akachi, and L.R. Juneja. "Improvement of Intestinal Microflora Balance and Prevention of Digestive and Respiratory Organ Diseases in Calves by Green Tea Extracts." *Livestock Production Science* 68 (2001): 217–229.

Lambert, Joshua D. and Chung S. Yang. "Cancer Chemopreventive Activity and Bioavailability of Tea and Tea Polyphenols." *Mutation Research* 523–524 (2003): 201–208.

Limsong, Jittra, E. Benjavongkulchai, and Jintakorn Kuvatanasuchati. "Inhibitory Effect of Some Herbal Extracts on Adherence of Streptococcus Mutans." *Journal of Ethnopharmacology* 92 (2004): 281–289.

Khan, Naghma and Hasan Mukhtar. "Tea Polyphenols for Health Promotion." *Life Sciences* 81 (2007): 519–533.

Santhosh, K.T., J. Swarnam, and K. Ramadasan. "Potent Suppressive Effect of Green Tea Polyphenols on Tobacco–Induced Mutagenicity." *Phytomedicine* 12 (2005): 216–220.

Weisburger, John H. "Tea and Health: a Historical Perspective." *Cancer Letters* 114 (1997): 315–317.

Yam, T.S., Saroj Shah, and J.M.T. Hamilton–Miller. "Microbiological Activity of Whole and Fractionated Crude Extracts of Tea (Camellia Sinensis), and of Tea Components." *FEMS Microbiology Letters* 152 (1997): 169–174.

Yang, Chung S., Joshua D. Lambert, Jihyeung Ju, Gang Lu, and Shengmin Sang. "Tea and Cancer Prevention: Molecular Mechanisms and Human Relevance." *Toxicology and Applied Pharmacology* 224 (2007): 265–273.

TEA TREE

Carson, C. F., T. V. Riley, and B. D. Cookson. "Efficacy and Safety of Tea Tree Oil as a Topical Antimicrobial Agent." *Journal of Hospital Infection* 40 (1998): 75–78.

Hammer, Katherine A., Christine F. Carson, and Thomas V. Riley. "Frequencies of Resistance to Melaleuca Alternifolia (Tea Tree) Oil and Rifampicin in Staphylococcus Aureus, Staphylococcus Epidermidis and Enterococcus Faecalis." *International Journal of Antimicrobial Agents* 32 (2008): 170–173.

Hammer, K.A., C.F. Carson, T.V. Riley, and J.B. Nielsen. "A Review of the Toxicity of Melaleuca Alternifolia (Tea Tree) Oil." *Food and Chemical Toxicology* 44 (2006): 616–625.

Traboulsi, Rana S., Pranab K. Mukherjee, and Mahmoud A. Ghannoum. "In Vitro Activity of Inexpensive Topical Alternatives Against Candida spp. Isolated from the Oral Cavity of HIV–Infected Patients." *International Journal of Antimicrobial Agents* 31 (2008): 272–276.

THUJA

Katoh, Takahiro, Taichi Akagi, Chie Noguchi, Tetsuya Kajimoto, Manabu Node, Reiko Tanaka, Manabu Nishizawa (nee Iwamoto), Hironori Ohtsu, Noriyuki Suzuki, and Koichi Saito. "Synthesis of DL–Standishinal and its Related Compounds for the Studies on Structure–Activity Relationship of Inhibitory Activity Against Aromatase." *Bioorganic & Medicinal Chemistry* 15 (2007): 2736–2748.

Kawai, Shingo, Kazuhiro Sugishita, and Hideo Ohashi. "Identification of Thuja Occidentalis Lignans and its Biosynthetic Relationship." *Phytochemistry* 51 (1999): 243–247.

Kawai, Shingo, Takao Hasegawa, Maiko Gotoh, and Hidea Oshashi. "4–O–Dethylyatein from the Branch Wood of Thuja Occidentalis." *Phytochemistry* 37, 6 (1994): 1699–1702.

Larson, D.W. "The Paradox of Great Longevity in a Short–Lived Tree Species." *Experimental Gerontology* 36 (2001): 651–673.

Yatagai, Mitsuyoshi, Toshiya Sato, and Toshio Takahashi. "Terpenes of Leaf Oils from Cupressaceae." *Biochemic Systematics and Ecology* 13, 4 (1985): 377–385.

TURMERIC

Aggarwal, Bharat B. and Kuzhuvelil B. Harikumar. "Potential Therapeutic Effects of Curcumin, the Anti–Inflammatory Agent, Against Neurodegenerative, Cardiovascular, Pulmonary, Metabolic, Autoimmune and Neoplastic Diseases." *The International Journal of Biochemistry & Cell Biology* xxx (2008): xxx–xxx (Article in Press).

Bosca', Ana Ramirez, Alfonso Soler, Miguel A. Carrion–Gutierrez, David Pamies Mira, Jose' Pardo Zapata, Joaquın Diaz–Alperi, August Bernd, Eliseo Quintanilla Almagro, and Jaime Miquel. "An Hydroalcoholic Extract of Curcuma Longa Lowers the Abnormally High Values of Human–Plasma Fibrinogen." *Mechanisms of Ageing and Development* 114 (2000): 207–210.

Gupta, Babita, Balaram Ghosh. "Curcuma Longa Inhibits TNF–a Induced Expression of Adhesion Molecules on Human Umbilical Vein Endothelial Cells." *International Journal of Immunopharmacology* 21 (1999): 745–757.

Jantan, I., S.M. Raweh, H.M. Sirat, S. Jamil, Y.H. Mohd Yasin, J. Jalil, and J.A. Jamal. "Inhibitory Effect of Compounds from Zingiberaceae Species on Human Platelet Aggregation." *Phytomedicine* 15 (2008): 306–309.

Johnson, Jeremy James and Hasan Mukhtar. "Curcumin for Chemoprevention of Colon Cancer." *Cancer Letters* 255 (2007): 170–181.

Peschel, Dieter, Ramona Koerting, Norbert Nass. "Curcumin Induces Changes in Expression of Genes Involved in Cholesterol Homeostasis." *Journal of Nutritional Biochemistry* 18 (2007): 113–119.

Wang, Li–Yao, Mian Zhang, Chao–Feng Zhang, and Zheng–Tao Wang. "Diaryl Derivatives from the Root Tuber of Curcuma Longa." *Biochemical Systematics and Ecology* 36 (2008): 476–480.

Watson, Jane L., Richard Hill, Patrick W. Lee, Carman A. Giacomantonio, and David W. Hoskin. "Curcumin Induces Apoptosis in HCT–116 Human Colon Cancer Cells in a p21–Independent Manner." *Experimental and Molecular Pathology* 84 (2008): 230–233.

Yodkeeree, Supachai, Wittaya haiwangyen, Spiridione Garbisa, Pornngarm Limtrakul. "Demethoxycurcumin and Bisdemethoxycurcumin Differentially Inhibit Cancer Cell Invasion Through the Down–Regulation of MMPs and uPA." *Journal of Nutritional Biochemistry* xx (2008): xxx–xxx (Article in Press).

Zhang, J.S., J. Guan, F.Q. Yang, H.G. Liu, X.J. Cheng, and S.P. Li. "Qualitative and Quantitative Analysis of Four Species of Curcuma Rhizomes Using Twice Development Thin Layer Chromatography." *Journal of Pharmaceutical and Biomedical Analysis* 48 (2008): 1024–1028.

UVA–URSI

Dykes, Gary A., Ryszard Amarowicz, and Ronald B. Pegg. "Enhancement of Nisin Antibacterial Activity by a Bearberry (Arctostaphylos Uva–ursi) Leaf Extract." *Food Microbiology* 20 (2003): 211–216.

Grases, F., G. Melero, A. Costa–Bauza, R. Prieto, and J.G. March. "Urolithiasis and Phytotherapy." *International Urology and Nephrology* 26, 5 (1994): 505–511

VALERIAN

Abourashed, E.A., U. Koetter, and A. Brattstrom. "In Vitro Binding Experiments with a Valerian, Hops and Their Fixed Combination Extract (Ze91019) to Selected Central Nervous System Receptors." *Phytomedicine* 11 (2004): 633–638.

Bent, Stephen, A. Padula, D. Moore, M. Patterson, and W. Mehling. "Valerian for Sleep: A Systematic Review and Meta–Analysis." *The American Journal of Medicine* 119 (2006): 1005–1012.

Fernandez, Sebastian P., C. Wasowski, A.C. Paladini, and M. Marder. "Synergistic Interaction Between Hesperidin, a Natural Flavonoid, and Diazepam." *European Journal of Pharmacology* 512 (2005): 189–198.

Francis, A.J.P. and R.J.W. Dempster. "Effect of Valerian, Valeriana Edulis, on Sleep Difficulties in Children with Intellectual Deficits: Randomised Trial." *Phytomedicine* 9 (2002):

273–279.

Lacher, Svenja K., R. Mayer, K. Sichardt, K. Nieber, and C.E. Muller. "Interaction of Valerian Extracts of Different Polarity with Adenosine Receptors: Identification of Isovaltrate as an Inverse Agonist at A1 Receptors. *Biochemical-pharmacology* 73 (2007): 248–258.

Leathwood, Peter D., F. Chauffard, E. Heck, and R. Munoz–Box. "Aqueous Extract of Valerian Root (Valeriana officinalis L.) Improves Sleep Quality in Man." *Pharmacology Biochemistry & Behavior* 17 (1982): 65–71.

Stevinson, Clare and E. Ernst. "Valerian for Insomnia: A Systematic Review of Randomized Clinical Trials." *Sleep Medicine* 1 (2000): 91–99.

WHITE WILLOW

Chrubasik, Sigrun, Elon Eisenberg, Edith Balan, Tuvia Weinberger, Rachel Luzzati, and Christian Conradt. "Treatment of Low Back Pain Exacerbations with Willow Bark Extract: A Randomized Double–Blind Study." *The American Journal of Medicine* 109 (2000): 9–14.

Orians, Colin M., Megan E. Griffiths, Bernadette M. Roche, and Robert S. Fritz. "Phenolic Glycosides and Condensed Tannins in Salix Sericea, S. Eriocephala and their F1 Hybrids: Not All Hybrids are Created Equal." *Biochemical Systematics and Ecology* 28 (2000): 619–632.

Tunón, H., C. Olavsdotter, and L. Bohlin. "Evaluation of Anti–Inflammatory Activity of some Swedish Medicinal Plants. Inhibition of Prostaglandin Biosynthesis and PAF–Induced Exocytosis." *Journal of Ethnopharmacology* 48 (1995): 61–76.

WILD INDIGO

Bodinet, C, U. Lindequist, E. Teuscher, and J. Freudenstein. "Effect of an Orally Applied Herbal Immunomodulator on Cytokine Induction and Antibody Response in Normal and Immunosuppressed Mice." *Phytomedi-cine* 9 (2002): 606–613.

Classena, B., S. Thude, W. Blaschek, M. Wack, and C. Bodinet. "Immunomodulatory Effects of Arabinogalactan–Proteins from Baptisia and Echinacea." *Phytomedicine* 13 (2006): 688–694.

Markham, K.R., T.J. Mabry, and W.T. Swift, Jr. "Distribution of Flavonoids in the Genus Baptisia (Leguminosae)." *Phytochemistry* 9 (1970): 2359–2364.

Naser, B., B. Lund, H.H. Henneicke–von Zepelin, G. Kohler, W. Lehmacher, and F. Scaglione. "A Randomized, Double–Blind, Placebo–Controlled, Clinical Dose–Response Trial of an Extract of Baptisia, Echinacea and Thuja for the Treatment of Patients with Common Cold." *Phytomedicine* 12 (2005): 715–722.

WILD YAM

Laveaga, Gabriela Soto. "Uncommon trajectories: Steroid Hormones, Mexican Peasants, and the Search for a Wild Yam." *Stud. Hist. Phil. Biol. & Biomed. Sci.* 36 (2005): 743–760.

Norton, Scott A. "Useful Plants of Dermatology. III. Corticosteroids, Strophanthus, and Dioscorea." *J Am Acad Dermatol* 38 (1998): 256–259.

Pedro, A. and Lehmann F. "Early History of Steroid Chemistry in Mexico: the Story of Three Remarkable Men." *Steroids* 57 (1992): 403–408.

Sautour, M., T. Miyamoto, and M.–A. Lacaille–Dubois. "Steroidal Saponins and Flavan–3–ol glycosides from Dioscorea Villosa." *Biochemical Systematics and Ecology* 34 (2006): 60–63.

WITCH HAZEL

Deters, Alexandra, Andreas Dauer, Esther Schnetz, Manige Fartasch, and Andreas Hensel. "High Molecular Compounds (Polysaccharides and Proanthocyanidins) from Hamamelis Virginiana Bark: Influence on Human Skin Keratinocyte Proliferation and Differentiation and Influence on Irritated Skin." *Phytochemistry* 58 (2001): 949–958.

WORMWOOD

Freitas, Mariana V. de, Rita de Cassia M. Netto, Juliana C. da Costa Huss, Tatiana Maria T. de Souza, Junia O. Costa, Cynthia B. Firmino, Nilson Penha–Silva. "Influence of Aqueous Crude Extracts of Medicinal Plants on the Osmotic Stability of Human Erythrocytes." *Toxicology in Vitro* 22 (2008): 219–224.

Gilani, Anwar–ul Hassan and Khalid Hussain Janbaz. "Effects of Acetaminophen Hepatotoxicity Preventive and Curative Artemisia Absinthium on and CC14–Induced Hepatotoxicity." *Gen. Pharmac* 26 2 (1995): 309–315.

Lutz, Daíse Lopes, Daniela S. Alviano, Celuta S. Alviano, and Paul P. Kolodziejczyk. "Screening of Chemical Composition, Antimicrobial and Antioxidant Activities of Artemisia Essential Oils." *Phytochemistry* 69 (2008): 1732–1738.

Meschler, Justin P. and Allyn C. Howlett. "Thujone Exhibits Low Affinity for Cannabinoid Receptors But Fails to Evoke Cannabimimetic Responses." *Pharmacology Biochemistry and Behavior* 62, 3 (1999): 473–480.

Omer, B., S. Krebs, H. Omer, and T.O. Noor. "Steroid–Sparing Effect of Wormwood (Artemisia Absinthium) in Crohn's Disease: A Double–Blind Placebo–Controlled Study." *Phytomedicine* 14 (2007): 87–95.

YARROW

Benedek, Birgit, B. Kopp, and M.F. Melzig. "Achillea millefolium L. s.l. – Is the Anti–inflammatory Activity Mediated by Protease Inhibition?" *Journal of Ethnopharmacology* 113 (2007): 312–317.

Benedek, B., N. Geisz, W. Jager, T. Thalhammer, and B. Kopp. "Choleretic Effects of Yarrow (Achillea millefolium s.l.) in the Isolated Perfused Rat Liver." *Phytomedicine* 13 (2006): 702–706.

Cavalcanti, A.M., C.H. Baggio, C.S. Freitas, and L. Rieck. " Safety and Antiulcer Efficacy Studies of Achillea Millefolium vL. After Chronic Treatment in Wistar Rats." *Journal of Ethnopharmacology* 107 (2006): 277–284.

Dalsenter, Paulo R., A.M. Cavalcanti, A.J.M. Andrade, S.L. Araújo, and M.C.A. Marques. "Reproductive Evaluation of Aqueous Crude Extract of Achillea Millefolium L. (Asteraceae) in Wistar Rats." *Reproductive Toxicology* 18 (2004): 819–823.

Guedon, Didier, P. Abbe, and J.L. Lamaison. "Leaf and Flower Head Flavonoids of Achillea Millefolium L. Subspecies." *Biochemical Systematics and Ecology* 21, 5 (1993): 607–611.

Innocentia, G., E. Vegetob, S. Dall'Acqua, P. Ciana, M. Giorgetti, E. Agradi, A. Sozzi, G. Fico, and F. Tome. "In Vitro Estrogenic Activity of Achillea Millefolium L." *Phytomedicine* 14 (2007): 147–152.

Kelley, Bruce D., Glenn D. Appelt, and Jennifer M. Appelt. "Pharmacological Aspects of Selected Herbs Employed in Hispanic Folk Medicine in the San Luis Valley of Colorado, USA: II Asclepias Asperula (Inmortal) and Achillea Lanulosa (Plumajillo)." *Journal of Ethnopharmacology* 22 (1988): l–9.

Kubelka, Wolfgang, U. Kastner, S. Glasl, J. Saukel, and J. Jurenitsch. "Chemotaxonomic Relevance of Sesquiterpenes Within the Achillea Millefolium Group." *Biochemical Systematics and Ecology* 27 (1999): 437–444.

Kültür, A."Medicinal Plants used in Kırklareli Province (Turkey)." *Journal of Ethnopharmacology* 111 (2007): 341–364.

Lans, Cheryl, N. Turner, T. Khan, and G. Brauer. "Ethnoveterinary Medicines Used to Treat Endoparasites and Stomach Problems in Pigs and Pets in British Columbia, Canada." *Veterinary Parasitology* 148 (2007): 325–340.

Lietave, Jan. "Medicinal Plants in a Middle Paleolithic Grave Shanidar IV?" *Journul of Ethnopharmacology* 35 (1992): 263–266.

Mockute, Danute and A. Judzentiene. "Variability of the Essential Oils Composition of Achillea Millefolium ssp. Millefolium Growing Wild in Lithuania." *Biochemical Systematics and Ecology* 31 (2003): 1033–1045.

YELLOWDOCK

Fairbairn, J. W. and F.J. El–Muhtadi. "Chemotaxonomy of Anthraquinones in Rumex." *Phytochemistry* 11 (1972): 263–268.

Saleh, Nabiel A.M., Mohamed N. El–Hadidi, and Raafat F.M. Arafa. "Flavonoids and Anthraquinones of some Egyptian Rumex Species (Polygonaceae)." *Biochemical Systematics and Ecology* 21, 2 (1993): 301–303.

YERBA SANTA

Bacon, John D., Gary L. Hannan, Nianbai Fang, and Tom J. Mabry. "Chemosystematics of the Hydrophyllaceae" Flavonoids of Three Species of Eriodictyon." *Biochemical Systematics and Ecology* 14, 6 (1986): 591–595.

Johnson, Nelson D. "Flavonoid Aglycones from Eriodictyon Californicum Resin and their Implications for Herbivory and UV Screening." *Biochemical Systematics and Ecology* 11, 3 (1963): 211–215.

Salle, A. J., Gregory J. Jarm, and Lawrence G. Wayne. "Studies on the Antibacterial Properties of Eriodictyon Californicum." From the Department of Baceriology, University of California, Los Angeles, California (1951).

YUCCA

Hussain, I., A.M. Ismail, and P.R. Cheeke. "Effects of Feeding Yucca Schidigera Extract in Diets Varying in Crude Protien and Urea Contents on Growth Performance and Cecum and Blood Urea and Ammonia Concentrations of Rabbits." *Animal Feed Science Technology* 62, (1996): 121–129.

Hussain, I. and P.R. Cheeke. "Effect of Dietary Yucca Schidigera Extract on Rumen and Blood Profiles of Steers Fed Concentrate or Roughage–Based Diets." *Animal Feed Science and Technology* 51 (1995): 231–242.

Wang, Y., T.A. McAllister, C.J. Newbold, L.M. Rode, P.R. Cheeke, and K–J. Cheng. "Effects of Yucca Schidigera Extract on Fermentation and Degradation of Steroidal Saponins in the Rumen Simulation Technique (RUSITEC)[1]." *Animal Feed Science and Technology* 74 (1998): 143–153.

GLOSSARY

Abscess

An accumulation of pus (defunct leukocytes, damaged tissue cells, and cellular wastes) within tissues or organs either resolving by coming to "a head" or diminishing internally.

Acetylcholine

Serves as a neurotransmitter throughout the central and peripheral nervous systems, though it is most closely associated with the parasympathetic branch of the autonomic nervous system.

Acetylcholinesterase (AChE)

An enzyme of the central nervous system that breaks down acetylcholine into choline and acetate.

Achene

A term used to describe a seed common to the Sunflower family.

Adaptogen

A somewhat vague term used widely in the herbal medicine field to describe a plant which is capable of increasing an individual's tolerance to stress. Actions of these plants often seem contradictory, at times providing stimulation and at others, sedation. Ginseng is considered a classic adaptogen.

Addison's disease

A life threatening disease caused by tuberculosis or autoimmune involvement. Symptoms of hypotension, abnormal skin pigmentation, weight loss, and weakness are caused by diminished levels of adrenal cortex hormones, cortisol and aldosterone.

Adrenal cortex

The outer layer of the adrenal gland; secretes mineralocorticoids and glucocorticoids.

Adrenal medulla

Inner layer of the adrenal gland; secrets catecholamines epinephrine and norepinephrine.

Adrenaline

(Epinephrine) Both a catecholamine hormone and a neurotransmitter. It is secreted by the adrenal medulla and is used by the sympathetic branch of the central nervous system. It is a prominent physiologic agent in flight or flight reactions and low–grade stress states.

Albumin

A plasma protein crucial in transporting many organic substances – bile acids, hormones, and fatty acids. It is also important in maintaining proper plasma osmotic pressure. Plasma albumin levels diminish in certain renal and hepatic diseases, and if dietary levels of protein are insufficient.

Aldosterone

A mineralocorticoid secreted by the adrenal cortex; it is involved in sodium/potassium dynamics and blood pressure.

Allopathic

Pertaining to present day conventional medicine when solely used to suppress or oppose symptoms, such as steroids for inflammation, analgesics for pain, etc.

Alterative

Pertaining to the quality, or a substance (usually an herbal medicine) that positively alters organs or functions of elimination, detoxification, or immunity.

Alveoli

(Pulmonary alveoli) Small sacs within the lungs where carbon dioxide and oxygen exchange takes place.

Alzheimer's disease

A progressive brain disease with a number of potential causative factors. Senile plaques, neurofibrillary tangles, and loss of acetyltransferase activity are common. Progressed effects are dementia and personality change.

Amebiasis

(Montezuma's revenge or Traveler's diarrhea) An intestinal infection involving Entamoeba histolytica from contaminated food or water. Usually the large intestine is affected but in severe cases infection can migrate to the liver, spleen, brain, lungs, and other areas.

Amenorrhea

The abnormal cessation of menses, often due to extreme weight loss, physical–emotional stress, or the alteration of ovarian hormones.

Amylase

Present in saliva and pancreatic juice this enzyme breaks down starches into simple sugars.

Anaphrodisiac

That which curbs libido.

Anaphylaxis

A potentially life threatening allergic reaction; shock and respiratory distress usually accompanies the episode.

Androgen

Any substance, but usually hormonal, that promotes masculinization. Testosterone and androstenedione are examples.

Anesthetic

An agent that causes numbness or reduces/eliminates pain sensations.

Angina pectoris

A particular spasmodic, suffocative pain due to heart tissue ischemia; radiating left arm pain is a common symptom. An episode may be precipitated by physical exertion and is caused by coronary artery obstruction from plaque buildup.

Annual

Any plant that germinates, then sets seed and dies in one year.

Anorexia

Simply the lack of appetite for food. Anorexia nervosa, more complex than a simple loss of appetite, is considered a mental disorder.

Anovulatory cycle

A menstrual cycle without ovulation.

Antibody

(See Immunoglobulin)

Anticholinergic

Inhibiting to the parasympathetic nervous system; pertaining to any substance whether pharmaceutical, herbal, or otherwise that lessens gastrointestinal tract, mucosal, and skin secretion and excretion.

Antigen

A substance capable of stimulating a specific acquired immune response. Bacteria and foreign particles are prime examples.

Antiseptic

Inhibiting to the growth and spread of microorganisms.

Antiviral

Inhibiting to virus reproduction or its cellular attachment.

Aphrodisiac

A sexual excitant.

Aphthous stomatitis

(Canker sore) A small white ulcer of the oral mucosa. Stress, immune deficiency, and allergic reaction are common underlying factors.

Apoptosis

The innate process of programed cell death. When operating properly this function is a key cancer inhibitor. Many illnesses are linked to an excess or lack of apoptosis.

Arachidonic acid (AA)

An essential fatty acid intrinsic to prostaglandin, leukotriene, and thromboxane synthesis. It holds a place in both normal cellular process and disease development.

Arrhythmia

Irregular rhythm of the heartbeat.

Asthenic

Weakness; deficiency.

Asthma

A condition of bronchial constriction due to spasm or autoimmune inflammation.

Asthma, humid

Asthma with copious expectoration.

Atherosclerosis

Arterial inflammation in conjunction with plaque deposits. Also known as "hardening of the arteries".

Atonic

Lacking normal tone.

Autonomic nervous system

Composed of the sympathetic and parasympathetic nervous systems; mainly involved with visceral function.

Ayurveda

Traditional Indian medicine. Thought to predate Traditional Chinese Medicine, the system describes herbs as having energetic qualities and people being of different constitutional types.

Basophil

A granular leukocyte involved in innate immunity.

Bedsore

Ulcer development from bed confinement; lack of circulation and continual pressure are factors in development.

Benign prostrate hypertrophy (BPH)

Prostrate enlargement associated with age and corresponding DHT levels.

Bifidobacteria

One of a number of gram–positive, anaerobic bacteria belonging to the Bifidobacterium genus. Common species found in the large bowel are B. adolescentis, B. eriksonii, and B. infantis.

Bile

An alkaline liquid secreted by the liver composed of cholesterol, bile salts, phospholipids, bilirubin diglucuronide, and electrolytes. It is essential for fat digestion.

Boil

(Furuncle) A painful, subcutaneous nodule with an enclosed core. Usually caused by Staphylococci entering through hair follicles, liver and immune deficiencies are common constitutional factors.

Bract

A modified leaf situated at the base of a flower.

Bradycardia

Slowed heart rate; slower than 60 beat per minute (common for athletes and young adults).

Bronchitis

Mechanical, bacterial, viral, or allergy induced inflammation of one or more bronchi.

Bronchorrhoea

Excessive lung airway discharge.

Canker sores

(See Aphthous stomatitis)

Cardiac glycoside

Glycosides found in some Cactus, Figwort, Dogbane, and Lily family plants. In therapeutic doses, they are slowing and strengthening to the heart.

Carminative

A term used to describe a medicine that relieves gas pains and bloating.

Catkin

(Ament) A compact male or female, spike–like inflorescence, typically found in Willow or Birch family plants.

Central nervous system

The segment of the nervous system consisting of the brain and spinal cord.

Cervical dysplasia

Cellular changes in the epithelium of the cervix; regarded as a precursor to carcinoma. HPV infection is thought to be the main inducer of tissue alteration.

Cervicitis

Inflammation of the cervix, either due to infection or injury.

Chicken pox

(Varicella–zoster) A contagious herpes virus causing reddened and itching vesicles.

Cholecystokinin (CCK)

Both a hormone secreted by the upper small intestine and by the hypothalamus as a neurotransmitter. It stimulates gallbladder contraction, secretion of pancreatic enzymes, and in response to food it is involved in feelings of satiety and fullness.

Cholesterol

A common sterol produced by the liver and obtained from the diet. It is involved in cell–membrane structure, is a base for steroidal hormones, and is the precursor in bile formation. It is a contributing factor in arterial plaques and in some gallstones.

Choleretic

Either an activity or an agent that stimulates bile production by the liver.

Cholinergic

(Parasympathomimetic) Referring to autonomic nerve fibers that use acetylcholine as a neurotransmitter.

Chologogue

Any substance that stimulates bile release from the gallbladder. Many of these herbs are choleretics as well.

Coccidioides immitis

The fungus responsible for Coccidioidomy-cosis or Valley fever.

Coccidioidomycosis

(Valley fever) The disease caused by Coccidioides immitis. Primary manifestations are cough, fever, and joint pain. The infection is usually self–resolving but can be serious in some racial groups and immune compromised individuals.

Collagenation

The process of collagen formation in cartilage or other tissues.

Colonic flora

Bacterial strains existing in the large intestine, many of which are necessary for gastrointestinal and systemic health.

Condyloma acuminatum

(Venereal or genital warts) caused by Human papillomavirus (HPV). Infectious and sexually transmitted, infection predisposes women to cervical dysplasia.

Conjunctivitis

An inflammation of the conjunctiva, typically involving redness, swelling, and discharge. There can be bacterial, viral, mechanical, or allergic involvement.

Corpus luteum

A temporary glandular mass located in the ovary; secretes progesterone during pregnancy and throughout part of the menstrual cycle.

Corticosteroids

Two groups of hormones secreted by the adrenal cortex: glucocorticoids (cortisol) and mineralocorticoids (aldosterone).

Cortisol

The main glucocorticoid secreted by the adrenal cortex. It is involved in glucose, protein, and fat metabolism, stress response, and immunity.

Cyclooxygenase

An enzyme or activity involved in prostaglandin synthesis, particularly inflammatory processes.

Cystitis

Inflammation of the urinary bladder.

Deciduous

Describing a plant that is not evergreen; herbage falling from the plant seasonally.

Dehydroepiandrosterone (DHEA)

An adrenal cortex steroid hormone. It plays a large role as an androgen precursor in premenopausal women and as a major androgen in postmenopausal women. Supplementation in women can often cause masculine tendencies.

Dementia

Loss of cognitive ability, memory, and judgement. Alzheimer's disease, stroke, or a variety of neurological diseases are common causes.

Demulcent

A quality or an agent that is soothing and allays irritation of surface tissues. Most in this class are mucilaginous or oily.

Diaphoresis

Perspiration or sweating.

Diaphoretic

A substance that promotes sweating (diaphoresis) or the activity of something that promotes sweating.

5–α–dihydrotestosterone (DHT)

Formed through 5–α–reductase's activity on testosterone, DHT is both an important androgen and one of the main causes of BPH and male pattern baldness.

Dioecious

Imperfect male and female flowers borne on different plants.

Diuretic

A substance that promotes urine excretion or the activity of increasing urine excretion.

Doctrine of Signatures

A philosophy of resemblance applied to herbal medicine popular up until the 17th century. Example: if in some way a plant resembles a heart it is a medicine for that organ.

Dopamine

A catecholamine–type neurotransmitter, widely acting throughout the central nervous system.

Duodenal ulcer

An ulcer of the upper small intestine or duodenum.

Dust cells

(Alveolar macrophage or Alveolar phagocyte) A phagocyte that resides within the lung's alveoli; they ingest inhaled particulate matter and are important in pulmonary immunity.

Dysmenorrhea

Painful menstruation.

Dyspepsia

Faulty digestion, resulting in discomfort, gas, and sometimes, gastrointestinal tract stasis.

Eclectics

A school of medicine existing up until the mid 20th century, devoted to potentiated plant medicines and treatment of the individual (not just the symptom).

Edema

Increased intercellular fluid buildup from numerous causes, but typically from kidney or heart dysfunction, or venous or lymphatic obstruction.

Emmenagogue

Something that induces menstruation.

Endometriosis

A condition where endometrial tissue develops in other than normal areas (ex pelvic cavity). Cyclic pain and inflammation are common symptoms.

Endometrium

Inner mucus membrane layer of the uterus.

Entamoeba histolytica

A common ameboid protozoa; the cause of amebiasis. Severe infections may affect the lungs, liver, spleen, and other organs.

Enteric

Of the small intestine.

Enteric coated

A coating applied to a tablet or capsule specially designed to breakdown in the small intestine.

Entire

Referring to the margin of a leaf; not toothed, lobed, or divided, but continuous.

Eosinophil

A granular leukocyte involved in innate immunity; it is specific to parasite defence.

Erythrocyte

(Red blood cell) A main component of blood; responsible for oxygen transport.

Escherichia coli

A gram negative, anaerobic bacterium normally found in the large intestine. The organism typically causes urinary tract infections. Colonization often takes place through poor hygiene and alkaline urine.

Essential oil

Non–polar, volatile oil content of an aromatic plant. Commonly extracted through distillation. Mint family plants are typical subjects.

Essential hypertension

(Idiopathic or primary hypertension) Elevated blood pressure without organic causes. It is largely a functional problem with sodium intake, weight, and stress being primary causative agents.

Estrogen

A hormone found in both sexes; necessary for proper female sexual development, reproductive health, and pregnancy.

Eupatory tribe

A division of the Sunflower family. Plants in this division are apt to contain either toxic or non–toxic pyrrolizidine alkaloids. The Brickellia and Eupatorium genera are both in this tribe.

Extracellular fluid

Pertaining to fluid outside of a cell, such as lymphatic fluid.

Fibroid

(Uterine leiomyoma) A benign tumor composed of smooth muscle usually developing in the myometrium of the uterus during a women's 30s or 40s.

Flavonoids

A group of phenolic compounds closely related to tannins; many have therapeutic effects on cell/tissue structure.

Follicle stimulating hormone (FSH)

A pituitary hormone necessary for women's follicle maturation and in men, proper spermatogenesis.

Fusarium

A genus of fungi; a number of species are pathogenic to man.

Gamma–aminobutyric acid (GABA)

A key inhibitory neurotransmitter found throughout the central nervous system.

Gastritis

Inflammation of the stomach often caused from stress, poor diet, mechanical insults, or pharmaceutical side effects.

Gastroenteritis

Inflammation of the stomach and intestinal lining. It can be viral or bacterial initiated, and in some cases, is triggered by intense adrenergic reaction. It is most commonly the result of food poisoning.

Genital warts

(See Condyloma acuminatum)

Giardia

A parasite in humans and in other vertebrates, commonly spread by contaminated food, water, and direct human/animal contact. Giardia lamblia is the most notorious species. The organism attaches itself to the microvilli of the intestinal walls causing diarrhea, nausea, weight loss, and fatigue among other symptoms.

Gingivitis

An acute or chronic inflammation of the gingivae or gums.

Glaucoma

A group of eye diseases caused by increased intraocular pressure. Changes in the optic disk and ultimately blindness occur if left untreated.

Glomerulonephritis

Inflammation of the capillary structures in the glomeruli of the kidney from a residual hemolytic infection or autoimmune involvement.

Glucose–6–phosphate–dehydrogenase deficiency (G6PD)

A genetic deficiency causing, to varying degrees, hemolytic anemia.

Glutathione

An important naturally occurring tripeptide involved in detoxification and antioxidant functions.

Glycogen

The primary storage carbohydrate found in liver and muscle tissue. It is broken down into glucose.

Gout, primary

Affecting 30–50 year old men and post–menopausal women, symptoms are due to improper purine metabolism resulting in urate crystals forming around the joints and as urinary deposits. If left unchecked it can be painful and debilitating.

Granulocyte

Typically a neutrophil, basophil, or eosinophil that contain immunologic granules that when released heighten inflammatory–defense processes.

Helicobacter pylori

(Campylobacter pylori) A gram–negative bacterium involved in gastric ulcer formation and gastritis.

Hematuria

Blood in the urine.

Hemolysis

The break down of red blood cell membranes resulting in the liberation of hemoglobin. This can be caused from a myriad of factors but most predominantly, it is triggered by autoimmune reaction, snake venom, micro-organisms, and some plant saponins.

Hemolysis, intravascular

Severe red blood cell breakdown within blood vessels.

Hemorrhoids

A varicosity affecting the anal region.

Hemostatic

An activity or something that slows or stops blood flow; typically astringents or other substances that have a localized or systemic vasoconstrictive effect.

Hepatitis C

Inflammation of the liver caused by the hepatitis C virus. This chronic infection is typically the result of contaminated blood transfusions or intravenous drug use.

Hepatocyte

A liver cell.

Herbaceous

Herb–like. Describing a plant or a portion of a plant that is non–woody.

Herpes zoster

(See Shingles)

Homeopathy

A system of medicine founded by Samuel Hahnemann. "Like treats like" and infinitesimal doses are hallmarks of this system.

Human papillomavirus (HPV)

A significant group of viruses responsible for common and genital warts, cervical dysplasia, and most cases of cervical cancer.

Hyaluronidase

A class of enzymes that breakdown hyaluronic acid. They occur naturally in various tissues and in bee and snake venoms. It is surmised one reason Echinacea is useful in limiting some of the deleterious effects of snakebite is through its antihyaluronidase activity.

Hydrochloric acid (HCL)

Solutions of hydrogen chloride secreted by gastric parietal cells in response to hormonal, local, or nervous system stimulation; necessary for initial protein breakdown in the stomach.

Hydrophilic

(See hygroscopic)

Hydrophobic

Insoluble in water; lacking polar constituents.

Hygroscopic

Absorbing water or having water–interacting polar groups.

Hyperglycemia

Elevated blood glucose levels.

Hyperglycemia, post–prandial

Elevated blood glucose levels after meals.

Hypertension

(See Essential hypertension)

Hypoglycemia

Lowered blood glucose levels.

Immunoglobulin

A specific immune system molecule that interacts only with a particular antigen. They are classed by individual function. (IgM, IgG, IgA, IgD, and IgE)

Immunoglobulin E (IgE)

An antibody that has a significant role in allergic process.

Influenza

(Flu) A highly variable group of RNA viruses belonging to a single sub–type. Affects both people (usually the young and old) and animals.

Insomnia

Inability to sleep.

Insulin dependent diabetes mellitus (IDDM)

(Juvenile onset or Type I) Onset usually occurs in late childhood or in the early teens and is characterized by the destruction of the pancreatic beta cells by viral infection or autoimmune reaction. There is some genetic predisposition as well. Lack of endogenous insulin is the hallmark of IDDM. Reliance upon exogenous insulin is necessary, otherwise hyperglycemia and corresponding problems result. IDDM is difficult to treat solely with natural therapies.

Interleukin

A broad group of immunologic compounds (cytokines); many are produced by T–lymphocytes and macrophages. They are involved in an array of immunologic activities, including inflammatory responses.

Intermittent claudication

Usually dependant upon atherosclerosis and/ or smoking this lack of circulation to the extremities causes pain, cramping, and numbness.

Interstitial cystitis

Chronic inflammation of urinary/bladder tissue; research points to bladder wall dysfunction/damage.

Interstitial fluid

Fluid between cells or tissue; as opposed to intracellular fluid.

Intraocular pressure

Pressure within the eye; when elevated it is associated with glaucoma.

Involucre

A whorl of bracts at the base of a flower.

Ischemia

Lack of blood in an area. Often due to blood vessel constriction or damage (atherosclerosis).

Isotonic

A solution that has the same tonicity as the tissues that are exposed to the solution. Most notable are eyewash solutions that have roughly the same tonicity/salinity as ocular membranes or tears.

Keratin

The main protein group that forms the skin, hair, and nails.

Keratinocyte

(Malpighian cell) A keratin producing epidermal cell.

Kupffer cell

A line of phagocytic cells residing in the liver.

Lactobacillus

A genus of naturally occurring bacteria found in the mouth, intestine, and vagina. In proper concentrations the bacteria plays a role in surrounding tissue health.

Lanceolate

Widest below the middle; narrow and tapering to the tip.

Latex

A milky sap from a plant.

Leukocyte

(White blood cell) A granular or nongranular type cell, largely involved in immunologic processes.

Leukotriene

A group of immunologically active compounds responsible for leucocyte movement and inflammatory responses.

Lipolysis

The breakdown of fat.

Lithiasis

The formation of urinary tract deposits/concretions.

Litholysis

The breakdown of urinary tract deposits.

Low density lipoprotein (LDL)

A group of lipoproteins involved in the transport of cholesterol from the liver to peripheral tissues. Elevated levels usually reflect poorly on cardiovascular health.

Luteinizing hormone (LH)

A pituitary hormone that promotes ovulation and progesterone secretion. In men, it is important in the formation of the teste's Leydig cells.

Lymphocyte

Divided into T–lymphocytes and B–lymphocytes they are responsible for humoral and cellular immunity. Closely associated with acquired immunity.

Macrophage

A mononuclear phagocyte widely distributed throughout varying tissues. It comprises one of the first lines of defense in response to pathogens; part of the body's innate cellular immunity.

Malaria

An infectious disease caused by the protozoa genus Plasmodium. It is transmitted through mosquito bites.

Mast cell

Intrinsic to the inflammatory–allergic response, these cells release histamine and heparin containing granules.

Melanocyte

Surface skin cells that synthesize the pigment melanin.

Menopause

The cessation of menstruation due to insufficient reproductive hormones. Naturally occurring in the 4th or 5th decade.

Menorrhagia

Excessive menstruation.

Menorrhalgia

(See Dysmenorrhea)

Menorrhea

Normal menstruation.

Micrococcus

A genus of gram–positive bacterial; found in soil, water, and dairy products.

Microsporum

A genus of ringworm–type fungi causing skin and hair infections.

Microvasculature

The finer circulatory vessels of the body.

Mineralocorticoids

Mainly aldosterone secreted by the adrenal cortex necessary in proper water and electrolyte balance. This group of adrenal hormones causes water and sodium retention and potassium loss.

Monoamine oxidase

Enzymes responsible for the breakdown of an array neurotransmitters or similar agents, i.e. serotonin, norepinephrine.

Monocyte

These phagocytic leukocytes are formed within bone marrow and eventually migrate to tissues where they develop into macrophages.

Monoecious

Separate male and female flowers borne on the same plant.

Montezuma's revenge

(See Amebiasis)

Mucin

The main component of mucus; composed of glycoproteins, glycolipids, and polysaccharides.

Mucor

A genus of fungi. Many species form on decaying bread; some are pathogenic to humans.

Mucus

Composed of mucin, inorganic salts, and leukocytes. Secreted by mucus membranes and is necessary for proper functioning of many organs and tissue groups.

Multiple sclerosis

A disease where demyelination of white (sometimes gray as well) matter in the central nervous system causes weakness, incoordination, and other CNS disturbances. There is a significant autoimmune component.

Mutagenic

Causing genetic change; applied especially to cancer–causing agents.

Myasthenia gravis

An autoimmune disorder affecting acetylcholine receptor sites. Symptoms of fatigue and muscular weakness, especially affecting the eyes, face, and throat are common.

Myobacterium

A large family of gram–positive bacteria. A number of species are pathogenic, causing diseases such as tuberculosis and leprosy.

Natural killer cells (NK cells)

Large, granular lymphocytes which play a significant part in innate immunity.

Nephritis

Inflammation of the kidneys.

Nephron

A functional unit of the kidney. The majority of renal activities are carried out by nephrons.

Nightshade alkaloids

Alkaloids found in the Nightshade family. Many of these compounds have profound anticholinergic effects. Atropine and scopolamine are two of these compounds that are still used in conventional medicine.

Nocturnal emission

(See Spermatorrhea)

Non–insulin dependent diabetes mellitus (NIDDM)

(Adult onset or Type II) Chronic hyperglycemia as a result of a sedentary lifestyle and poor dietary choices (although there is some genetic predisposition). Typically, insulin levels are normal or even elevated. The situation is closely related to the notorious "Syndrome X". If insulin sensitivity is left impaired, cardiovascular and peripheral nervous system disturbances can ensue.

Norepinephrine

(Noradrenaline) A catecholamine acting as a hormone and neurotransmitter. Secreted by the adrenal medulla and the sympathetic nervous system, it is largely involved in stress (fight or flight) reactions.

Oblanceolate
Lance shaped, but slightly rounded towards the end of the leaf and narrower towards the leaf stem.

Obovate
Egg–shaped.

Oncotic pressure
The force that counterbalances capillary blood pressure.

Orthostatic hypotension
A fall in blood pressure and associated sensations when quickly standing or moving from a static position.

Panicles
Flowers maturing in branched groupings from the bottom of the cluster, up.

Parasympathetic
The cholinergic branch of the autonomic nervous system involved in rest, repair, and nutritive functions of the body.

Parenchymal cells
Functional cells of an organ or group of tissues, as opposed to structural cells.

Pelvic inflammatory disease (PID)
A description of general inflammation of the reproductive area in women. STDs are the most common cause. Associated with endometriosis and infertility.

Pepsin
A proteolytic enzyme derived from pepsinogen by hydrochloric acid. It is responsible for the bulk of gastric protein breakdown.

Perennial
A plant that lives three years or more.

Perimenopause
The period before menopause when reproductive hormones and their effects within the body become irregular.

Periodontitis
Inflammation of the tissues surrounding the teeth. Often a progression of chronic gingivitis, it can ultimately cause tooth and bone loss.

Peripheral
Away from the center.

Peripheral vascular disease
Vascular disturbance of the larger non–truck circulatory vessels. Usually associated with atherosclerosis, ischemia, and thrombosis.

Peristalsis
The wave–like contraction of the alimentary canal and other tubular organs/ducts which serve to move contents.

Petiole
A leaf stalk.

Phagocytosis
A process by which white blood cells – macrophages and neutrophils – engulf and eliminate particulate material or microorganisms deemed harmful to the internal environment.

Pharyngitis
Inflammation of the pharynx.

Pimple
A pustule usually on the upper parts of the body, commonly a result of Acne vulgaris.

Pinnae
(Pinna) a leaflet of a pinnate leaf.

Pinnate
A compound leaf with leaflets arranged on both sides of the axis.

Pinnatifid
Pinnately cleft, narrow lobes of a leaf not reaching the mid–vein.

Pinworms
(Enterobius vermicularis, formally called Ascaris vermicularis or Oxyuris vermicularis) Nematode type worms that can colonize the upper large intestine; common in children and causes anal itching. Infection can occasionally spread to female genitals and bladder.

Pistillate
Used to describe a female flower. A flower lacking stamens.

Placenta
A temporary organ that forms between the mother and fetus. It provides blood borne nutrients, hormones, and other necessary substances for the fetus's development.

Plasmodium falciparum
The main protozoa that causes malaria.

Platelet activating factor (PAF)

A compound produced by an array of immunologic and tissue cells designed to stimulate certain immune functions, platelet aggregation, inflammation, and allergic response.

Platelet aggregation

The clumping together of platelets often triggered by injury or a number of metabolic syndromes.

Pleurisy

An acute or chronic inflammation of the lung and thoracic cavity's serous membrane or pleura. Fever, dry cough, and stitch in the side are common symptoms.

Portal vein

The vein that carries enriched blood from the digestive organs to the liver.

Postpartum

(Postnatal) The period following birth. During this time (4–6 weeks) the mother's body is returning to pre–pregnancy conditions while the newborn adapts to external life.

Progesterone

A reproductive hormone secreted by the corpus luteum, placenta, and in small quantities, by the adrenal cortex. Aside from uterine preparatory and pregnancy sustaining effects, altered circulating levels of the hormone is a factor in premenstrual discomforts and menstrual cycle irregularities.

Prolactin

Traditionally defined as a hormone secreted by the anterior pituitary responsible for lactation. Research suggests the hormone has a broader role in chronic stress states.

Prostaglandin

A diverse group of naturally occurring compounds involved in a wide array of physiological responses. Many are pro–inflammatory, cellular excitants.

Prostatitis

Inflammation of the prostate.

Proteolytic enzyme

An enzyme that breaks down protein into smaller polypeptides by splitting peptide bonds. In supplement form they are used as digestive aids and as antiinflammatories.

Protozoa

Simple, single celled organisms; many are parasitic.

Psoriasis

A syndrome of inflammation and excessive cellular production affecting the skin, joints, and even nails. Red, scaly patches of skin called psoriatic plaques are common. Cause of the disease is an issue of debate. Both autoimmune reaction and excessive growth of skin cells have been implicated as possible factors.

Psychosomatic

Having physical symptoms that originate from the mind or emotions.

Pubescent

Hair–like quality.

Pyorrhea

(See Periodontitis)

Pyrrolizidine alkaloids

A group of compounds common in the Sunflower and Borage families responsible for liver inflammation and subsequent hepatocyte breakdown.

Raceme

An unbranched, elongated group of flowers with pedicels.

Raynaud's syndrome and disease

Severity seems to be the main dividing line between the two types. Vasoconstriction of the smaller vessels in the extremities, resulting in discolored, painful, and cold fingers and/or toes. In severe cases ulceration and infection can develop. Smoking and stress are the main aggravations.

5–α–reductase

The enzyme responsible for the conversion of testosterone into DHT.

Reye's syndrome

Usually occurring as a result of an acute viral infection (often respiratory centered or associated with chicken pox). Fever, vomiting, elevated liver enzyme levels, and brain swelling are common. This childhood syndrome is rare, but can result in seizures and death.

Aspirin use in febrile conditions has been linked as a possible factor.

Rheumatoid arthritis
Chronic joint inflammation usually affecting the hands and feet. It is autoimmune mediated and if left untreated leads to lack of mobility and joint deformation.

Rhinitis
Inflammation of nasal mucus membranes; a typical hayfever response.

Ringworm
A non–specific term for a fungal infection affecting the skin. Often developing in a ring–like pattern, numerous fungal strains are causative agents.

Roundworm
(Nematode) An organism from the nematode class; many are intestinal parasites.

Rubefacient
Something that reddens the skin, usually through vasodilation.

Salmonella
A genus of gram–negative bacteria. Many species cause food poisoning.

Samara
A winged fruit, common in the Fraxinus and the Ailanthus genera.

Scrofula (Scrofuloderma)
A tuberculous or similar infection affecting the skin and underlying lymph nodes particularly of the neck area.

Scrofulous
A somewhat antiquated term; afflicted with scrofula or having a scrofula–like appearance.

Seborrheic dermatitis
(Cradle cap, seborrheic eczema, or seborrhea) A chronic skin condition characterized by redness and yellow scaly patches on the trunk, groin, face, and/or scalp. Allergic and constitutional factors are involved.

Seminal vesicle
A pair of glands situated next to the urinary bladder; their secretions comprise approximately 60% of semen.

Sequela
A complication or condition arising from an initial disease or injury.

Serrate
Designating a toothed margin; saw–like.

Shigella
A gram–negative bacteria in the Enterobacteria family. Many cause severe diarrhea/dysentery.

Shingles
(Herpes zoster) More common in the elderly and in immune compromised individuals, shingles manifests as nerve pain and corresponding vesicles over affected dermatomes. Occurrence is normally on only one side of the body and is thought to involve expression of latent varicella–zoster virus – called H. ophthalmicus when the virus affects the trigeminal nerve.

Simple
An undivided leaf that is not separated into leaflets. Describing an herb used singly, not in formula.

Sinusitis
Inflammation of the sinuses. Typical causes are allergic reaction or bacterial, viral, or fungal infections. Poor tissue health and local immunity are predisposing factors.

Spasmolytic
Antispasmodic.

Spermatorrhea
Involuntary and excessive discharge of semen without copulation; excessive wet dreams or nocturnal emission.

Spikelet
The flower cluster of grasses and sedges, or a secondary spike.

Staminate
Used to describe a male flower bearing only stamens, not pistils.

Staphylococcus
A genus of gram–positive, anaerobic bacteria; many are pathogenic.

Strep throat
Streptococcus infection affecting the throat.

Streptococcus
A gram–positive genus of bacteria. Most spe-

cies are pathogenic, notably S. pyogenes.

Streptomycetes

A genus of fungus–like aerobic bacterial. Many conventional antibiotics are derived from this group. A number of species are pathogenic.

Succus entericus

Secretions of the small intestine containing enzymes, hormones, and mucus.

Sudorific

Diaphoretic; an agent that causes sweating.

Sympathetic nervous system

A branch of the autonomic nervous system closely associated with fight or flight/stress responses.

Sympathomimetic

(Adrenergic) Having sympathetic nervous system–like effects (postganglionic fibers).

Tachycardia

Accelerated heartbeat; usually greater than 100 beat per minute.

Taiga

Meaning forest in Russian. A circumboreal forest zone existing below the tundra.

Tepal

A specialized sepal or petal; common in the Passionflower family.

Testosterone

A major male sex hormone produced in the testes. It is crucial for bone and muscle growth and sperm formation in the male.

Thyroid stimulating hormone (TSH)

(Thyrotropin) a pituitary hormone that is necessary in the thyroid's normal functioning. Low levels can be an indicator of hyperthyroidism.

Thyroxine (T4)

A pro–hormone secreted by the thyroid gland; transformed into T3 at tissue sites.

Thromboxane

An eicosanoid responsible for platelet aggregation and vasoconstriction.

Thrush

(Candidiasis or yeast infection) Called oral thrush when limited to the mouth region.

Tinnitus

Ringing in the ear. Causes range from local injury to cardiovascular disease.

Tobacco heart

Cardiovascular weakness caused from years of smoking.

Tomentose

Covered by soft, matted hair.

Tonsillitis

Inflammation of the small rounded masses of lymph tissue (palatine tonsils) located near the back of the tongue. This normally occurs through heightened leukocyte activity.

Traveler's diarrhea

(See Amebiasis)

Trichophyton

A genus of fungi known to cause skin, nail, and hair infections.

Trifoliate

Three–leaved.

Triiodothyronine (T3)

A thyroid hormone responsible for the majority of that gland's cellular effects.

Ulcerative colitis

(Crone's disease) Chronic inflammation affecting the mucosa and submucosa of the colon wall. Symptoms of abdominal pain, diarrhea, and ulceration. Autoimmune involvement is typical.

Ureter

The urinary tube arising from the kidney leading to the bladder.

Ureteritis

Inflammation of the ureter.

Urethra

The urinary tube leading from the bladder to the body's exterior.

Urethritis

Inflammation of the urethra.

Uric acid

The end result of purine (RNA–DNA) catabolism in primates. Gout is a disorder of excess uric acid.

Vaginitis

Inflammation of the vagina. There is usually a bacterial/fungal/viral component.

Vagus nerve

A key parasympathetic cranial nerve involved in viscera innervation. It affects the digestive tract, lungs, heart, liver, and other areas. Certain herbs (Asclepias) stimulate vagus nerve function, particularly when digestive function is depressed by stress.

Vasoconstriction

Blood vessel constriction.

Vasodilation

Blood vessel dilation.

Vermifuge

An agent that kills or expels parasites.

Verruca vulgaris

Common wart. A member of the larger HPV group.

Vertigo

The illusionary sensation of the body or surroundings revolving. Often associated with inner ear or CNS disorders.

Very low density lipoprotein (VLDL)

Transports triglycerides from the intestine and liver to adipose and muscle tissues. High levels of VLDLs are associated with atherosclerosis.

Vitiligo

A chronic pigmentary disorder resulting in depigmented skin. A hyperpigmented border may surround these white patches. It is possibly autoimmune mediated with some genetic predisposition.

Volatile oil

Non–polar aromatics that disperse easily through sun exposure or through other forms of heat such as boiling.

Vulnerary

An agent that encourages wound healing.

White blood cell

(See leukocyte)

INDEX

M

Nyctaginaceae 243
Nymphaea alba 233
  odorata 233
Nymphaeaceae 243

O

Oak 174, 177, 184, 204, 241, 242. See Quercus
Oatgrass 200
Oatstraw 200
Ocotillo 169, 204. See Fouquieria splendens
Oenothera 233
Ohio 95, 127
  buckeye 127
Oil of bay. See Pimenta racemosa
ointment 35
Ojibwa Indians 179
Oklahoma 47, 95, 141
Oleaceae 243
Olea europaea 233
Olive. See Olea europaea
Oman 153
Onagraceae 243
Ontario 114
Oolong tea 185
opiates 73, 160
Opium lettuce 200
Oplopanax horridum 233
Opuntia 233
Orchidaceae 243
Oregon 164, 209
Oregongrape 57, 65, 105, 107, 115, 145, 157–158,
    169, 215, 216, 217, 218, 219, 221, 241
Oregon myrtle. See Umbellularia californica
Orobanchaceae 243
Orobanche 233
Orris root. See Iris florentina
Oshá 138
Osmorhiza 233
osteoporosis 129
Oxydendrum arboreum 233
oxytocin 67
Oxytropis 56

P

Pacific Northwest 90, 158
Paeonia 233
Paeoniaceae 243
Paiute 139
Pakistan 84, 175
Pale echinacea 94
Palm family. See Arecaceae
Panama 77
Panax ginseng 47, 49, 99, 110, 233
  quinquefolia 47
  quinquefolium 47
  quinquefolius 47, 233
pancreatic juice 53, 288
Papaveraceae 243
Papoose root 66
Papua New Guinea 131
Paraguay 146
  tea 146
parasites 54, 206, 291, 292, 298, 300
Parietaria 233
Parsley root. See Petroselinum crispum
Parthenium incanum 233
Partidgeberry 180
Passiflora 233
  foetida 159
  incarnata 159
  mexicana 159
Passifloraceae 159
Passionflower 80, 104, 159–161, 194, 215, 217, 218,
    299
Passionflower family. See Passifloraceae
Pau d'arco 188. See Tabebuia
Paullinia 233
  cupana 120
  cupana var. sorbilis 120
Pausinystalia yohimbe 233
Pea family. See Fabaceae
Pectis 233
Pedicularis 233
Pegaga 116
Peganum harmala. See Syrian rue
Pellitory of the wall. See Parietaria
pelvic inflammatory disease 66
Peniocereus greggii 233
Pennsylvania 62
Pennyroyal 76, 161–162, 215, 216, 220, 221

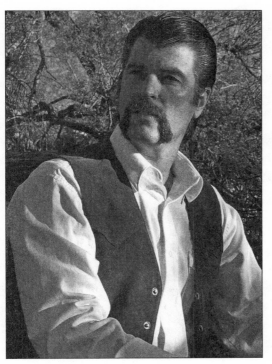

Active in the field for over 20 years, Charles W. Kane continues to write, teach, and see patients. Committed to helping people through the usage of medicinal plants, he is well regarded for his no–nonsense approach in a field known for the opposite. Kane has also written *Herbal Medicine of the American Southwest*. He is a veteran of the war on terrorism and lives in southern Arizona.

If interested in applying for Kane's 5 month program, *Studies in Western Herbal Medicine*, or to schedule an office visit, he can be reached at PO Box 5472 Oracle, AZ 85623. For more information go to www.tcbmed.com.